ain Management

Pain Management

Edited by **Pam Kellner**

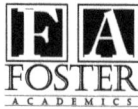

FOSTER
ACADEMICS

New Jersey

Published by Foster Academics,
61 Van Reypen Street,
Jersey City, NJ 07306, USA
www.fosteracademics.com

Pain Management
Edited by Pam Kellner

International Standard Book Number: 978-1-63242-309-2 (Hardback)

The publisher's policy is to use permanent paper from mills that operate a sustainable forestry policy. Furthermore, the publisher ensures that the text paper and cover boards used have met acceptable environmental accreditation standards.

Trademark Notice: Registered trademark of products or corporate names are used only for explanation and identification without intent to infringe.

Printed in the United States of America.

Contents

Preface

In my initial years as a student, I used to run to the library at every possible instance to grab a book and learn something new. Books were my primary source of knowledge and I would not have come such a long way without all that I learnt from them. Thus, when I was approached to edit this book; I became understandably nostalgic. It was an absolute honor to be considered worthy of guiding the current generation as well as those to come. I put all my knowledge and hard work into making this book most beneficial for its readers.

International experts and veterans have contributed significant information in this book which encompasses several topics regarding the present pain management problems, and provides the readers with a glimpse into the future of pain treatment. This book comprises both original research works as well as clinical information categorized under the sections: pain science, acute pain and opioids. The aim of this book is to serve as a valuable source of reference for a broad spectrum of readers including the pain clinicians as well as the common masses.

I wish to thank my publisher for supporting me at every step. I would also like to thank all the authors who have contributed their researches in this book. I hope this book will be a valuable contribution to the progress of the field.

Editor

Part 1

Pain Science

Intrathecal Studies on Animal Pain Models

Jen-Kun Cheng
Mackay Memorial Hospital/Mackay Medical College
Taiwan

1. Introduction

Spinal and epidural anesthesia have been widely used in clinical settings for the management of peri-operative, neuropathic and cancer pain (Dureja et al., 2010; Hong, 2010; Mercadante, 1999). They provide another route for the analgesic administration in addition to oral or systemic absorption. Since the pain pathway initiate with primary and secondary neurons located in dorsal root ganglion and spinal cord, respectively, the *intrathecal* (spinal) route may provide an effective alternative for less drug dosage and fewer side effects, compared with systemic administration.

In recent decades, many animal pain models have been developed to explore the possible mechanisms involved in the pathogenesis of clinically relevant pain statuses, such as postoperative (Brennan et al., 1996), neuropathic (Kim & Chung, 1992), inflammatory (Wheeler-Aceto et al., 1990) and cancer pain (Clohisy & Mantyh, 2003). These studies not only help to extent our understanding on pain mechanisms but also provide novel promising agents or targets for the management of different pain situations (Mogil et al., 2010). In this chapter, we present various animal pain models, emphasizing on *intrathecal* studies, and potential therapeutic molecular targets and analgesics found in latest years. In addition, the related neurotoxicity studies and morphine-induced tolerance will be mentioned.

2. Intrathecal animal pain studies

The first mentioned *intrathecal* study using rat animal model was reported by Yaksh, beginning with the study of *intrathecal* morphine (Yaksh et al., 1977). For *intrathecal* drug administration, a polyethylene catheter is inserted *intrathecally* in rats during inhalation anesthesia (LoPachin et al., 1981). The catheter is passed caudally from the cisterna magnum to the level of lumbar enlargement. Since the development of *intrathecal* catheterization, lots of studies explored the pharmacology and pain pathways using *intrathecal* space as a route of drug administration, either in basic researches or clinical studies. The *intrathecal* studies on various pain models provide a lot of promising analgesics for the management of different pain statuses.

2.1 Postoperative pain model

The postoperative or incisional pain model was proposed by Brennan in 1996 (Brennan et al., 1996). A 1-cm longitudinal incision is made through skin, fascia and muscle of the plantar aspect of the hindpaw in anesthetized rats. The lesion produced reliable and quantifiable mechanical allodynia and thermal hyperalgesia around the wound and spontaneous nociceptive behaviors for about one week, which mimics the clinical course of postoperative pain. Selective denervations of the rat hindpaw prior to foot incision reveal both the sural and tibial nerves are responsible for the nociception transmission from the incision. This model helps to better understand mechanisms of sensitization caused by surgery and provide promising therapeutics for postoperative pain management (Kang & Brennan, 2009).

2.2 Inflammatory formalin pain model
The formalin test involves subcutaneous injection of 5% formaldehyde (50 µl) at the plantar surface of the rat hindpaw, using a 27-gauge needle. After injection, the rat displays characteristic nociceptive behaviors, flinching, shaking, biting and licking of the injected paw. Two phases of nociceptive behaviors are observed after formalin injection as described previously (Abbott et al., 1995). Phase 1 is initiated within seconds after injection and it lasts for about 5–10min. After several minutes quiescent, a second phase of flinching occurs and peaks at 25–35 min after injection.

The formalin-induced nociceptive response in rats is believed to be an inflammatory pain and involves central sensitization in the spinal cord (Abbott et al., 1995). The hindpaw injection of formalin induces tissue injury leading to acute (phase 1) and facilitated (phase 2) states of pain. The phase 2 response is believed to be a persistent input-induced nociceptive behavior mediated through central sensitization (Coderre & Melzack, 1992). LTP of C-fiber-evoked field potentials in the spinal superficial dorsal horn has been reported in the formalin-injected rats (Sandkuhler & Liu, 1998). *Intrathecal* injection of T-type Ca^{2+} channel blockers (mibefradil and Ni^{2+}) has been reported to attenuate formalin-induced pain behaviours, either phase 1 or 2, indicating the important role of T-type Ca^{2+} channel in the spinal central sensitization (Cheng et al., 2007). Other chemical irritants, such as complete Freund's adjuvant (CFA), carrageenan or capsaicin, could also be used to be injected subcutaneously into the plantar surface of rat hindpaw to induce pain behaviors (Duarte et al., 2011; Thorpe et al., 2011; Yu et al., 2011).

2.3 Nerve injury-induced neuropathic pain model
Nerve injuries due to trauma, chemotherapy, diabetic mellitus or tumor invasion may induce neuropathic pain, which is usually refractory to conventional analgesic agents, including opioids and non-steroid anti-inflammatory agents. For the past decades, several animal models have been developed to mimic the clinical conditions and explore the possible mechanisms underlying neuropathic pain. Among these neuropathic pain models, nerve injury-induced neuropathic pain (NINP) models, such as spinal nerve ligation, spared nerve injury and chronic constriction injury, are most often studied (Ji & Strichartz, 2004).

Several targets have been proposed to be involved in the pathogenesis of NINP, such as NMDA receptors (Szekely et al., 2002) and ion channels (Rogers et al., 2006). Recently, new molecules have been emerging as promising targets for the treatment of NINP, such as purinergic receptors (Donnelly-Roberts et al., 2008), cannabinoid receptors (Lynch & Campbell, 2011), transient receptor potential V1 (TRPV1) receptor (Facer et al., 2007), chemokine receptors (White et al., 2007), acid-sensing ion channel (Mazzuca et al., 2007; Poirot et al., 2006), annexin 2 light chain p11 (Foulkes et al., 2006) and matrix metalloproteinase (Kawasaki et al., 2008a).

The L5/6 spinal nerve ligation neuropathic pain model was reported by Kim and Chung in 1992 (Kim & Chung, 1992). This model involves a tight ligation of L5 and L6 spinal nerves of animals under anesthesia. The nociceptive behavioral assessments also consist of von Frey hair test (Chaplan et al., 1994) and radiant heat test (Hargreaves et al., 1988) for the quantification of mechanical allodynia and thermal hyperalgesia, respectively, on the affected hindpaw. Compared with postoperative pain model and formalin inflammatory pain model, this model induced chronic nociceptive behaviors lasting for several weeks. This chronic pain model helps to reveal the possible mechanisms involved in the development and maintenance of nerve injury-induced pain, either the neuronal components or glial components.

Spared nerve injury pain model was developed by Decosterd and Woolf in 2000 (Decosterd & Woolf, 2000). An adaptation of spared nerve injury surgery was later developed in the mouse (Bourquin et al., 2006). This model involves a lesion of two of the three terminal branches of the sciatic nerve (tibial and common peroneal nerves) leaving the remaining sural nerve intact. The spared nerve injury model differs from the L5/6 spinal ligation pain model in that the co-mingling of distal intact axons with degenerating axons is restricted, and it permits behavioral testing of the non-injured skin territories adjacent to the denervated areas. The mechanical (von Frey and pinprick) sensitivity and thermal (hot and cold) responsiveness is increased in the ipsilateral sural territory.

2.4 Cancer pain model

Cancer pain significantly affects the diagnosis, quality of life and survival of patients with cancer. Tumor growth may produce inflammation in tumor bearing tissues, which will release inflammatory mediators to stimulate nociceptors. Tumor growth may also compress the peripheral nerves in tumor bearing tissues, inducing nerve injury. Therefore, cancer pain is likely to share mechanisms of inflammatory pain and neuropathic pain, although this pain may have distinct mechanisms (Ghilardi et al., 2010). Whether inflammation or nerve injury dominates during tumor growth may depend on the interactions between tumor cells and surrounding tissues (Cain et al., 2001).

In recent years, several laboratories have developed cancer pain models by inoculation of tumor cells into a hindpaw of mouse (Constantin et al., 2008). Animals inoculated with melanoma cells into the plantar of the hindpaw show marked pain hypersensitivity and peripheral nerve degeneration (Gao et al., 2009a). We have used this melanoma cancer pain model to test the anti-tumor growth and analgesic effects of JNK inhibitor (Gao et al., 2009a). Other cancer pain models include breast, prostate and bone cancer pain models (Bloom et al., 2011; Ghilardi et al., 2010; Jimenez-Andrade et al., 2010). These cancer pain models may possess different pathophysiologies for pain induction. For example, intramedullary injection of breast cancer cells could induce periosteal sprouting of CGRP(+) sensory fibers and pain, both of which could be blocked by anti-nerve growth factor (NGF) (Bloom et al., 2011). Inhibitor of NGF receptor TrkA has been shown to attenuate bone cancer pain and tumor-induced sprouting of sensory nerve fibers (Ghilardi et al., 2010). Similarly, NGF also plays an important role in the induction of prostate cancer-induced sensory fiber sprouting and bone pain (Jimenez-Andrade et al., 2010).

3. Potential therapeutic molecular targets for pain management

Voltage-gated ion channels and glial cells have all been found to be promising therapeutic targets for pain management. Voltage-gated ion channels are a class of transmembrane ion channels that are activated by changes in membrane potential; these types of ion channels are especially critical in excitable cells, including neuronal, cardiac and skeletal cells (Szu-Yu Ho & Rasband, 2011), or even cancer cell migration (Cuddapah & Sontheimer, 2011). Since voltage-gated ion channels are important for neuronal excitability, conduction and transmission, they have long been the targets of interest in the field of pain research.

3.1 Voltage-gated Na$^+$ channels

Voltage-gated Na$^+$ channels are essential for the initiation of action potentials which are crucial for nerve conduction. Their activation and inactivation are strongly gated by the membrane potential of neuronal cells, but their properties can also be modulated by G-proteins or protein kinases (Kakimura et al., 2010). Voltage-gated Na$^+$ channels are constituted by the pore-forming α−subunit and auxiliary β-subunits. Up to now, nine α−subunits (Nav1.1-1.9) and four β-subunits (β1-4) have been identified (Catterall et al., 2005). The Na$^+$ channels can be either sensitive (Nav1.1, Nav1.2, Nav1.3, Nav1.6) or resistant (Nav1.4, Nav1.5, Nav1.7, Nav1.8, Nav1.9) to tetrodotoxin (TTX), a toxin found in the liver of puffer fish. Neuronal cells contain most of the Na$^+$ channel subtypes but Nav1.4 and Nav1.5, respectively, are mainly in skeletal and cardiac muscles (Jarecki et al., 2010). Nav1.1, Nav1.3, Nav1.6, Nav1.7, Nav1.8 and Nav1.9 have been found in adult dorsal root ganglion (DRG) sensory neurons and these isoforms can be important for the firing properties of sensory neurons (Hunanyan et al., 2011). After spared nerve injury in rats, altered neuronal electrogenesis in DRG neurons, such as accelerated re-priming of TTX-sensitive Na$^+$ currents, was observed and may be due to a complex regulation of voltage-gated Na$^+$ channels (Berta et al., 2008; Wang et al., 2011).

Several lines of evidence indicate that Nav1.7, and Nav1.8 are involved in pain regulation, especially NINP (Lampert et al., 2010). Nav1.7 and Nav1.8 channels have been shown to accumulate in neuroma endings in humans with neuropathic pain (Kretschmer et al., 2002). This accumulation may be due to a loss of myelin inhibition or target determined transfer of Na$^+$ channels (Aurilio et al., 2008). Loss of Nav1.7 function may lead to complete insensitivity to pain in humans (Cox et al., 2010). Compounds possessing Nav1.7 blocking effects have been reported to reverse nerve injury-induced mechanical allodynia (Tyagarajan et al., 2010). Nav1.8 is increased in sciatic nerve after nerve injury and *intrathecal* antisense oligoneucleotide directed against Nav1.8 is effective in neuropathic pain models (Joshi et al., 2006). A μΩ-conotoxin MrVIB was found to be a preferential Nav1.8 blocker and could reverse partial sciatic nerve ligation-induced mechanical allodynia and thermal hyperalgesia, when given *intrathecally* (Ekberg et al., 2006). Intraperitoneal administration of A-803467, a selective Nav1.8 blocker, has been reported to attenuate nerve injury-induced mechanical allodynia (Jarvis et al., 2007). Nonetheless, Nassar et al. found that mice lacking Nav1.7 and Nav1.8 still develop neuropathic pain after spinal nerve ligation (Nassar et al., 2005). Recent studies also revealed a role of Nav1.3 (Mo et al., 2011) and Nav1.9 (Leo et al., 2010) in the development of neuropathic pain. For normal nerve conduction, Nav1.1 family is involved (Catterall et al., 2010). Therefore, the selective Nav1.3, Nav1.7, Nav1.8 and Nav1.9 channel blockers will have clinical potential in the treatment of neuropathic pain since they do not affect normal neuronal conduction.

Besides the pore-forming α-subunit, β2 subunit was reported to be up-regulated in injured and non-injured sensory neurons after peripheral nerve injuries (Pertin et al., 2005) and the development of spared nerve injury-induced mechanical allodynia is attenuated in β2-null mice (Lopez-Santiago et al., 2006), suggesting the important role of β2 subunit in NINP. The involvement of Na^+ channel β2 subunit in neuropathic and inflammatory pain has been extensively reviewed (Brackenbury & Isom, 2008).

In addition to changes in protein expression, phosphorylation-induce change of conductance or gating property of Na^+ channels may also lead to enhanced neuronal excitability and NINP (Aurilio et al., 2008). The activation of presynaptic delta-opioid receptor by enkephalin has been reported to prevent the increase in neuronal $Na_V1.7$ in DRG through inhibition of PKC and p38 (Chattopadhyay et al., 2008). Tumor necrosis factor-α (TNF-α), a pro-inflammatory cytokine involved in NINP formation (Schafers et al., 2003), was found to enhance TTX-resistant Na^+ currents in isolated DRG neurons *via* a TNF receptor 1- and p38-dependent mechanism (Jin & Gereau, 2006). The Na^+ currents of isolated sensory neurons can be enhanced by protein kinase A and protein kinase C (Gold et al., 1998; Mo et al., 2011), both of which are involved in NINP (Gao et al., 2005; Song et al., 2006). Phosphorylation of TTX-S and TTX-R sodium channels involving both serine/threonine and tyrosine sites has been reported to contribute to painful diabetic neuropathy (Hong et al., 2004). Further studies are required to reveal the exact role of Na^+ channel phosphorylation in the pathogenesis of NINP.

3.2 Voltage-gated Ca^{2+} channels

Voltage-gated Ca^{2+} channels are involved in neuron excitability, neurotransmitter release, synaptic transmission and gene expression (Dolmetsch et al., 2001). Ca^{2+} channels are constituted by the pore-forming α-subunit and auxiliary subunits, β- and α2δ□subunits. They are classified into Cav1, Cav2 and Cav3 families based on their structure homology, but are categorized as L- (Cav1.1, Cav1.2 and Cav1.3), P/Q- (Cav2.1), N- (Cav2.2), R- (Cav2.3), and T- (Cav3.1, Cav3.2 and Cav3.3) type based on their sensitivity to specific blockers, activation/inactivation characteristics and current conductance (Catterall et al., 2002). Various Ca^{2+} channel blockers have been tested in the postoperative, inflammatory and neuropathic pain models (Cheng et al., 2007). The potential use of Ca^{2+} channel blockers for neuropathic pain treatment and roles of Ca^{2+} channels in ascending pain pathway have been well reviewed (Yaksh, 2006; Zamponi et al., 2009).

3.2.1 N-type Ca^{2+} channels

N-type Ca^{2+} channels are distributed in the dorsal root ganglia and spinal dorsal horn. It is generally believed that N-type Ca^{2+} channels are involved in the neurotransmitter release of spinal dorsal horn (Smith et al., 2002). Substance P, one of the neurotransmitter of primary sensory neurons, has been found to be mostly co-localized with N-type Ca^{2+} channels in the spinal dorsal horn (Westenbroek et al., 1998).

Several lines of evidence indicate that N-type Ca^{2+} channels play an important role in NINP. Mice lacking N-type Ca^{2+} channels exhibit reduced signs of neuropathic pain after spinal nerve ligation (Saegusa et al., 2001). *Intrathecal* small interference RNA knockdown of N-type Ca^{2+} channels reversed sciatic nerve constriction-induced tactile allodynia and thermal hyperalgesia (Altier et al., 2007).

New non-peptide compounds with N-type Ca^{2+} channel blocking property have been recently developed in pharmaceutical companies for the treatment of neuropathic pain (Knutsen et al., 2007). A highly reversible ω-conotoxin FVIA, a potent N-type Ca2+ channel blocker with fewer side effects, was found to possess analgesic effect in the formalin test and neuropathic pain models (Lee et al., 2010). Recent findings suggest that diminished Ca^{2+}

influx through N-type Ca^{2+} channels may contribute to sensory neuron dysfunction and pain after nerve injury (McCallum et al., 2011).

3.2.2 T-type Ca^{2+} channels

T-type Ca^{2+} channels are low-voltage activated Ca^{2+} channels. It can serve as an initiator to trigger the opening of high-voltage activated ion channels. In spinal dorsal horn, it may be involved in spontaneous neurotransmitter release and long term potentiation (LTP) (Ikeda et al., 2003). LTP, a form of synaptic plasticity, in the spinal dorsal horn is believed to contribute to the central sensitization of pain transmission (Ji et al., 2003), a wiring phenomenon usually observed in neuropathic pain (Romanelli & Esposito, 2004).

Among three subtypes of T-type Ca^{2+} channels, $Ca_V3.1$, $Ca_V3.2$ and $Ca_V3.3$, $Ca_V3.2$ mRNAs are mostly abundant in the spinal dorsal horn and are limited to the superficial layers (Talley et al., 1999). *Intrathecal* injection of the antisense oligonucleotide targeted to the α1-subunit of $Ca_V3.2$, but not $Ca_V3.3$ or $Ca_V3.1$, produced analgesic effect in both acute and neuropathic pain states (Bourinet et al., 2005), suggesting that $Ca_V3.2$ is much more involved in spinal nociceptive pathway than $Ca_V3.1$ and $Ca_V3.3$.

Subtype-specific blockers of T-type Ca^{2+} channels are not commercially available. However, mibefradil, a non-selective T-type Ca^{2+} channel blocker, when given systemically or intraplantarly, can reverse mechanical allodynia and thermal hyperalgesia induced by L5/6 spinal nerve ligation (Dogrul et al., 2003). Our recent work on *intrathecal* T-type Ca^{2+} channel blockers (mibefradil or Ni^{2+}) revealed their effectiveness in the second phase of formalin test (Cheng et al., 2007). In these years, small molecules with potent blocking effect on T-type Ca^{2+} channels, such as KYS05090, have been developed (Doddareddy et al., 2007; Seo et al., 2007). Recent studies revealed spinal T-type Ca^{2+} (Cav3.2 and Cav3.3 but not Cav3.1) channels may play an important role in the pathogenesis of chronic compression of DRG-induced neuropathic pain (Wen et al., 2010). In addition, Cav3.2-dependent activation of extracellular signal-regulated kinase in the anterior nucleus of paraventricular thalamus was found to contribute to the development of acid-induced chronic mechanical hyperalgesia (Chen et al., 2010).

3.2.3 P/Q- and R-type Ca^{2+} channels

Compared with N-type Ca^{2+} channel, it seems P/Q type is much less important in NINP. Only one study using transgenic mice revealed its involvement in chronic constriction injury-induced mechanical allodynia (Luvisetto et al., 2006). The hypoalgesic behaviors of P/Q-type Ca^{2+} channel mutant mouse suggest P/Q-type Ca^{2+} channel has a pro-nociceptive role (Fukumoto et al., 2009). As for R-type Ca^{2+} channel, its blocker SNX-482 could inhibit C-fiber and Aδ-fiber-mediated neuronal responses after L5/6 spinal nerve ligation, when administered *intrathecally* (Matthews et al., 2007). Moreover, the responses to innocuous mechanical and thermal stimuli were more sensitive to SNX-482 in nerve-ligated rats than control animals (Matthews et al., 2007). These findings suggest spinal R-type Ca^{2+} channel could be a potential therapeutic target for NINP. Blocking the R-type Ca^{2+} channel has been reported to enhance morphine analgesia and reduce morphine-induced tolerance (Yokoyama et al., 2004).

3.2.4 α2δ subunit of Ca^{2+} channels

α2δ subunit is one of the modulatory subunits of Ca^{2+} channels, which could modulate the membrane targeting and conductance of α1 subunit of Ca^{2+} channel (Felix, 1999). Four isoforms (α2δ-1~4) were identified (Qin et al., 2002). The α2δ-1 subunit is up-regulated in dorsal root ganglion and dorsal spinal cord after peripheral nerve injury (Li et al., 2004). *Intrathecal* injection of α2δ-1 antisense oligonucleotide could block this up-regulation in spinal dorsal horn and diminish injury-induced tactile allodynia (Li et al., 2004). Over expression of α2δ-1 in spinal dorsal horn neurons could enhance Ca^{2+} currents, exaggerate dorsal horn neuronal responses to external stimuli and increase the nociceptive responses in neuropathic pain models (Li et al., 2006).

α2δ subunit is the specific binding site in the central nervous system of gabapentin and its analogue pregabalin (Klugbauer et al., 2003), both of which have been shown to be effective in preclinical and clinical studies of neuropathic pain (Cheng & Chiou, 2006). Gabapentin was first designed as a chemical analogue of γ-aminobutyric acid, an inhibitory neurotransmitter, to treat spasticity and was later found to have anticonvulsant and antinociceptive activities in various seizure and pain models. A point mutation of the arginine 217 of α2δ-1 subunit, which is critical for gabapentin binding (Wang et al., 1999), was found to cause a loss of gabapentin-induced analgesia (Field et al., 2006). Recently, chronic *intrathecal* infusion of gabapentin was found to prevent nerve ligation-induced mechanical allodynia and thermal hyperalgesia without causing obvious neuropathological changes in spinal cord and cauda equine (Chu et al., 2011).

Gabapentin has been found to attenuate morphine-induced tolerance (Lin et al., 2005) and this finding may encourage the combined use of gabapentin with morphine in the treatment of neuropathic pain. It is interesting to note that α2δ-1 subunit was identified to be a receptor involved in excitatory synapse formation and gabapentin may act by blocking new synapse formation (Eroglu et al., 2009).

3.3 Voltage-gated K$^+$ channels

The opening of K$^+$ channel may lead to cell repolarization and make the neuron less excitable and down-regulation of K$^+$ channel in nociceptive neurons may decrease pain threshold. There are 12 different families of voltage-gated K$^+$ channels (Kv1 to Kv12) and all Kv channels are tetramers of α subunits (Ocana et al., 2004). A-type K$^+$ channel (A-channels) is a group of Kv channels that are activated transiently and inactivated rapidly. Five A-channels Kv1.4, Kv3.4, Kv4.1, Kv4.2, and Kv4.3 were found in mammals (Chien et al., 2007; Mienville et al., 1999; Serodio et al., 1996). Except for Kv3.4 with high-voltage activation, the other four are activated at low voltages (Coetzee et al., 1999). Kv1.4 proteins in the somata of DRG neurons are greatly reduced in the L5/6 spinal nerve ligation pain model (Rasband et al., 2001). The expression of Kv1.4 is also reduced in the small-/medium sized (Aδ-/C-) trigeminal ganglion neurons after temporomandibular joint inflammation (Takeda et al., 2008). Gene expressions of Kv1.2, Kv1.4, and Kv4.2 are down-regulated in the DRG following sciatic nerve transection (Park et al., 2003). Recent study also revealed the Kv1.2 expression is decreased in DRG neurons from rats with irritable bowel syndrome, a visceral pain model (Luo et al., 2011). The expression of Kv3.4 and Kv4.3 in DRG neurons were found to be also decreased after spinal nerve ligation and *intrathecal* injections of antisense oligodeoxynucleotides against Kv3.4 or Kv4.3 in naïve rats could induce mechanical hypersensitivity (Chien et al., 2007). New compounds with A-type K$^+$ channel opening activity, such as KW-7158 (Sculptoreanu et al., 2004), may prove to be effective for the treatment of NINP.

The Kv7 channel (also known as KCNQ) opener retigabine has been reported to be effective in sciatic chronic constrict injury (Blackburn-Munro & Jensen, 2003) and L5 spinal nerve ligation (Dost et al., 2004) pain models. It is important to note that the antiallodynic effect of retigabine could be inhibited by linopirdine, a selective KCNQ channel blocker, indicating the involvement of KCNQ channel opening in the effect of retigabine (Dost et al., 2004). When directly applied to the spinal cord, retigabine inhibited the Aδ and C fiber-mediated response of dorsal horn neurons to noxious stimuli (Passmore et al., 2003). Recently, the selective cyclooxygenase-2 (COX-2) inhibitor celecoxib was found to enhance Kv7.2-7.4, Kv7.2/7.3 and Kv7.3/7.5 currents expressed in HEK 293 cells, providing a novel mechanism for its antinociceptive effect (Du et al., 2011b). Based on these reports, further efforts may be needed to develop subtype-specific K^+ channel openers and to test their effects in NINP models.

Just as voltage-gated Na^+ channels, K^+ channels could also be modulated by phosphorylation (Sergeant et al., 2005). The Kv4.2 current of spinal dorsal horn neurons could be inhibited by extracellular signal-regulated kinase (ERK)-induced phosphorylation (Hu et al., 2003). Genetic elimination of Kv4.2 increases excitability of dorsal horn neurons and sensitivity to tactile and thermal stimuli (Hu et al., 2006). This modulation of Kv4.2 by ERK may underlie the induction of central sensitization, a cellular mechanism of NINP (Ji et al., 2003). The role of Kv channels in different trigeminal neuropathic and inflammatory pain models was recently reviewed (Takeda et al., 2011).

3.4 Other K^+ channels

In addition to Kv channels, there are other K^+ channels that are important for pain modulation, such as G-protein coupled inwardly rectifying (GIRK or Kir3), ATP-sensitive (K_{ATP} or Kir6), Ca^{2+}-activated (KCa) and two-pore (K_{2P}) K^+ channels (Gutman et al., 2003). Activation of K_{ATP} channels was recently found to antagonize nociceptive behavior and hyper-excitability of DRG neurons from rats (Du et al., 2011a). Following partial sciatic nerve ligation, elevated tyrosine phosphorylation (pY12) of Kir3.1 was observed in the spinal superficial dorsal horn of wild type, but not Kir3.1 knock-out, mice (Ippolito et al., 2005). This phosphorylation may suppress channel conductance and accelerate channel deactivation (Ippolito et al., 2002), leading to enhanced neuronal excitability and could possibly contribute to the genesis of NINP. It is interesting to note that induced expression of Kir2.1 in chronically compressed DRG neurons can effectively suppress the neuronal excitability and, if induced at the beginning of the chronic compression, prevent the development of compression-induced hyperalgesia (Ma et al., 2010).

The TREK-1 channel is a member of mechano-gated K_{2P} family, one of the targets of inhalation anesthetics (Patel et al., 1999). TREK-1 is highly expressed in small sensory neurons and extensively co-localized with TRPV1 (Alloui et al., 2006). Mice with a disrupted TREK-1 gene are more sensitive to painful heat and low threshold mechanical stimuli and display an increased thermal and mechanical hyperalgesia in conditions of inflammation (Alloui et al., 2006). On the other hand, the TREK-1 null mice showed decreased sensitivity to acetone (less cold allodynia) after sciatic nerve ligation (Alloui et al., 2006). The chemotherapy drug oxaliplatin, which induces cold hypersensitivity, could lower the expression of TREK-1 (Descoeur et al., 2011). Future studies are needed to elucidate the role of TREK-1 channels in NINP. Similar as TREK-1, TREK-2 is also a member of the K_{2P} family. TREK-2 provide the major background K^+ conductance in cell body of small to medium-sized DRG neurons (Mathie, 2007), which are the major component of nociceptors. Based on these findings, it is also intriguing to investigate the role of TREK-2 in NINP (Huang & Yu, 2008).

Changes in the expression and function of voltage-gated ion channels in the pain pathway may contribute to the development and maintenance of NINP. Manipulations aiming at voltage-gated ion channels may provide novel strategies for the treatment of NINP. In addition to ion channel modulators, recent studies also reveal the promising roles of glial inhibitors, such as minocycline, and morphine in the management of NINP.

3.5 Microglia and astrocyte activation in nerve injury-induced neuropathic pain

During the last decade, the neuroimmune system, such as spinal glial cells, has been found to be critical for the development and maintenance of nerve injury-induced neuropathic pain (Watkins et al., 2007). Nerve injury not only induces morphological changes of microglia but also biochemical changes to induce pain. Nerve injury results in a up-regulation of P2X4 receptor (Tsuda et al., 2003) and CX3CR1 receptor in spinal cord microglia (Verge et al., 2004; Zhuang et al., 2007). *Intrathecal* blockade of P2X4 and CX3CR1 signaling attenuates NINP (Tsuda et al., 2003; Zhuang et al., 2007). The chemokine receptor CCR2 and the Toll-like recepotor-4 (TLR4) are also important for the formation of neuropathic pain *via* microglial activation (Abbadie et al., 2003; Tanga et al., 2005). Phosphorylation of p38 in microglia via activation of P2X4 receptor could increase the synthesis and release of the neurotrophin BDNF and pro-inflammatory cytokines (IL-1β, IL-6, and TNF-α), all of which could enhance nociceptive transmission in the spinal cord (Coull et al., 2005; Ji & Suter, 2007; Kawasaki et al., 2008b; Wang et al., 2010)

Our study using continuous *intrathecal* infusion of minocycline, a microglia inhibitor, revealed its effectiveness in attenuating the development of nerve injury-induced pain and no obvious spinal neurotoxicity was observed after the infusion (Lin et al., 2007). Other glial modulators, such as AV-411 (Ledeboer et al., 2006) and pentoxifylline (Mika et al., 2007), also possessed analgesic effect in NINP models. In addition to glial activation, compliment activation was recently found to participate in spinal nerve ligation-induced pain (Levin et al., 2008). Similar with gabapentin, minocycline could also attenuate morphine-induced tolerance (Cui et al., 2008) and this made itself a promising drug to be co-administered with morphine in the treatment of neuropathic pain. It is worthwhile to note that the attenuation effect of minocycline on morphine-induced tolerance is associated with inhibition of p38 activation in spinal microglia caused by chronic morphine (Cui et al., 2008).

In contrast to microglia, which is important for the development phase of NINP (Ji & Suter, 2007), astrocytes activation was critical for the maintenance phase of NINP (Zhuang et al., 2006). JNK-induced MCP-1 production and JAK-STAT3 pathway in spinal cord astrocytes was found to contribute to the maintenance of NINP (Gao et al., 2009b; Tsuda et al., 2011). The role of astrocyte activation and kinases involved in glial activation after nerve injury have been well reviewed (Gao & Ji, 2010; Ji et al., 2009).

4. Morphine in nerve injury-induced neuropathic pain

Morphine is the main drug used in pain clinics, especially in cancer pain. Recent animal studies also revealed the effectiveness of morphine in NINP models (Mika et al., 2007; Zhang et al., 2005). However, acute and chronic use of morphine can induce hyperalgesia and analgesia tolerance (Mao et al., 1994), which often lead to increased drug consumption and unwanted side-effects.

4.1 Glial non-opioid/p38 pathway in morphine-induced analgesia and tolerance

Using the tail flick test, Tseng's group has shown that morphine could induce anti-analgesia, which could be prevented by *levo-*, *dextro*naloxone **(a non-opioid ligand)** and p38 inhibitor *via* a glial non-opioid mechanism (Wu et al., 2006a; Wu et al., 2006b; Wu et al., 2005). From the works of Tseng's group, it could be summarized that 1) both *dextro-* and *levo*-morphine and lipopolysaccharide (LPS), a toll-like receptor (TLR)-4 agonist, could induce anti-analgesia, which could be prevented by *dextro-*, *levo*-naloxone and p38 inhibitor; 2) the anti-analgesia-inducing potency is: *dextro*-morphine > *levo*-morphine, and the reversal potency is: *levo*-naloxone > *dextro*-naloxone, which may imply the different binding affinities of *dextro*/*levo*- morphine and naloxone to the putative non-opioid receptor or TLR-4 (Hutchinson et al., 2007).

Inspired by the studies of Hong's group showing naloxone could attenuate LPS-induced microglial activation and neuronal damage (Liu et al., 2000), Watkin's group further tested the possible involvement of the putative nonopioid/TLR-4 pathway in NINP. They found *dextro*-naloxone, *levo*-naltrexone, and LPS-antagonist possess analgesic effects in chronic constriction neuropathic pain model (Hutchinson et al., 2007). Taken together with the role of glial p38 activation in NINP (Jin et al., 2003) and morphine-induced tolerance (Cui et al., 2006), it is possible that the putative glia non-opioid/TLR-4 pathway is important for the development of NINP and morphine-induced tolerance (Cui et al., 2006).

4.2 Intrathecal studies on morphine tolerance

Morphine has long been used *intrathecally* in the management of cancer and non-cancer chronic pain (Plummer et al., 1991; Roberts et al., 2001). However, the long-term use of morphine is associated with severe side-effects and tolerance (Osenbach & Harvey, 2001). Recently, many studies have revealed that *intrathecal* morphine could induce glial activation and neuro-inflammation in the spinal cord (Muscoli et al., 2010; Zhang et al., 2011). Several therapeutic targets have been found, including cytokine receptors, kappa-opioid receptors, N-methyl-D-aspartate receptors, and Toll-like receptors (Hameed et al., 2010; Lewis et al., 2010). Recently, tumor necrosis factor (TNF)-α antagonist etanercept was found to reverse morphine-induced tolerance and block morphine-induced neuroinflammation in the microglia (Shen et al., 2011). *Intrathecal* gabapentin and minocycline could also enhance the antinociceptive effects of morphine and attenuate morphine-induced tolerance (Habibi-Asl et al., 2009; Hutchinson et al., 2008; Lin et al., 2005). These promising agents may be co-administered with *intrathecal* morphine to improve the pain management for cancer patients (Christo & Mazloomdoost, 2008; Mercadante et al., 2004).

5. Intrathecal neurotoxicity studies

For a drug to be tested *intrathecally* in clinical trials, it is imperative to examine its neurotoxic effects first in animals (Bennett et al., 2000; Smith et al., 2008). For instance, *intrathecal* lidocaine has been found to induce neuropathological changes in the spinal cord and cauda equina (Kirihara et al., 2003). Other analgesics, such as adenosine, sufentanil, alfentanil and morphine have all been tested *intrathecally* in animal studies to examine their potential neurotoxicity (Chiari et al., 1999; Sabbe et al., 1994; Westin et al., 2010). Recently, chronic *intrathecal* infusion of minocycline or gabapentin has been reported to cause no grossly neurotoxicity in animal studies (Chu et al., 2011; Lin et al., 2007), supporting the *intrathecal* use of these agents for pain management.

6. Conclusion

Intrathecal space has been a route for spinal anesthesia and analgesics. This space also provides us a way to explore the possible mechanisms involved in pain transmission. Since pain is a major world-wide issue in clinical settings, more and more *intrathecal* animal studies have been undertaken to explore the possible mechanisms involved in the formation of different pain statuses and help to develop promising analgesics to alleviate the suffering of pain patients. These efforts will eventually help to provide better pain managements in clinical settings.

7. Acknowledgment

This chapter was supported by a John J. Bonica Trainee Fellowship from the International Association for the Study of Pain (IASP), a grant of NSC 98-2314-B-195-002-MY3 from National Science Council, Taipei, Taiwan and grants MMH 10015 and 10044 from Mackay Memorial Hospital, Taipei, Taiwan to J.K.C.

8. References

Abbadie, C., Lindia, J.A., Cumiskey, A.M., Peterson, L.B., Mudgett, J.S., Bayne, E.K., DeMartino, J.A., MacIntyre, D.E. & Forrest, M.J. (2003). Impaired neuropathic pain responses in mice lacking the chemokine receptor CCR2. *Proc Natl Acad Sci U S A*, Vol.100, No.13, pp. 7947-7952.

Abbott, F.V., Franklin, K.B. & Westbrook, R.F. (1995). The formalin test: scoring properties of the first and second phases of the pain response in rats. *Pain*, Vol.60, No.1, pp. 91-102.

Alloui, A., Zimmermann, K., Mamet, J., Duprat, F., Noel, J., Chemin, J., Guy, N., Blondeau, N., Voilley, N., Rubat-Coudert, C., Borsotto, M., Romey, G., Heurteaux, C., Reeh, P., Eschalier, A. & Lazdunski, M. (2006). TREK-1, a K+ channel involved in polymodal pain perception. *EMBO J*, Vol.25, No.11, pp. 2368-2376.

Altier, C., Dale, C.S., Kisilevsky, A.E., Chapman, K., Castiglioni, A.J., Matthews, E.A., Evans, R.M., Dickenson, A.H., Lipscombe, D., Vergnolle, N. & Zamponi, G.W. (2007). Differential role of N-type calcium channel splice isoforms in pain. *J Neurosci*, Vol.27, No.24, pp. 6363-6373.

Aurilio, C., Pota, V., Pace, M.C., Passavanti, M.B. & Barbarisi, M. (2008). Ionic channels and neuropathic pain: physiopathology and applications. *J Cell Physiol*, Vol.215, No.1, pp. 8-14.

Bennett, G., Deer, T., Du Pen, S., Rauck, R., Yaksh, T. & Hassenbusch, S.J. (2000). Future directions in the management of pain by intraspinal drug delivery. *J Pain Symptom Manage*, Vol.20, No.2, pp. S44-50.

Berta, T., Poirot, O., Pertin, M., Ji, R.R., Kellenberger, S. & Decosterd, I. (2008). Transcriptional and functional profiles of voltage-gated Na(+) channels in injured and non-injured DRG neurons in the SNI model of neuropathic pain. *Mol Cell Neurosci*, Vol.37, No.2, pp. 196-208.

Blackburn-Munro, G. & Jensen, B.S. (2003). The anticonvulsant retigabine attenuates nociceptive behaviours in rat models of persistent and neuropathic pain. *Eur J Pharmacol*, Vol.460, No.2-3, pp. 109-116.

Bloom, A.P., Jimenez-Andrade, J.M., Taylor, R.N., Castaneda-Corral, G., Kaczmarska, M.J., Freeman, K.T., Coughlin, K.A., Ghilardi, J.R., Kuskowski, M.A. & Mantyh, P.W. (2011). Breast Cancer-Induced Bone Remodeling, Skeletal Pain and Sprouting of Sensory Nerve Fibers. *J Pain*, pp.

Bourinet, E., Alloui, A., Monteil, A., Barrere, C., Couette, B., Poirot, O., Pages, A., McRory, J., Snutch, T.P., Eschalier, A. & Nargeot, J. (2005). Silencing of the $Ca_v3.2$ T-type calcium channel gene in sensory neurons demonstrates its major role in nociception. *EMBO J*, Vol.24, No.2, pp. 315-324.

Bourquin, A.F., Suveges, M., Pertin, M., Gilliard, N., Sardy, S., Davison, A.C., Spahn, D.R. & Decosterd, I. (2006). Assessment and analysis of mechanical allodynia-like behavior induced by spared nerve injury (SNI) in the mouse. *Pain*, Vol.122, No.1-2, pp. 14 e11-14.

Brackenbury, W.J. & Isom, L.L. (2008). Voltage-gated Na^+ channels: potential for beta subunits as therapeutic targets. *Expert Opin Ther Targets*, Vol.12, No.9, pp. 1191-1203.

Brennan, T.J., Vandermeulen, E.P. & Gebhart, G.F. (1996). Characterization of a rat model of incisional pain. *Pain*, Vol.64, No.3, pp. 493-501.

Cain, D.M., Wacnik, P.W., Turner, M., Wendelschafer-Crabb, G., Kennedy, W.R., Wilcox, G.L. & Simone, D.A. (2001). Functional interactions between tumor and peripheral nerve: changes in excitability and morphology of primary afferent fibers in a murine model of cancer pain. *J Neurosci*, Vol.21, No.23, pp. 9367-9376.

Catterall, W.A., Goldin, A.L. & Waxman, S.G. (2005). International Union of Pharmacology. XLVII. Nomenclature and structure-function relationships of voltage-gated sodium channels. *Pharmacol Rev*, Vol.57, No.4, pp. 397-409.

Catterall, W.A., Kalume, F. & Oakley, J.C. (2010). $Na_v1.1$ channels and epilepsy. *J Physiol*, Vol.588, No.Pt 11, pp. 1849-1859.

Catterall, W.A., Striessnig, J., Snutch, T.P. & Perez-Reyes, E. (2002). Voltage-gated calcium channels. *The IUPHAR compendium of voltage-gated ion channels*, pp. 32-56.

Chaplan, S.R., Bach, F.W., Pogrel, J.W., Chung, J.M. & Yaksh, T.L. (1994). Quantitative assessment of tactile allodynia in the rat paw. *J Neurosci Methods*, Vol.53, No.1, pp. 55-63.

Chattopadhyay, M., Mata, M. & Fink, D.J. (2008). Continuous delta-opioid receptor activation reduces neuronal voltage-gated sodium channel (NaV1.7) levels through activation of protein kinase C in painful diabetic neuropathy. *J Neurosci*, Vol.28, No.26, pp. 6652-6658.

Chen, W.K., Liu, I.Y., Chang, Y.T., Chen, Y.C., Chen, C.C., Yen, C.T. & Shin, H.S. (2010). Ca(v)3.2 T-type Ca^{2+} channel-dependent activation of ERK in paraventricular thalamus modulates acid-induced chronic muscle pain. *J Neurosci*, Vol.30, No.31, pp. 10360-10368.

Cheng, J.K. & Chiou, L.C. (2006). Mechanisms of the antinociceptive action of gabapentin. *J Pharmacol Sci*, Vol.100, No.5, pp. 471-486.

Cheng, J.K., Lin, C.S., Chen, C.C., Yang, J.R. & Chiou, L.C. (2007). Effects of intrathecal injection of T-type calcium channel blockers in the rat formalin test. *Behav Pharmacol*, Vol.18, No.1, pp. 1-8.

Chiari, A., Yaksh, T.L., Myers, R.R., Provencher, J., Moore, L., Lee, C.S. & Eisenach, J.C. (1999). Preclinical toxicity screening of intrathecal adenosine in rats and dogs. *Anesthesiology*, Vol.91, No.3, pp. 824-832.

Chien, L.Y., Cheng, J.K., Chu, D., Cheng, C.F. & Tsaur, M.L. (2007). Reduced expression of A-type potassium channels in primary sensory neurons induces mechanical hypersensitivity. *J Neurosci*, Vol.27, No.37, pp. 9855-9865.

Christo, P.J. & Mazloomdoost, D. (2008). Interventional pain treatments for cancer pain. *Ann N Y Acad Sci*, Vol.1138, pp. 299-328.

Chu, L.C., Tsaur, M.L., Lin, C.S., Hung, Y.C., Wang, T.Y., Chen, C.C. & Cheng, J.K. (2011). Chronic intrathecal infusion of gabapentin prevents nerve ligation-induced pain in rats. *Br J Anaesth*, Vol.106, No.5, pp. 699-705.

Clohisy, D.R. & Mantyh, P.W. (2003). Bone cancer pain. *Cancer*, Vol.97, No.3 Suppl, pp. 866-873.

Coderre, T.J. & Melzack, R. (1992). The contribution of excitatory amino acids to central sensitization and persistent nociception after formalin-induced tissue injury. *J Neurosci*, Vol.12, No.9, pp. 3665-3670.

Coetzee, W.A., Amarillo, Y., Chiu, J., Chow, A., Lau, D., McCormack, T., Moreno, H., Nadal, M.S., Ozaita, A., Pountney, D., Saganich, M., Vega-Saenz de Miera, E. & Rudy, B. (1999). Molecular diversity of K+ channels. *Ann N Y Acad Sci*, Vol.868, pp. 233-285.

Constantin, C.E., Mair, N., Sailer, C.A., Andratsch, M., Xu, Z.Z., Blumer, M.J., Scherbakov, N., Davis, J.B., Bluethmann, H., Ji, R.R. & Kress, M. (2008). Endogenous tumor necrosis factor alpha (TNFalpha) requires TNF receptor type 2 to generate heat hyperalgesia in a mouse cancer model. *J Neurosci*, Vol.28, No.19, pp. 5072-5081.

Coull, J.A., Beggs, S., Boudreau, D., Boivin, D., Tsuda, M., Inoue, K., Gravel, C., Salter, M.W. & De Koninck, Y. (2005). BDNF from microglia causes the shift in neuronal anion gradient underlying neuropathic pain. *Nature*, Vol.438, No.7070, pp. 1017-1021.

Cox, J.J., Sheynin, J., Shorer, Z., Reimann, F., Nicholas, A.K., Zubovic, L., Baralle, M., Wraige, E., Manor, E., Levy, J., Woods, C.G. & Parvari, R. (2010). Congenital insensitivity to pain: novel SCN9A missense and in-frame deletion mutations. *Hum Mutat*, Vol.31, No.9, pp. E1670-1686.

Cuddapah, V.A. & Sontheimer, H. (2011). Ion Channels and the Control of Cancer Cell Migration. *Am J Physiol Cell Physiol*, pp.

Cui, Y., Chen, Y., Zhi, J.L., Guo, R.X., Feng, J.Q. & Chen, P.X. (2006). Activation of p38 mitogen-activated protein kinase in spinal microglia mediates morphine antinociceptive tolerance. *Brain Res*, Vol.1069, No.1, pp. 235-243.

Cui, Y., Liao, X.X., Liu, W., Guo, R.X., Wu, Z.Z., Zhao, C.M., Chen, P.X. & Feng, J.Q. (2008). A novel role of minocycline: attenuating morphine antinociceptive tolerance by inhibition of p38 MAPK in the activated spinal microglia. *Brain Behav Immun*, Vol.22, No.1, pp. 114-123.

Decosterd, I. & Woolf, C.J. (2000). Spared nerve injury: an animal model of persistent peripheral neuropathic pain. *Pain*, Vol.87, No.2, pp. 149-158.

Descoeur, J., Pereira, V., Pizzoccaro, A., Francois, A., Ling, B., Maffre, V., Couette, B., Busserolles, J., Courteix, C., Noel, J., Lazdunski, M., Eschalier, A., Authier, N. & Bourinet, E. (2011). Oxaliplatin-induced cold hypersensitivity is due to remodelling of ion channel expression in nociceptors. *EMBO Mol Med*, Vol.3, No.5, pp. 266-278.

Doddareddy, M.R., Choo, H., Cho, Y.S., Rhim, H., Koh, H.Y., Lee, J.H., Jeong, S.W. & Pae, A.N. (2007). 3D pharmacophore based virtual screening of T-type calcium channel blockers. *Bioorg Med Chem*, Vol.15, No.2, pp. 1091-1105.

Dogrul, A., Gardell, L.R., Ossipov, M.H., Tulunay, F.C., Lai, J. & Porreca, F. (2003). Reversal of experimental neuropathic pain by T-type calcium channel blockers. *Pain*, Vol.105, No.1-2, pp. 159-168.

Dolmetsch, R.E., Pajvani, U., Fife, K., Spotts, J.M. & Greenberg, M.E. (2001). Signaling to the nucleus by an L-type calcium channel-calmodulin complex through the MAP kinase pathway. *Science*, Vol.294, No.5541, pp. 333-339.

Donnelly-Roberts, D., McGaraughty, S., Shieh, C.C., Honore, P. & Jarvis, M.F. (2008). Painful purinergic receptors. *J Pharmacol Exp Ther*, Vol.324, No.2, pp. 409-415.

Dost, R., Rostock, A. & Rundfeldt, C. (2004). The anti-hyperalgesic activity of retigabine is mediated by KCNQ potassium channel activation. *Naunyn Schmiedebergs Arch Pharmacol*, Vol.369, No.4, pp. 382-390.

Du, X., Wang, C. & Zhang, H. (2011a). Activation of ATP-sensitive potassium channels antagonize nociceptive behavior and hyperexcitability of DRG neurons from rats. *Mol Pain*, Vol.7, No.1, pp. 35.

Du, X., Zhang, X., Qi, J., An, H., Li, J., Wan, Y., Fu, Y., Gao, H., Gao, Z., Zhan, Y. & Zhang, H. (2011b). Characteristics and molecular basis of celecoxib modulation on Kv7 potassium channels. *Br J Pharmacol*, pp.

Duarte, D.B., Duan, J.H., Nicol, G.D., Vasko, M.R. & Hingtgen, C.M. (2011). Reduced expression of SynGAP, a neuronal GTPase activating protein, enhances capsaicin-induced peripheral sensitization. *J Neurophysiol*, pp.

Dureja, G.P., Usmani, H., Khan, M., Tahseen, M. & Jamal, A. (2010). Efficacy of intrathecal midazolam with or without epidural methylprednisolone for management of post-herpetic neuralgia involving lumbosacral dermatomes. *Pain Physician*, Vol.13, No.3, pp. 213-221.

Ekberg, J., Jayamanne, A., Vaughan, C.W., Aslan, S., Thomas, L., Mould, J., Drinkwater, R., Baker, M.D., Abrahamsen, B., Wood, J.N., Adams, D.J., Christie, M.J. & Lewis, R.J. (2006). muO-conotoxin MrVIB selectively blocks Nav1.8 sensory neuron specific sodium channels and chronic pain behavior without motor deficits. *Proc Natl Acad Sci U S A*, Vol.103, No.45, pp. 17030-17035.

Eroglu, C., Allen, N.J., Susman, M.W., O'Rourke, N.A., Park, C.Y., Ozkan, E., Chakraborty, C., Mulinyawe, S.B., Annis, D.S., Huberman, A.D., Green, E.M., Lawler, J., Dolmetsch, R., Garcia, K.C., Smith, S.J., Luo, Z.D., Rosenthal, A., Mosher, D.F. & Barres, B.A. (2009). Gabapentin receptor alpha2delta-1 is a neuronal thrombospondin receptor responsible for excitatory CNS synaptogenesis. *Cell*, Vol.139, No.2, pp. 380-392.

Facer, P., Casula, M.A., Smith, G.D., Benham, C.D., Chessell, I.P., Bountra, C., Sinisi, M., Birch, R. & Anand, P. (2007). Differential expression of the capsaicin receptor TRPV1 and related novel receptors TRPV3, TRPV4 and TRPM8 in normal human tissues and changes in traumatic and diabetic neuropathy. *BMC Neurol*, Vol.7, pp. 11.

Felix, R. (1999). Voltage-dependent Ca^{2+} channel $\alpha_2\delta$ auxiliary subunit: structure, function and regulation. *Receptors Channels*, Vol.6, No.5, pp. 351-362.

Field, M.J., Cox, P.J., Stott, E., Melrose, H., Offord, J., Su, T.Z., Bramwell, S., Corradini, L., England, S., Winks, J., Kinloch, R.A., Hendrich, J., Dolphin, A.C., Webb, T. & Williams, D. (2006). Identification of the alpha2-delta-1 subunit of voltage-dependent calcium channels as a molecular target for pain mediating the analgesic actions of pregabalin. *Proc Natl Acad Sci U S A*, Vol.103, No.46, pp. 17537-17542.

Foulkes, T., Nassar, M.A., Lane, T., Matthews, E.A., Baker, M.D., Gerke, V., Okuse, K., Dickenson, A.H. & Wood, J.N. (2006). Deletion of annexin 2 light chain p11 in nociceptors causes deficits in somatosensory coding and pain behavior. *J Neurosci*, Vol.26, No.41, pp. 10499-10507.

Fukumoto, N., Obama, Y., Kitamura, N., Niimi, K., Takahashi, E., Itakura, C. & Shibuya, I. (2009). Hypoalgesic behaviors of P/Q-type voltage-gated Ca^{2+} channel mutant mouse, rolling mouse Nagoya. *Neuroscience*, Vol.160, No.1, pp. 165-173.

Gao, X., Kim, H.K., Chung, J.M. & Chung, K. (2005). Enhancement of NMDA receptor phosphorylation of the spinal dorsal horn and nucleus gracilis neurons in neuropathic rats. *Pain*, Vol.116, No.1-2, pp. 62-72.

Gao, Y.J., Cheng, J.K., Zeng, Q., Xu, Z.Z., Decosterd, I., Xu, X. & Ji, R.R. (2009a). Selective inhibition of JNK with a peptide inhibitor attenuates pain hypersensitivity and tumor growth in a mouse skin cancer pain model. *Exp Neurol*, Vol.219, No.1, pp. 146-155.

Gao, Y.J. & Ji, R.R. (2010). Targeting astrocyte signaling for chronic pain. *Neurotherapeutics*, Vol.7, No.4, pp. 482-493.

Gao, Y.J., Zhang, L., Samad, O.A., Suter, M.R., Yasuhiko, K., Xu, Z.Z., Park, J.Y., Lind, A.L., Ma, Q. & Ji, R.R. (2009b). JNK-induced MCP-1 production in spinal cord astrocytes contributes to central sensitization and neuropathic pain. *J Neurosci*, Vol.29, No.13, pp. 4096-4108.

Ghilardi, J.R., Freeman, K.T., Jimenez-Andrade, J.M., Mantyh, W.G., Bloom, A.P., Kuskowski, M.A. & Mantyh, P.W. (2010). Administration of a tropomyosin receptor kinase inhibitor attenuates sarcoma-induced nerve sprouting, neuroma formation and bone cancer pain. *Mol Pain*, Vol.6, pp. 87.

Gold, M.S., Levine, J.D. & Correa, A.M. (1998). Modulation of TTX-R INa by PKC and PKA and their role in PGE2-induced sensitization of rat sensory neurons in vitro. *J Neurosci*, Vol.18, No.24, pp. 10345-10355.

Gutman, G.A., Chandy, K.G., Adelman, J.P., Aiyar, J., Bayliss, D.A., Clapham, D.E., Covarriubias, M., Desir, G.V., Furuichi, K., Ganetzky, B., Garcia, M.L., Grissmer, S., Jan, L.Y., Karschin, A., Kim, D., Kuperschmidt, S., Kurachi, Y., Lazdunski, M., Lesage, F., Lester, H.A., McKinnon, D., Nichols, C.G., O'Kelly, I., Robbins, J., Robertson, G.A., Rudy, B., Sanguinetti, M., Seino, S., Stuehmer, W., Tamkun, M.M., Vandenberg, C.A., Wei, A., Wulff, H. & Wymore, R.S. (2003). International Union of Pharmacology. XLI. Compendium of voltage-gated ion channels: potassium channels. *Pharmacol Rev*, Vol.55, No.4, pp. 583-586.

Habibi-Asl, B., Hassanzadeh, K. & Charkhpour, M. (2009). Central administration of minocycline and riluzole prevents morphine-induced tolerance in rats. *Anesth Analg*, Vol.109, No.3, pp. 936-942.

Hameed, H., Hameed, M. & Christo, P.J. (2010). The effect of morphine on glial cells as a potential therapeutic target for pharmacological development of analgesic drugs. *Curr Pain Headache Rep*, Vol.14, No.2, pp. 96-104.

Hargreaves, K., Dubner, R., Brown, F., Flores, C. & Joris, J. (1988). A new and sensitive method for measuring thermal nociception in cutaneous hyperalgesia. *Pain*, Vol.32, No.1, pp. 77-88.

Hong, R.W. (2010). Less is more: the recent history of neuraxial labor analgesia. *Am J Ther*, Vol.17, No.5, pp. 492-497.

Hong, S., Morrow, T.J., Paulson, P.E., Isom, L.L. & Wiley, J.W. (2004). Early painful diabetic neuropathy is associated with differential changes in tetrodotoxin-sensitive and -resistant sodium channels in dorsal root ganglion neurons in the rat. *J Biol Chem*, Vol.279, No.28, pp. 29341-29350.

Hu, H.J., Carrasquillo, Y., Karim, F., Jung, W.E., Nerbonne, J.M., Schwarz, T.L. & Gereau, R.W.t. (2006). The kv4.2 potassium channel subunit is required for pain plasticity. *Neuron*, Vol.50, No.1, pp. 89-100.

Hu, H.J., Glauner, K.S. & Gereau, R.W.t. (2003). ERK integrates PKA and PKC signaling in superficial dorsal horn neurons. I. Modulation of A-type K+ currents. *J Neurophysiol*, Vol.90, No.3, pp. 1671-1679.

Huang, D. & Yu, B. (2008). Recent advance and possible future in TREK-2: a two-pore potassium channel may involved in the process of NPP, brain ischemia and memory impairment. *Med Hypotheses*, Vol.70, No.3, pp. 618-624.

Hunanyan, A.S., Alessi, V., Patel, S., Pearse, D.D., Matthews, G. & Arvanian, V.L. (2011). Alterations of action potentials and the localization of Nav1.6 sodium channels in spared axons after hemisection injury of the spinal cord in adult rats. *J Neurophysiol*, Vol.105, No.3, pp. 1033-1044.

Hutchinson, M.R., Bland, S.T., Johnson, K.W., Rice, K.C., Maier, S.F. & Watkins, L.R. (2007). Opioid-induced glial activation: mechanisms of activation and implications for opioid analgesia, dependence, and reward. *ScientificWorldJournal*, Vol.7, pp. 98-111.

Hutchinson, M.R., Northcutt, A.L., Chao, L.W., Kearney, J.J., Zhang, Y., Berkelhammer, D.L., Loram, L.C., Rozeske, R.R., Bland, S.T., Maier, S.F., Gleeson, T.T. & Watkins, L.R. (2008). Minocycline suppresses morphine-induced respiratory depression, suppresses morphine-induced reward, and enhances systemic morphine-induced analgesia. *Brain Behav Immun*, Vol.22, No.8, pp. 1248-1256.

Ikeda, H., Heinke, B., Ruscheweyh, R. & Sandkuhler, J. (2003). Synaptic plasticity in spinal lamina I projection neurons that mediate hyperalgesia. *Science*, Vol.299, No.5610, pp. 1237-1240.

Ippolito, D.L., Temkin, P.A., Rogalski, S.L. & Chavkin, C. (2002). N-terminal tyrosine residues within the potassium channel Kir3 modulate GTPase activity of Galphai. *J Biol Chem*, Vol.277, No.36, pp. 32692-32696.

Ippolito, D.L., Xu, M., Bruchas, M.R., Wickman, K. & Chavkin, C. (2005). Tyrosine phosphorylation of K(ir)3.1 in spinal cord is induced by acute inflammation, chronic neuropathic pain, and behavioral stress. *J Biol Chem*, Vol.280, No.50, pp. 41683-41693.

Jarecki, B.W., Piekarz, A.D., Jackson, J.O., 2nd & Cummins, T.R. (2010). Human voltage-gated sodium channel mutations that cause inherited neuronal and muscle channelopathies increase resurgent sodium currents. *J Clin Invest*, Vol.120, No.1, pp. 369-378.

Jarvis, M.F., Honore, P., Shieh, C.C., Chapman, M., Joshi, S., Zhang, X.F., Kort, M., Carroll, W., Marron, B., Atkinson, R., Thomas, J., Liu, D., Krambis, M., Liu, Y.,

McGaraughty, S., Chu, K., Roeloffs, R., Zhong, C., Mikusa, J.P., Hernandez, G., Gauvin, D., Wade, C., Zhu, C., Pai, M., Scanio, M., Shi, L., Drizin, I., Gregg, R., Matulenko, M., Hakeem, A., Gross, M., Johnson, M., Marsh, K., Wagoner, P.K., Sullivan, J.P., Faltynek, C.R. & Krafte, D.S. (2007). A-803467, a potent and selective Nav1.8 sodium channel blocker, attenuates neuropathic and inflammatory pain in the rat. *Proc Natl Acad Sci U S A*, Vol.104, No.20, pp. 8520-8525.

Ji, R.R., Gereau, R.W.t., Malcangio, M. & Strichartz, G.R. (2009). MAP kinase and pain. *Brain Res Rev*, Vol.60, No.1, pp. 135-148.

Ji, R.R., Kohno, T., Moore, K.A. & Woolf, C.J. (2003). Central sensitization and LTP: do pain and memory share similar mechanisms? *Trends Neurosci*, Vol.26, No.12, pp. 696-705.

Ji, R.R. & Strichartz, G. (2004). Cell signaling and the genesis of neuropathic pain. *Sci STKE*, Vol.252 pp. reE14.

Ji, R.R. & Suter, M.R. (2007). p38 MAPK, microglial signaling, and neuropathic pain. *Mol Pain*, Vol.3, pp. 33.

Jimenez-Andrade, J.M., Bloom, A.P., Stake, J.I., Mantyh, W.G., Taylor, R.N., Freeman, K.T., Ghilardi, J.R., Kuskowski, M.A. & Mantyh, P.W. (2010). Pathological sprouting of adult nociceptors in chronic prostate cancer-induced bone pain. *J Neurosci*, Vol.30, No.44, pp. 14649-14656.

Jin, S.X., Zhuang, Z.Y., Woolf, C.J. & Ji, R.R. (2003). p38 mitogen-activated protein kinase is activated after a spinal nerve ligation in spinal cord microglia and dorsal root ganglion neurons and contributes to the generation of neuropathic pain. *J Neurosci*, Vol.23, No.10, pp. 4017-4022.

Jin, X. & Gereau, R.W.t. (2006). Acute p38-mediated modulation of tetrodotoxin-resistant sodium channels in mouse sensory neurons by tumor necrosis factor-alpha. *J Neurosci*, Vol.26, No.1, pp. 246-255.

Joshi, S.K., Mikusa, J.P., Hernandez, G., Baker, S., Shieh, C.C., Neelands, T., Zhang, X.F., Niforatos, W., Kage, K., Han, P., Krafte, D., Faltynek, C., Sullivan, J.P., Jarvis, M.F. & Honore, P. (2006). Involvement of the TTX-resistant sodium channel Nav 1.8 in inflammatory and neuropathic, but not post-operative, pain states. *Pain*, Vol.123, No.1-2, pp. 75-82.

Kakimura, J., Zheng, T., Uryu, N. & Ogata, N. (2010). Regulation of the spontaneous augmentation of Na(V)1.9 in mouse dorsal root ganglion neurons: effect of PKA and PKC pathways. *Mar Drugs*, Vol.8, No.3, pp. 728-740.

Kang, S. & Brennan, T.J. (2009). Chemosensitivity and mechanosensitivity of nociceptors from incised rat hindpaw skin. *Anesthesiology*, Vol.111, No.1, pp. 155-164.

Kawasaki, Y., Xu, Z.Z., Wang, X., Park, J.Y., Zhuang, Z.Y., Tan, P.H., Gao, Y.J., Roy, K., Corfas, G., Lo, E.H. & Ji, R.R. (2008a). Distinct roles of matrix metalloproteases in the early- and late-phase development of neuropathic pain. *Nat Med*, Vol.14, No.3, pp. 331-336.

Kawasaki, Y., Zhang, L., Cheng, J.K. & Ji, R.R. (2008b). Cytokine mechanisms of central sensitization: distinct and overlapping role of interleukin-1beta, interleukin-6, and tumor necrosis factor-alpha in regulating synaptic and neuronal activity in the superficial spinal cord. *J Neurosci*, Vol.28, No.20, pp. 5189-5194.

Kim, S.H. & Chung, J.M. (1992). An experimental model for peripheral neuropathy produced by segmental spinal nerve ligation in the rat. *Pain*, Vol.50, No.3, pp. 355-363.

Kirihara, Y., Saito, Y., Sakura, S., Hashimoto, K., Kishimoto, T. & Yasui, Y. (2003). Comparative neurotoxicity of intrathecal and epidural lidocaine in rats. *Anesthesiology*, Vol.99, No.4, pp. 961-968.

Klugbauer, N., Marais, E. & Hofmann, F. (2003). Calcium channel alpha2delta subunits: differential expression, function, and drug binding. *J Bioenerg Biomembr*, Vol.35, No.6, pp. 639-647.

Knutsen, L.J., Hobbs, C.J., Earnshaw, C.G., Fiumana, A., Gilbert, J., Mellor, S.L., Radford, F., Smith, N.J., Birch, P.J., Russell Burley, J., Ward, S.D. & James, I.F. (2007). Synthesis and SAR of novel 2-arylthiazolidinones as selective analgesic N-type calcium channel blockers. *Bioorg Med Chem Lett*, Vol.17, No.3, pp. 662-667.

Kretschmer, T., Happel, L.T., England, J.D., Nguyen, D.H., Tiel, R.L., Beuerman, R.W. & Kline, D.G. (2002). Accumulation of PN1 and PN3 sodium channels in painful human neuroma-evidence from immunocytochemistry. *Acta Neurochir (Wien)*, Vol.144, No.8, pp. 803-810; discussion 810.

Lampert, A., O'Reilly, A.O., Reeh, P. & Leffler, A. (2010). Sodium channelopathies and pain. *Pflugers Arch*, Vol.460, No.2, pp. 249-263.

Ledeboer, A., Liu, T., Shumilla, J.A., Mahoney, J.H., Vijay, S., Gross, M.I., Vargas, J.A., Sultzbaugh, L., Claypool, M.D., Sanftner, L.M., Watkins, L.R. & Johnson, K.W. (2006). The glial modulatory drug AV411 attenuates mechanical allodynia in rat models of neuropathic pain. *Neuron Glia Biol*, Vol.2, No.4, pp. 279-291.

Lee, S., Kim, Y., Back, S.K., Choi, H.W., Lee, J.Y., Jung, H.H., Ryu, J.H., Suh, H.W., Na, H.S., Kim, H.J., Rhim, H. & Kim, J.I. (2010). Analgesic effect of highly reversible omega-conotoxin FVIA on N type Ca^{2+} channels. *Mol Pain*, Vol.6, pp. 97.

Leo, S., D'Hooge, R. & Meert, T. (2010). Exploring the role of nociceptor-specific sodium channels in pain transmission using Nav1.8 and Nav1.9 knockout mice. *Behav Brain Res*, Vol.208, No.1, pp. 149-157.

Levin, M.E., Jin, J.G., Ji, R.R., Tong, J., Pomonis, J.D., Lavery, D.J., Miller, S.W. & Chiang, L.W. (2008). Complement activation in the peripheral nervous system following the spinal nerve ligation model of neuropathic pain. *Pain*, Vol.137, No.1, pp. 182-201.

Lewis, S.S., Hutchinson, M.R., Rezvani, N., Loram, L.C., Zhang, Y., Maier, S.F., Rice, K.C. & Watkins, L.R. (2010). Evidence that intrathecal morphine-3-glucuronide may cause pain enhancement via toll-like receptor 4/MD-2 and interleukin-1beta. *Neuroscience*, Vol.165, No.2, pp. 569-583.

Li, C.Y., Song, Y.H., Higuera, E.S. & Luo, Z.D. (2004). Spinal dorsal horn calcium channel $\alpha_2\delta$-1 subunit upregulation contributes to peripheral nerve injury-induced tactile allodynia. *J Neurosci*, Vol.24, No.39, pp. 8494-8499.

Li, C.Y., Zhang, X.L., Matthews, E.A., Li, K.W., Kurwa, A., Boroujerdi, A., Gross, J., Gold, M.S., Dickenson, A.H., Feng, G. & Luo, Z.D. (2006). Calcium channel alpha2delta1 subunit mediates spinal hyperexcitability in pain modulation. *Pain*, Vol.125, No.1-2, pp. 20-34.

Lin, C.S., Tsaur, M.L., Chen, C.C., Wang, T.Y., Lin, C.F., Lai, Y.L., Hsu, T.C., Pan, Y.Y., Yang, C.H. & Cheng, J.K. (2007). Chronic intrathecal infusion of minocycline prevents the development of spinal-nerve ligation-induced pain in rats. *Reg Anesth Pain Med*, Vol.32, No.3, pp. 209-216.

Lin, J.A., Lee, M.S., Wu, C.T., Yeh, C.C., Lin, S.L., Wen, Z.H. & Wong, C.S. (2005). Attenuation of morphine tolerance by intrathecal gabapentin is associated with suppression of morphine-evoked excitatory amino acid release in the rat spinal cord. *Brain Res*, Vol.1054, No.2 pp. 167-173.

Liu, B., Du, L. & Hong, J.S. (2000). Naloxone protects rat dopaminergic neurons against inflammatory damage through inhibition of microglia activation and superoxide generation. *J Pharmacol Exp Ther*, Vol.293, No.2, pp. 607-617.

LoPachin, R.M., Rudy, T.A. & Yaksh, T.L. (1981). An improved method for chronic catheterization of the rat spinal subarachnoid space. *Physiol Behav*, Vol.27, No.3, pp. 559-561.

Lopez-Santiago, L.F., Pertin, M., Morisod, X., Chen, C., Hong, S., Wiley, J., Decosterd, I. & Isom, L.L. (2006). Sodium channel beta2 subunits regulate tetrodotoxin-sensitive sodium channels in small dorsal root ganglion neurons and modulate the response to pain. *J Neurosci*, Vol.26, No.30, pp. 7984-7994.

Luo, J.L., Qin, H.Y., Wong, C.K., Tsang, S.Y., Huang, Y. & Bian, Z.X. (2011). Enhanced Excitability and Down-Regulated Voltage-Gated Potassium Channels in Colonic DRG Neurons from Neonatal Maternal Separation Rats. *J Pain*, Vol.12, No.5, pp. 600-609.

Luvisetto, S., Marinelli, S., Panasiti, M.S., D'Amato, F.R., Fletcher, C.F., Pavone, F. & Pietrobon, D. (2006). Pain sensitivity in mice lacking the Ca(v)2.1alpha1 subunit of P/Q-type Ca^{2+} channels. *Neuroscience*, Vol.142, No.3, pp. 823-832.

Lynch, M.E. & Campbell, F. (2011). Cannabinoids for Treatment of Chronic Non-Cancer Pain; a Systematic Review of Randomized Trials. *Br J Clin Pharmacol*, pp.

Ma, C., Rosenzweig, J., Zhang, P., Johns, D.C. & LaMotte, R.H. (2010). Expression of inwardly rectifying potassium channels by an inducible adenoviral vector reduced the neuronal hyperexcitability and hyperalgesia produced by chronic compression of the spinal ganglion. *Mol Pain*, Vol.6, pp. 65.

Mao, J., Price, D.D. & Mayer, D.J. (1994). Thermal hyperalgesia in association with the development of morphine tolerance in rats: roles of excitatory amino acid receptors and protein kinase C. *J Neurosci*, Vol.14, No.4, pp. 2301-2312.

Mathie, A. (2007). Neuronal two-pore-domain potassium channels and their regulation by G protein-coupled receptors. *J Physiol*, Vol.578, No.Pt 2, pp. 377-385.

Matthews, E.A., Bee, L.A., Stephens, G.J. & Dickenson, A.H. (2007). The Cav2.3 calcium channel antagonist SNX-482 reduces dorsal horn neuronal responses in a rat model of chronic neuropathic pain. *Eur J Neurosci*, Vol.25, No.12, pp. 3561-3569.

Mazzuca, M., Heurteaux, C., Alloui, A., Diochot, S., Baron, A., Voilley, N., Blondeau, N., Escoubas, P., Gelot, A., Cupo, A., Zimmer, A., Zimmer, A.M., Eschalier, A. & Lazdunski, M. (2007). A tarantula peptide against pain via ASIC1a channels and opioid mechanisms. *Nat Neurosci*, Vol.10, No.8, pp. 943-945.

McCallum, J.B., Wu, H.E., Tang, Q., Kwok, W.M. & Hogan, Q.H. (2011). Subtype-specific reduction of voltage-gated calcium current in medium-sized dorsal root ganglion neurons after painful peripheral nerve injury. *Neuroscience*, Vol.179, pp. 244-255.

Mercadante, S. (1999). Neuraxial techniques for cancer pain: an opinion about unresolved therapeutic dilemmas. *Reg Anesth Pain Med*, Vol.24, No.1, pp. 74-83.

Mercadante, S., Villari, P. & Ferrera, P. (2004). Dialogues on complex analgesic strategies for difficult pain syndromes. *Support Care Cancer*, Vol.12, No.8, pp. 599-603.

Mienville, J.M., Maric, I., Maric, D. & Clay, J.R. (1999). Loss of IA expression and increased excitability in postnatal rat Cajal-Retzius cells. *J Neurophysiol*, Vol.82, No.3, pp. 1303-1310.

Mika, J., Osikowicz, M., Makuch, W. & Przewlocka, B. (2007). Minocycline and pentoxifylline attenuate allodynia and hyperalgesia and potentiate the effects of morphine in rat and mouse models of neuropathic pain. *Eur J Pharmacol*, Vol.560, No.2-3, pp. 142-149.

Mo, G., Grant, R., O'Donnell, D., Ragsdale, D.S., Cao, C.Q. & Seguela, P. (2011). Neuropathic Nav1.3-mediated sensitization to P2X activation is regulated by protein kinase C. *Mol Pain*, Vol.7, pp. 14.

Mogil, J.S., Davis, K.D. & Derbyshire, S.W. (2010). The necessity of animal models in pain research. *Pain*, Vol.151, No.1, pp. 12-17.

Muscoli, C., Doyle, T., Dagostino, C., Bryant, L., Chen, Z., Watkins, L.R., Ryerse, J., Bieberich, E., Neumman, W. & Salvemini, D. (2010). Counter-regulation of opioid analgesia by glial-derived bioactive sphingolipids. *J Neurosci*, Vol.30, No.46, pp. 15400-15408.

Nassar, M.A., Levato, A., Stirling, L.C. & Wood, J.N. (2005). Neuropathic pain develops normally in mice lacking both Na(v)1.7 and Na(v)1.8. *Mol Pain*, Vol.1, pp. 24.

Ocana, M., Cendan, C.M., Cobos, E.J., Entrena, J.M. & Baeyens, J.M. (2004). Potassium channels and pain: present realities and future opportunities. *Eur J Pharmacol*, Vol.500, No.1-3, pp. 203-219.

Osenbach, R.K. & Harvey, S. (2001). Neuraxial infusion in patients with chronic intractable cancer and noncancer pain. *Curr Pain Headache Rep*, Vol.5, No.3, pp. 241-249.

Park, S.Y., Choi, J.Y., Kim, R.U., Lee, Y.S., Cho, H.J. & Kim, D.S. (2003). Downregulation of voltage-gated potassium channel alpha gene expression by axotomy and neurotrophins in rat dorsal root ganglia. *Mol Cells*, Vol.16, No.2, pp. 256-259.

Passmore, G.M., Selyanko, A.A., Mistry, M., Al-Qatari, M., Marsh, S.J., Matthews, E.A., Dickenson, A.H., Brown, T.A., Burbidge, S.A., Main, M. & Brown, D.A. (2003). KCNQ/M currents in sensory neurons: significance for pain therapy. *J Neurosci*, Vol.23, No.18, pp. 7227-7236.

Patel, A.J., Honore, E., Lesage, F., Fink, M., Romey, G. & Lazdunski, M. (1999). Inhalational anesthetics activate two-pore-domain background K^+ channels. *Nat Neurosci*, Vol.2, No.5, pp. 422-426.

Pertin, M., Ji, R.R., Berta, T., Powell, A.J., Karchewski, L., Tate, S.N., Isom, L.L., Woolf, C.J., Gilliard, N., Spahn, D.R. & Decosterd, I. (2005). Upregulation of the voltage-gated sodium channel beta2 subunit in neuropathic pain models: characterization of expression in injured and non-injured primary sensory neurons. *J Neurosci*, Vol.25, No.47, pp. 10970-10980.

Plummer, J.L., Cherry, D.A., Cousins, M.J., Gourlay, G.K., Onley, M.M. & Evans, K.H. (1991). Long-term spinal administration of morphine in cancer and non-cancer pain: a retrospective study. *Pain*, Vol.44, No.3, pp. 215-220.

Poirot, O., Berta, T., Decosterd, I. & Kellenberger, S. (2006). Distinct ASIC currents are expressed in rat putative nociceptors and are modulated by nerve injury. *J Physiol*, Vol.576, No.Pt 1, pp. 215-234.

Qin, N., Yagel, S., Momplaisir, M.L., Codd, E.E. & D'Andrea, M.R. (2002). Molecular cloning and characterization of the human voltage-gated calcium channel $\alpha_2\delta$-4 subunit. *Mol Pharmacol*, Vol.62, No.3, pp. 485-496.

Rasband, M.N., Park, E.W., Vanderah, T.W., Lai, J., Porreca, F. & Trimmer, J.S. (2001). Distinct potassium channels on pain-sensing neurons. *Proc Natl Acad Sci U S A*, Vol.98, No.23, pp. 13373-13378.

Roberts, L.J., Finch, P.M., Goucke, C.R. & Price, L.M. (2001). Outcome of intrathecal opioids in chronic non-cancer pain. *Eur J Pain*, Vol.5, No.4, pp. 353-361.

Rogers, M., Tang, L., Madge, D.J. & Stevens, E.B. (2006). The role of sodium channels in neuropathic pain. *Semin Cell Dev Biol*, Vol.17, No.5, pp. 571-581.

Romanelli, P. & Esposito, V. (2004). The functional anatomy of neuropathic pain. *Neurosurg Clin N Am*, Vol.15, No.3, pp. 257-268.

Sabbe, M.B., Grafe, M.R., Mjanger, E., Tiseo, P.J., Hill, H.F. & Yaksh, T.L. (1994). Spinal delivery of sufentanil, alfentanil, and morphine in dogs. Physiologic and toxicologic investigations. *Anesthesiology*, Vol.81, No.4, pp. 899-920.

Saegusa, H., Kurihara, T., Zong, S., Kazuno, A., Matsuda, Y., Nonaka, T., Han, W., Toriyama, H. & Tanabe, T. (2001). Suppression of inflammatory and neuropathic pain symptoms in mice lacking the N-type Ca^{2+} channel. *EMBO J*, Vol.20, No.10, pp. 2349-2356.

Sandkuhler, J. & Liu, X. (1998). Induction of long-term potentiation at spinal synapses by noxious stimulation or nerve injury. *Eur J Neurosci*, Vol.10, No.7, pp. 2476-2480.

Schafers, M., Svensson, C.I., Sommer, C. & Sorkin, L.S. (2003). Tumor necrosis factor-alpha induces mechanical allodynia after spinal nerve ligation by activation of p38 MAPK in primary sensory neurons. *J Neurosci*, Vol.23, No.7, pp. 2517-2521.

Sculptoreanu, A., Yoshimura, N. & de Groat, W.C. (2004). KW-7158 [(2S)-(+)-3,3,3-trifluoro-2-hydroxy-2-methyl-N-(5,5,10-trioxo-4,10-dihydro thieno[3,2-c][1]benzothiepin-9-yl)propanamide] enhances A-type K^+ currents in neurons of the dorsal root ganglion of the adult rat. *J Pharmacol Exp Ther*, Vol.310, No.1, pp. 159-168.

Seo, H.N., Choi, J.Y., Choe, Y.J., Kim, Y., Rhim, H., Lee, S.H., Kim, J., Joo, D.J. & Lee, J.Y. (2007). Discovery of potent T-type calcium channel blocker. *Bioorg Med Chem Lett*, Vol.17, No.21, pp. 5740-5743.

Sergeant, G.P., Ohya, S., Reihill, J.A., Perrino, B.A., Amberg, G.C., Imaizumi, Y., Horowitz, B., Sanders, K.M. & Koh, S.D. (2005). Regulation of Kv4.3 currents by Ca^{2+}/calmodulin-dependent protein kinase II. *Am J Physiol Cell Physiol*, Vol.288, No.2, pp. C304-313.

Serodio, P., Vega-Saenz de Miera, E. & Rudy, B. (1996). Cloning of a novel component of A-type K^+ channels operating at subthreshold potentials with unique expression in heart and brain. *J Neurophysiol*, Vol.75, No.5, pp. 2174-2179.

Shen, C.H., Tsai, R.Y., Shih, M.S., Lin, S.L., Tai, Y.H., Chien, C.C. & Wong, C.S. (2011). Etanercept restores the antinociceptive effect of morphine and suppresses spinal neuroinflammation in morphine-tolerant rats. *Anesth Analg*, Vol.112, No.2, pp. 454-459.

Smith, H.S., Deer, T.R., Staats, P.S., Singh, V., Sehgal, N. & Cordner, H. (2008). Intrathecal drug delivery. *Pain Physician*, Vol.11, No.2 Suppl, pp. S89-S104.

Smith, M.T., Cabot, P.J., Ross, F.B., Robertson, A.D. & Lewis, R.J. (2002). The novel N-type calcium channel blocker, AM336, produces potent dose-dependent antinociception after intrathecal dosing in rats and inhibits substance P release in rat spinal cord slices. *Pain*, Vol.96, No.1-2, pp. 119-127.

Song, X.J., Wang, Z.B., Gan, Q. & Walters, E.T. (2006). cAMP and cGMP contribute to sensory neuron hyperexcitability and hyperalgesia in rats with dorsal root ganglia compression. *J Neurophysiol*, Vol.95, No.1, pp. 479-492.

Szekely, J.I., Torok, K. & Mate, G. (2002). The role of ionotropic glutamate receptors in nociception with special regard to the AMPA binding sites. *Curr Pharm Des*, Vol.8, No.10, pp. 887-912.

Szu-Yu Ho, T. & Rasband, M.N. (2011). Maintenance of neuronal polarity. *Dev Neurobiol*, Vol.71, No.6, pp. 474-482.

Takeda, M., Tanimoto, T., Nasu, M. & Matsumoto, S. (2008). Temporomandibular joint inflammation decreases the voltage-gated K+ channel subtype 1.4-immunoreactivity of trigeminal ganglion neurons in rats. *Eur J Pain*, Vol.12, No.2, pp. 189-195.

Takeda, M., Tsuboi, Y., Kitagawa, J., Nakagawa, K., Iwata, K. & Matsumoto, S. (2011). Potassium channels as a potential therapeutic target for trigeminal neuropathic and inflammatory pain. *Mol Pain*, Vol.7, pp. 5.

Talley, E.M., Cribbs, L.L., Lee, J.H., Daud, A., Perez-Reyes, E. & Bayliss, D.A. (1999). Differential distribution of three members of a gene family encoding low voltage-activated (T-type) calcium channels. *J Neurosci*, Vol.19, No.6, pp. 1895-1911.

Tanga, F.Y., Nutile-McMenemy, N. & DeLeo, J.A. (2005). The CNS role of Toll-like receptor 4 in innate neuroimmunity and painful neuropathy. *Proc Natl Acad Sci U S A*, Vol.102, No.16, pp. 5856-5861.

Thorpe, L.B., Goldie, M. & Dolan, S. (2011). Central and Local Administration of Gingko Biloba Extract EGb 761(R) Inhibits Thermal Hyperalgesia and Inflammation in the Rat Carrageenan Model. *Anesth Analg*, Vol.112, No.5, pp. 1226-1231.

Tsuda, M., Kohro, Y., Yano, T., Tsujikawa, T., Kitano, J., Tozaki-Saitoh, H., Koyanagi, S., Ohdo, S., Ji, R.R., Salter, M.W. & Inoue, K. (2011). JAK-STAT3 pathway regulates spinal astrocyte proliferation and neuropathic pain maintenance in rats. *Brain*, Vol.134, No.Pt 4, pp. 1127-1139.

Tsuda, M., Shigemoto-Mogami, Y., Koizumi, S., Mizokoshi, A., Kohsaka, S., Salter, M.W. & Inoue, K. (2003). P2X4 receptors induced in spinal microglia gate tactile allodynia after nerve injury. *Nature*, Vol.424, No.6950, pp. 778-783.

Tyagarajan, S., Chakravarty, P.K., Zhou, B., Taylor, B., Eid, R., Fisher, M.H., Parsons, W.H., Wyvratt, M.J., Lyons, K.A., Klatt, T., Li, X., Kumar, S., Williams, B., Felix, J., Priest, B.T., Brochu, R.M., Warren, V., Smith, M., Garcia, M., Kaczorowski, G.J., Martin, W.J., Abbadie, C., McGowan, E., Jochnowitz, N., Weber, A. & Duffy, J.L. (2010). Discovery of a novel class of biphenyl pyrazole sodium channel blockers for treatment of neuropathic pain. *Bioorg Med Chem Lett*, Vol.20, No.24, pp. 7479-7482.

Verge, G.M., Milligan, E.D., Maier, S.F., Watkins, L.R., Naeve, G.S. & Foster, A.C. (2004). Fractalkine (CX3CL1) and fractalkine receptor (CX3CR1) distribution in spinal cord and dorsal root ganglia under basal and neuropathic pain conditions. *Eur J Neurosci*, Vol.20, No.5, pp. 1150-1160.

Wang, M., Offord, J., Oxender, D.L. & Su, T.Z. (1999). Structural requirement of the calcium-channel subunit $\alpha_2\delta$ for gabapentin binding. *Biochem J*, Vol.342 (Pt 2), pp. 313-320.

Wang, W., Gu, J., Li, Y.Q. & Tao, Y.X. (2011). Are voltage-gated sodium channels on the dorsal root ganglion involved in the development of neuropathic pain? *Mol Pain*, Vol.7, pp. 16.

Wang, Z., Ma, W., Chabot, J.G. & Quirion, R. (2010). Calcitonin gene-related peptide as a regulator of neuronal CaMKII-CREB, microglial p38-NFkappaB and astroglial ERK-Stat1/3 cascades mediating the development of tolerance to morphine-induced analgesia. *Pain*, Vol.151, No.1, pp. 194-205.

Watkins, L.R., Hutchinson, M.R., Ledeboer, A., Wieseler-Frank, J., Milligan, E.D. & Maier, S.F. (2007). Norman Cousins Lecture. Glia as the "bad guys": implications for improving clinical pain control and the clinical utility of opioids. *Brain Behav Immun*, Vol.21, No.2, pp. 131-146.

Wen, X.J., Xu, S.Y., Chen, Z.X., Yang, C.X., Liang, H. & Li, H. (2010). The roles of T-type calcium channel in the development of neuropathic pain following chronic compression of rat dorsal root ganglia. *Pharmacology*, Vol.85, No.5, pp. 295-300.

Westenbroek, R.E., Hoskins, L. & Catterall, W.A. (1998). Localization of Ca^{2+} channel subtypes on rat spinal motor neurons, interneurons, and nerve terminals. *J Neurosci*, Vol.18, No.16, pp. 6319-6330.

Westin, B.D., Walker, S.M., Deumens, R., Grafe, M. & Yaksh, T.L. (2010). Validation of a preclinical spinal safety model: effects of intrathecal morphine in the neonatal rat. *Anesthesiology*, Vol.113, No.1, pp. 183-199.

Wheeler-Aceto, H., Porreca, F. & Cowan, A. (1990). The rat paw formalin test: comparison of noxious agents. *Pain*, Vol.40, No.2, pp. 229-238.

White, F.A., Jung, H. & Miller, R.J. (2007). Chemokines and the pathophysiology of neuropathic pain. *Proc Natl Acad Sci U S A*, Vol.104, No.51, pp. 20151-20158.

Wu, H.E., Sun, H.S., Cheng, C.W., Terashvili, M. & Tseng, L.F. (2006a). dextro-Naloxone or levo-naloxone reverses the attenuation of morphine antinociception induced by lipopolysaccharide in the mouse spinal cord via a non-opioid mechanism. *Eur J Neurosci*, Vol.24, No.9, pp. 2575-2580.

Wu, H.E., Sun, H.S., Cheng, C.W. & Tseng, L.F. (2006b). p38 mitogen-activated protein kinase inhibitor SB203580 reverses the antianalgesia induced by dextro-morphine or morphine in the mouse spinal cord. *Eur J Pharmacol*, Vol.550, No.1-3, pp. 91-94.

Wu, H.E., Thompson, J., Sun, H.S., Terashvili, M. & Tseng, L.F. (2005). Antianalgesia: stereoselective action of dextro-morphine over levo-morphine on glia in the mouse spinal cord. *J Pharmacol Exp Ther*, Vol.314, No.3, pp. 1101-1108.

Yaksh, T.L. (2006). Calcium channels as therapeutic targets in neuropathic pain. *J Pain*, Vol.7, No.1 Suppl 1, pp. S13-30.

Yaksh, T.L., Kohl, R.L. & Rudy, T.A. (1977). Induction of tolerance and withdrawal in rats receiving morphine in the spinal subarachnoid space. *Eur J Pharmacol*, Vol.42, No.3, pp. 275-284.

Yokoyama, K., Kurihara, T., Saegusa, H., Zong, S., Makita, K. & Tanabe, T. (2004). Blocking the R-type (Cav2.3) Ca^{2+} channel enhanced morphine analgesia and reduced morphine tolerance. *Eur J Neurosci*, Vol.20, No.12, pp. 3516-3519.

Yu, Y.Q., Zhao, F., Guan, S.M. & Chen, J. (2011). Antisense-Mediated Knockdown of Na(V)1.8, but Not Na(V)1.9, Generates Inhibitory Effects on Complete Freund's Adjuvant-Induced Inflammatory Pain in Rat. *PLoS One*, Vol.6, No.5, pp. e19865.

Zamponi, G.W., Lewis, R.J., Todorovic, S.M., Arneric, S.P. & Snutch, T.P. (2009). Role of voltage-gated calcium channels in ascending pain pathways. *Brain Res Rev*, Vol.60, No.1, pp. 84-89.

Zhang, Y., Conklin, D.R., Li, X. & Eisenach, J.C. (2005). Intrathecal morphine reduces allodynia after peripheral nerve injury in rats via activation of a spinal A1 adenosine receptor. *Anesthesiology*, Vol.102, No.2, pp. 416-420.

Zhang, Y., Li, H., Li, Y., Sun, X., Zhu, M., Hanley, G., Lesage, G. & Yin, D. (2011). Essential role of toll-like receptor 2 in morphine-induced microglia activation in mice. *Neurosci Lett*, Vol.489, No.1, pp. 43-47.

Zhuang, Z.Y., Kawasaki, Y., Tan, P.H., Wen, Y.R., Huang, J. & Ji, R.R. (2007). Role of the CX3CR1/p38 MAPK pathway in spinal microglia for the development of neuropathic pain following nerve injury-induced cleavage of fractalkine. *Brain Behav Immun*, Vol.21, No.5, pp. 642-651.

Zhuang, Z.Y., Wen, Y.R., Zhang, D.R., Borsello, T., Bonny, C., Strichartz, G.R., Decosterd, I. & Ji, R.R. (2006). A peptide c-Jun N-terminal kinase (JNK) inhibitor blocks mechanical allodynia after spinal nerve ligation: respective roles of JNK activation in primary sensory neurons and spinal astrocytes for neuropathic pain development and maintenance. *J Neurosci*, Vol.26, No.13, pp. 3551-3560.

2

Neuroprotection and Pain Management

Kambiz Hassanzadeh and Esmael Izadpanah
Kurdistan University of Medical Sciences, Sanandaj
Iran

1. Introduction

Pain, as a sub modality of somatic sensation, has been defined as a complex constellation of unpleasant sensory, emotional and cognitive experiences provoked by real or perceived tissue damage and manifested by certain autonomic, psychological, and behavioral reactions. The benefit of these unpleasant sensations, however, is underscored by extreme cases: patients lacking the ability to perceive pain due to hereditary neuropathies often maintain unrealized infections; self mutilate, and have curtailed life spans. Normally, nociception and the perception of pain are evoked only at pressures and temperatures extreme enough to potentially injured tissues and by toxic molecules and inflammatory mediators. As opposed to the relatively more objective nature of other senses, pain is highly individual and subjective and the translation of nociception into pain perception can be curtailed by stress or exacerbated by anticipation (Woolf).

Chronic pain is estimated to affect millions of people worldwide and is one of the most common reasons for physician visits (Scascighini et al. 2008). Inflammation may cause direct painful stimuli as well as sensitize nociceptors to stimulation (McMahon et al. 2005). Thus, there are multiple points along the pain pathway that represent opportunities for therapeutic intervention. Despite this, there are only a limited number of mechanisms through which current pain medications work. Major classes of analgesics include opioids, non-steroidal anti-inflammatory drugs, antidepressants, and anticonvulsants. Although these treatments provide relief, the effects are often incomplete and complicated by serious side effects and/or tolerance. Thus, therapeutics with novel mechanisms of actions are desperately needed (Finnerup et al. 2005).

What exactly, from a neurobiological perspective, is pain? Pain is actually three quite different things, although it is difficult to make the distinction; nociceptive pain, inflammatory pain and neuropathic pain. Nociceptive pain is not a clinical problem, except in the specific context of surgery and other clinical procedures that necessarily involve noxious stimuli, where it must be suppressed by local and general anesthetics or high-dose opioids (Woolf).

Nociception involves multiple steps from the peripheral receptor, the afferent nerve transmitting the impulse to the spinal cord, the signal processing in the dorsal horn, with inhibitory and facilitatory elements and finally transmission to higher cerebral centers where the peripheral nociceptive stimulus is perceived as pain (Arendt-Nielsen and Sumikura 2002).

The second kind of pain is also adaptive and protective. By heightening sensory sensitivity after unavoidable tissue damage, this pain assists in the healing of the injured body part by creating a situation that discourages physical contact and movement. Pain hypersensitivity, or tenderness, reduces further risk of damage and promotes recovery, as after a surgical wound or in an inflamed joint, where normally innocuous stimuli now elicit pain. This pain is caused by activation of the immune system by tissue injury or infection, and is therefore called inflammatory pain.

Finally, there is the pain that is not protective, but maladaptive, resulting from abnormal functioning of the nervous system. This pathological pain, which is not a symptom of some disorder but rather a disease state of the nervous system, can occur after damage to the nervous system (neuropathic pain), but also in conditions in which there is no such damage or inflammation (dysfunctional pain) (Woolf).

The incidence of pain rises as people get older and women are more likely to be in pain than men. Pain management strategies include pain relieving medications, physical or occupational therapy and complementary therapies (such as acupuncture and massage).

Pharmacologic therapies are the foundation of chronic pain management. These therapies include nonopioids, opioids, and adjuvant analgesics, physical techniques physical measures, such as physical activity, physical and occupational therapy, orthotics, and assistive devices can serve as adjuncts to analgesics in the management of chronic pain (Paice and Ferrell).

On the other hand in recent years, we and others have focused on the relationship between neuroprotection and pain mechanism and management. Thus in this chapter we will review recent progress related to neuronal mechanism for using neuroprotective agents alone or in combination with antinociceptive drugs to reduce the pain. In addition we will focus on the effect of neuroprotective agents on prevention of tolerance to the analgesic effect of opiates.

2. Neuroprotection

Neuroprotection is the mechanism and strategies used to protect against neural injury or degeneration in the central nervous system (CNS). There is a wide range of neuroprotective products available or under investigation. Some products with neuroprotective effects are grouped into the following categories:

- Free radical scavengers
- Anti excitotoxic agents
- Anti apoptotic agents
- Anti inflammatory agents
- Neurotrophic factors

To better understand, we first discuss the mechanism by which neurotoxins induce toxicity.

3. Glutamate

Glutamate is a neurotransmitter with roles such as long-term potentiation and synaptic plasticity of the brain (Harris et al. 1984) and is also a exitotoxin whose neurotoxicity has been associated with numerous neurodegenerative diseases, such as Alzheimer disease (AD), (Kihara et al. 2002) vascular dementia, (Martinez et al. 1993) Parkinson disease (Greenamyre 2001) and amyotrophic lateral sclerosis (Cid et al. 2003).

Glutamatergic synapses are the key excitatory synapses within the brain, and mechanisms of both hyperglutamatergic and hypoglutamatergic functioning have been implicated in the pathophysiology of CNS disorders (Olney et al. 1999).

Glutamatergic receptors include both iontropic and metabotropic receptor subtypes. The iontropic receptors include N-Methyl-D-Aspartat (NMDA), α-amino-3-hydroxy-5-methyl-4-isoxazole propionic acid (AMPA), and kainate receptors. Binding of glutamate to these receptors causes Ca^{2+} and Na^+ entry into neurons, resulting in excitatory postsynaptic potentials and membrane depolarization. In addition, increased intracellular Ca^{2+} levels activate a number of signaling cascades (Berridge 1998). The NMDA receptor forms a channel allowing for ion influx, whereas the AMPA and kainate receptors open voltage-sensitive ion channels on the cell membrane. The NMDA receptor is voltage-gated and is blocked by magnesium and modulated by two coagonists, glycine and d-serine, as well as by several intracellular and extracellular mediators (Millan 2005)). It has been proposed that NMDA receptor hypofunction may lead to excessive stimulation of other iontropic receptors, causing a cascade of excitotoxic events including oxidative stress and apoptosis (Deutsch et al. 2001). Dysregulation of glutamateric functioning has been observed across many components of the glutamate neurotransmission system.

The mechanism of glutamate-induced neuronal death has been extensively studied: glutamate induces neuronal death *via* stimulation of NMDA receptor through which Ca^{2+} enters the cell and activates Ca^{2+}-dependent nitric oxide (NO) synthase, resulting in excessive nitric oxide formation, production of radicals, mitochondrial dysfunction and cell death (Kaneko et al. 1997). It has been shown that glutamate induces neuronal death associated with necrosis and apoptosis. Necrosis is caused by catastrophic cell damage and is characterized by cell swelling, injury to cytoplasmic organelles and rapid collapse of internal homeostasis, leading to the lysis of membranes and the release of cellular contents, resulting in inflammation. On the other hand, apoptosis is a process characterized by cell shrinkage, membrane blebbing, nuclear pyknosis, chromatin condensation and genomic fragmentation (Kerr et al. 1972; Schulte-Hermann et al. 1992; Takada-Takatori et al. 2009).

In rodents, blocking of NMDA receptors is associated with increased release of glutamate within the cerebral cortex (Moghaddam et al. 1997), (Adams and Moghaddam 1998) and nucleus accumbens (Razoux et al. 2007). However, elevations in glutamate within the prefrontal cortex of rodents occurs during short-term administration of NMDA antagonists, whereas long-term administration over 7 consecutive days actually results in a trend for lower basal levels and lower dialysate levels of glutamate upon challenge (Zuo et al. 2006). Thus, excitotoxic events associated with NMDA antagonists may be reflected by initial increases in glutamatergic neurotransmission that are followed subsequently and chronically by lower levels.

4. Apoptosis and *N*-Methyl-*D*-Aspartate antagonist-induced neurodegeneration

As noted before glutamate can induce apoptosis via NMDA receptor activation. Apoptosis or programmed cell death is a process normally associated with the elimination of redundant neurons during neurodevelopment (Johnson et al. 1995). Apoptosis involves the regulation of a complex molecular cascade controlling the activation of a family of cysteine proteases known as caspase proteins (Glantz et al. 2006). Caspases are responsible for breaking down important structural and functional proteins, leading to cellular degradation and eventually death. Apoptosis results from a cascade of gene activation and involves genes that both promote (i.e., Bax) (Schlesinger et al. 1997), (Gross et al. 1998) and oppose the process (i.e., Bcl-2) (Craig 1995), (Schlesinger et al. 1997), (Adams and Cory 1998). In a study we showed that there is a relation between glutamate increase and apoptosis promotion and increase in proapoptotic agent activity in both cerebral cortex and lumbar spinal cord of rat (Hassanzadeh et al.).

A vast array of stimuli can activate apoptosis in neurons (Sastry and Rao 2000). Many of these stimuli have been implicated in the pathophysiology of opioid–induced tolerance including glutamate excitotoxicity, increased calcium flux and mitochondria dysfunction and these mechanisms are discussed in detail later in this chapter.

5. Neuroactive steroids are neuroprotective

Neuroactive steroids are endogenous neuromodulators synthesized either within the brain (neurosteroids) or in the periphery by the adrenal glands and gonads. In addition to the classic effect of steroids on gene transcription via binding to intracellular steroid receptors, neuroactive steroids can alter neuronal excitability via nongenomic effects by acting at inhibitory Gama Amino Butiric Acid A (GABA$_A$) receptors and/or excitatory NMDA receptors, among others (Shulman and Tibbo 2005), (Marx et al. 2006). There is also evidence for a potential role of these neurosteroids in controlling GABA and glutamate release. Neuroactive steroids have also been implicated in neuroprotection, myelination, and modulation of the stress response. A number of neuroactive steroids are present in human postmortem brain at physiologically relevant nanomolar concentrations and serve as allosteric modulators of the GABA$_A$ receptor (Marx et al. 2006). Neuroactive steroids that are effective modulators of GABA$_A$ and/or T-type Ca2+ channels are promising tools for studying the role of these channels in peripheral pain perception. They appear to be very effective in alleviating peripheral Nociception in rat models of acute and chronic pain (Jevtovic-Todorovic et al. 2009).

6. Acetyl Choline Receptors (AChRs) and neuroprotection

Agonists and antagonist selective for AChR subtypes have been used in experimental and clinical research. Some of those compounds are potential candidates for the treatment of neurodegenerative disease such as Alzheimer's disease, Parkinson's disease and others. A growing list of *in vivo* and *in vitro* research suggest that AChRs modulators are gaining importance as clinically relevant neuroprotective drugs (Mudo et al. 2007).

The inhibition of α7 AChRs decreases the GABAergic tone causing increased ACh release into the synaptic cleft (Giorgetti et al. 2000), which then activates the α4β2 AChRs located post-synaptically. The selective α7 inhibitor methyllycaconitine (Ivy Carroll et al. 2007) mimics, at least in part, the neuroprotective effect of 4R (Ferchmin et al. 2003). Other *in vivo* and *in vitro* studies confirm that α7 inhibition can be neuroprotective (de Fiebre and de Fiebre 2005), (Laudenbach et al. 2002), (Martin et al. 2004).

Protection of neurons from neuronal damage and cell death in neurodegenerative disease is a major challenge in neuroscience research. Donepezil, galantamine and tacrine are acetylcholinesterase inhibitors used for the treatment of Alzheimer's disease, and were believed to be symptomatic drugs whose therapeutic effects are achieved by slowing the hydrolysis of acetylcholine at synaptic termini. However, recent accumulated evidence strongly suggests that these acetylcholinesterase inhibitors also possess neuroprotective properties whose mechanism is independent of acetylcholinesterase inhibition. It has been shown that acetylcholinesterase inhibitors protect neurons from glutamate-induced neurotoxicity in the primary culture of rat cortical neurons.

The long-standing belief was that acetylcholinesterase inhibitors are symptomatic agents that ameliorate cholinergic deficits by slowing the hydrolysis of acetylcholinesterase at synaptic nerve termini; however, recent studies have shown that acetylcholinesterase inhibitors have other pharmacological properties, for example, neuroprotection against toxic insults, such as glutamate and up-regulation of nicotinic receptors (Akaike 2006), (Takada-Takatori et al. 2009).

Several reports have indicated that activation of cholinergic neurons in the central nervous system produces antinociception and analgesia in a variety of animals, including humans (Harte et al. 2004) provide evidence supporting the involvement of the intralaminar thalamus in muscarinic induced antinociception. Pharmacological experiments have shown that the microinjection of acetylcholine or carbachol into specific brainstem nuclei can produce antinociception and can be reversed by muscarinic receptor antagonists (Brodie and Proudfit 1984), (Yaksh et al. 1985). Meanwhile some other types of receptors or drugs produce analgesia by mediation of ACh. Sumatriptan (5- HT1agonist) is able to induce antinociception by increasing cholinergic neurotransmission (Ghelardini et al. 1997). D2 antagonist prochlorperazine exerts an antinocicptive effect mediated by a central cholinergic mechanism (Ghelardini et al. 2004), (Yang et al. 2008). In addition, more recently we showed that an acethylcolinesterase inhibitor, donepezil, could prevent tolerance to the analgesic effect of morphine (unpublished data).

7. Cannabinoids, pain and neuroprotection

Pain severely impairs quality of life. Currently available treatments, generally opioids and anti-inflammatory drugs, are not always effective for certain painful conditions. The discovery of the cannabinoid receptors in the 1990s led to the characterization of the endogenous cannabinoid system in terms of its components and numerous basic physiologic functions. Cannabinoid$_1$ (CB1) receptors are present in nervous system areas involved in modulating nociception and evidence supports a role of the endocannabinoids in pain modulation. Cannabinoids have antinociceptive mechanisms different from that of other drugs currently in use, which thus opens a new line of promising treatment to mitigate pain that fails to respond to the pharmacologic treatments available, especially for neuropathic and inflammatory pains (Manzanares et al. 2006).

Cannabis extracts and synthetic cannabinoids are still widely considered illegal substances. The Cannabis sativa plant has been exploited for medicinal, agricultural and spiritual purposes in diverse cultures over thousands of years. Cannabis has been used recreationally for its psychotropic properties, while effects such as stimulation of appetite, analgesia and anti-emesis have lead to the medicinal application of cannabis. Indeed, reports of medicinal efficacy of cannabis can been traced back as far as 2700 BC, and even at that time reports also suggested a neuroprotective effect of the cultivar (Scotter et al.).

Preclinical and clinical studies have suggested that they may result useful to treat diverse diseases, including those related with acute or chronic pain. The discovery of cannabinoid receptors, their endogenous ligands, and the machinery for the synthesis, transport, and degradation of these retrograde messengers, has equipped us with neurochemical tools for novel drug design. Agonist-activated cannabinoid receptors, modulate nociceptive thresholds, inhibit release of pro-inflammatory molecules, and display synergistic effects with other systems that influence analgesia, especially the endogenous opioid system. Cannabinoid receptor agonists have shown therapeutic value against inflammatory and neuropathic pains, conditions that are often refractory to therapy. Although the psychoactive effects of these substances have limited clinical progress to study cannabinoid actions in pain mechanisms, preclinical research is progressing rapidly.

There has been anecdotal and preliminary scientific evidence of cannabis affording symptomatic relief in diverse neurodegenerative disorders. These include multiple sclerosis, Huntington's, Parkinson's and Alzheimer's diseases, and amyotrophic lateral sclerosis. This evidence implied that hypofunction or dysregulation of the endocannabinoid system may be responsible for some of the symptomatology of these diseases.

In Huntington's disease, Alzheimer's disease, as well as in ALS, pathologic changes in endocannabinoid levels and CB2 expression are induced by the inflammatory environment. CB1 activation has been shown to be effective in limiting cell death following excitotoxic lesions, while CB2 is involved in dampening inflammatory immune cell response to disease. These two targets may therefore work together to provide both neuroprotection to acute injury and immune suppression during more chronic responses (Scotter et al.).

During the last two decades, a large number of research papers have demonstrated the efficacy of cannabinoids and modulators of the endocannabinoid system in suppressing neuropathic pain in animal models. Cannabinoids suppress hyperalgesia and allodynia (i.e. mechanical allodynia, mechanical hyperalgesia, thermal hyperalgesia and, where evaluated, cold allodynia), induced by diverse neuropathic pain states through CB1 and CB2-specific mechanisms (Rahn and Hohmann 2009).

On the other hand, responses to cannabinoid (CB) receptor activation include opening of potassium channels, inhibition of calcium currents, and stimulation of various protein kinases (Deadwyler et al. 1995; Gomez del Pulgar et al. 2000; Galve-Roperh et al. 2002; Karanian et al. 2005b; Molina-Holgado et al. 2005; Karanian et al. 2007). Some of the many such signaling elements activated by endocannabinoids play important roles in neuronal maintenance (Bahr et al. 2006; Galve-Roperh et al. 2008). CB receptor transmission elicits modulatory effects on calcium channels, resulting in reduced neurotransmitter (e.g., GABA, glutamate) release (Hajos et al. 2000; Kreitzer and Regehr 2001; Wilson et al. 2001). One particular mitogen-activated protein kinase, extracellular signal-regulated kinase (ERK), is involved in cannabinergic signaling, as are focal adhesion kinase (FAK) and phosphatidylinositol 3'-kinase (PI3K). These signaling elements appear to play key roles in the neuroprotective nature of the endocannabinoid system, and the associated signaling pathways are disrupted by blocking CB receptor activation (Hwang et al.; Wallace et al. 2003; Khaspekov et al. 2004; Karanian et al. 2005a; Karanian et al. 2005b).

Together, these studies indicate that the neuroprotectant cannabinoids have antinociceptive properties.

8. Neuroprotection and tolerance to the analgesic effect

8.1 Opioid tolerance

Many types of neuronal cells and brain nuclei have the property of changing, acutely or chronically, their regular behavior by the action of pharmacological agents, such as psychoactive drugs. Acute changes, those that cease in a short time, would not be important to the chronic altered behavior if the cell recovered its original drug-free state, but it is observed that some adaptation occurs that impairs such a recovery. In fact, the disturbed cell under the influence of a drug tries to compensate for its acute effects by promoting changes in the opposite direction, transiently restoring its homeostasis. However, when the acute action of the drug is finished, the cell is imbalanced by its own reactive response(Sharma SK et al. 1975). As a consequence, the phenomenon of tolerance develops, that is, the need for an increased dose of the drug to produce the same effect (McQuay 1999). After tolerance is established, the withdrawal of the drug may produce physical or psychological symptoms opposed to the acute pharmacological actions of the drug itself. Opioid drugs are used clinically as unsurpassed analgesic agents but are also illegally abused on the street to induce a sense of well-being and euphoria. Tolerance to opioids, defined as a loss of effect following repeated treatments such that a higher dose is required for equivalent effect, limits the analgesic efficacy of these drugs and contributes to the social problems surrounding recreational opioid abuse.

In order to safely use morphine in clinic, we need to know how morphine tolerance and dependence are developed and what kinds of medicines could inhibit or prevent such mechanisms. In line with this, various approaches have been attempted to clarify the mechanisms underlying morphine tolerance and dependence. Here we summarize various proposed hypotheses and introduce our new approaches in this area.

8.2 Mechanisms for acute morphine tolerance

Prolonged and repeated exposures to opioid agonists reduce the responsiveness of G protein coupled opioid receptors. This reduction in receptor function is hypothesized to contribute to opioid tolerance, dependence, and addiction in humans (Nestler 1992). Substantial experimental evidence has divided this reduced function into separate but correlated receptor traffickings, 1) desensitization, 2) internalization, 3) sequestration/recycling, 4) down regulation (Law et al. 2000). The molecular events underlying opioid tolerance are currently discussed in relation to all these receptor trafficking mechanisms. According to current understanding, opioid receptors are desensitized on the cell surface through a phosphorylation process in the C-terminal (Afify et al. 1998) and/or third intracellular loop. On the other hand, receptor internalization or receptor disappearance from the cell surface, is now believed to contribute to resensitization through dephosphorylation during endosomal stages (Krueger et al. 1997; Zhang et al. 1997). Down-regulation is a loss of receptor protein in cells through increased degradation or decreased synthesis of the receptor. Little is known, however, regarding the regulation of this mechanism and involvement in opioid tolerance. Thus, much research has been done on the molecular basis of events in receptor phosphorylation in the membranes and internalization. Recent studies revealed that cAMP-dependent protein kinase A (PKA) (Harada et al. 1990), protein kinase C (PKC) (Ueda et al. 1995), Ca^{2+}/calmodulin-dependent protein kinases (Koch et al. 1997), G protein-coupled receptor kinases (GRKs) (Zhang et al. 1998), and mitogen-activated protein kinase (Polakiewicz et al. 1998) have roles in opioid receptor phosphorylation. PKC and GRK mechanisms are likely candidates for opioid desensitization and internalization (Ueda et al. 1995; Zhang et al. 1998).

8.3 PKC hypothesis

A number of reports have demonstrated that PKC is involved in the opioid tolerance or desensitization. Most of recent reports have demonstrated that PKC activators or inhibitors modulate opioid signaling in cells expressing opioid receptors. A series of reports have demonstrated the involvement of PKC in opioid tolerance by correlating both in vitro and in vivo studies.

8.4 Mechanisms for chronic morphine tolerance and dependence

Clear difference between acute morphine tolerance and chronic one has not been demonstrated for a long time. In algogenic-induced nociceptive flexion (ANF) test in mice the peripheral morphine analgesia developed the acute tolerance by 4 h pretreatment with morphine (Ueda et al. 2001). However, the peripheral analgesia had no change in mice that were given morphine for 5 days, a treatment which caused a marked chronic tolerance to systemic morphine analgesia (Ueda and Inoue 1999). Thus, it is evident that acute morphine tolerance mediates distinct mechanisms from the chronic one, and chronic tolerance is likely mediated through a complicated neuronal network present in the central nervous system.

8.5 cAMP hypothesis

Since the report by Sharma et al. (1975), it has been accepted that cAMP may play a key role in the morphine tolerance and dependence. According to this so-called cAMP hypothesis, a morphine-induced decrease in cAMP production is getting disappeared during long-period exposure to morphine (Sharma SK et al. 1975). As the naloxone application causes an abrupt increase in cAMP production, some unidentified mechanisms are supposed to mediate an increase in cAMP production through specific gene expressions during chronic morphine treatment. A candidate could be a cAMP-responsive element binding protein (CREB), which is involved in the gene expression of adenylyl cyclase. In vivo study using knockout mice demonstrates that CREB plays roles in the development of morphine dependence (Maldonado et al. 1996). Although several compounds possessing the antagonistic activity are reported to inhibit morphine tolerance and dependence, they have serious side effects at the same time (Trujillo and Akil 1991; Mao et al. 1992; Trujillo 1995; Mao 1999; Habibi-Asl and Hassanzadeh 2004; Habibi-Asl 2005; Asl et al. 2008).

8.6 Anti-opioid hypothesis

In addition to mechanisms at the single cellular level, the plasticity through neuronal networks would be involved in the development of morphine tolerance and dependence, as above-mentioned. One of approaches to cut in the mechanisms is based on the view that enhanced anti-opioid neuronal activity during chronic morphine treatments might suppress the acute morphine actions. The candidates include cholecystokinin (Mitchell et al. 2000), neuropeptide FF (Lake et al. 1992), nociceptin (Ueda et al. 2000) and glutamate, as an NMDA receptor ligand (Ueda et al. 2000; Mao and Mayer 2001). Among them the nociceptin (N/OFQ) system has been extensively characterized to be involved in the development of morphine tolerance and dependence. NMDA receptor has been long supposed to play important roles in the development of morphine tolerance and dependence (Trujillo and Akil 1991). Although several compounds possessing the antagonistic activity are reported to inhibit morphine tolerance and dependence, they have serious side effects at the same time (Trujillo and Akil 1991; Mao et al. 1992; Trujillo 1995; Mao 1999; Habibi-Asl and Hassanzadeh 2004; Habibi-Asl 2005; Asl et al. 2008).

8.7 Apoptosis hypothesis

Apoptosis, or programmed cell death, is an active process of normal cell death during development and also occurs as a consequence of the cytotoxic effect of various neurotoxins (e.g., MPTP/MPP+, MDMA, ethanol and cocaine) (Sastry and Rao 2000). Among the drugs of abuse, cocaine has been shown to cause a direct cytotoxic effect on the foetal rat heart, and to induce apoptosis in foetal rat myocardial cells in a dose-dependent manner (Xiao et al. 2000).

The induction of apoptosis in neurons has been demonstrated to share the same basic mechanisms with all other cell types (Sastry and Rao 2000). In vitro studies also indicate that exposure to μ- and/or κ-opioid receptor agonists of neuronal cultures from embryonic chick brain (Goswami et al. 1998) and specific cell lines (Dawson et al. 1997; Singhal et al. 1998; Singhal et al. 1999) increases their vulnerability to death by apoptotic mechanisms. The molecular mechanisms of apoptosis (i.e., the detailed cascade of events from the cell surface to final changes in the nucleus) have not been established yet, but various key proteins are involved in the regulation of programmed cell death (Sastry and Rao 2000). Some members of the Bcl-2 family of proteins, such as Bcl-2 and Bcl-xL, suppresses apoptosis, while the expression of other, such as the homologues Bax and Bak, are pro-apoptotic (Adams and Cory 1998). Specifically, the Bcl-2 oncoprotein, localized mainly to the mitochondrial membranes, has been shown to play an important role in protecting neurons from apoptotic cell death (Hockenbery et al. 1990), probably by preventing the release of cytochrome c (induced by Bax) and the subsequent activation of specific proteases termed caspases, the proteolytic enzymes which are crucial for the execution of nuclear fragmentation and apoptosis (Adams and Cory 1998; Sastry and Rao 2000). In fact, Bax mRNA and Bax protein are increased in the substantia nigra of MPTP-treated mice (degeneration of dopamine neurons by apoptosis) (Hassouna et al. 1996), and the release of cytochrome c from the mitochondria and the subsequent activation of caspases-3/9 was shown to play a key role in cocaine-induced apoptosis in foetal rat myocardial cells (Xiao et al. 2000). The results of our studies demonstrated that chronic morphine administration in rat, induced apoptosis; decrease in Bcl-2 and increase in caspase3 activity in both cerebral cortex and lumbar spinal cord in rat (Hassanzadeh et al.). Another key element involved in the regulation of apoptosis is the Fas glycoprotein (also known as CD95 or Apo1), a cell surface receptor that belongs to the tumor necrosis factor receptor family (death receptors) and that is expressed abundantly in various tissues (Nagata 1999). In contrast to Bcl-2 mitochondrial protein, the Fas receptor triggers cell apoptosis when it binds to its ligand, Fas, and Fas-mediated death bypasses the usual long sequence of signaling enzymes and immediately activates a pre-existing caspase cascade (Nagata 1999). In the context of the induction of aberrant apoptosis in opioid addiction, it was of great interest the in vitro study demonstrating the ability of morphine to increase, through a naloxone-sensitive mechanism, the expression (mRNA) of the pro-apoptotic receptor Fas in mouse splenocytes and in human blood lymphocytes (Yin et al. 1999). A relevant consequence of the morphine-induced potentiation of apoptosis in lymphocytes (Singhal et al. 1999; Yin et al. 1999) is the reduction of the immune response (and the increase in recurrent infections) observed in heroin addicts (Govitrapong et al. 1998).

On the other hand, over a decade, the NMDA receptor (NMDAR), a subgroup of glutamate receptors, has been implicated in the development of opioid tolerance (Trujillo and Akil 1991; Mao et al. 1994). Activation of NMDARs can lead to neurotoxicity under many circumstances (Rothman and Olney 1986; Moncada et al. 1992; Catania et al. 1993) For instance, peripheral nerve injury has been shown to activate spinal cord NMDARs, which results in not only intractable neuropathic pain but also neuronal cell death by means of apoptosis (Mao et al. 1997; Whiteside and Munglani 2001). Furthermore, cross talk between the cellular mechanisms of opioid tolerance and neuropathic pain has been proposed, suggesting that a common cellular mechanism may be involved in both neuropathic pain and opioid tolerance (Mayer et al. 1999). Thus, it is possible that the cellular process leading to the development of opioid tolerance may also cause neurotoxic changes in response to prolonged opioid administration. More recently, we examined the hypothesis that neurotoxicity in the form of apoptotic cell death would be induced in association with the development of morphine tolerance. In confirmation of Mao et al. findings, we demonstrated that chronic opioid injection leads to apoptosis in the CNS which was in association with the development of tolerance to the analgesic effect (Habibi-Asl et al. 2009a). Figure1 shows the possible mechanisms of opioid-induced neuronal apoptosis and its association with opioid tolerance.

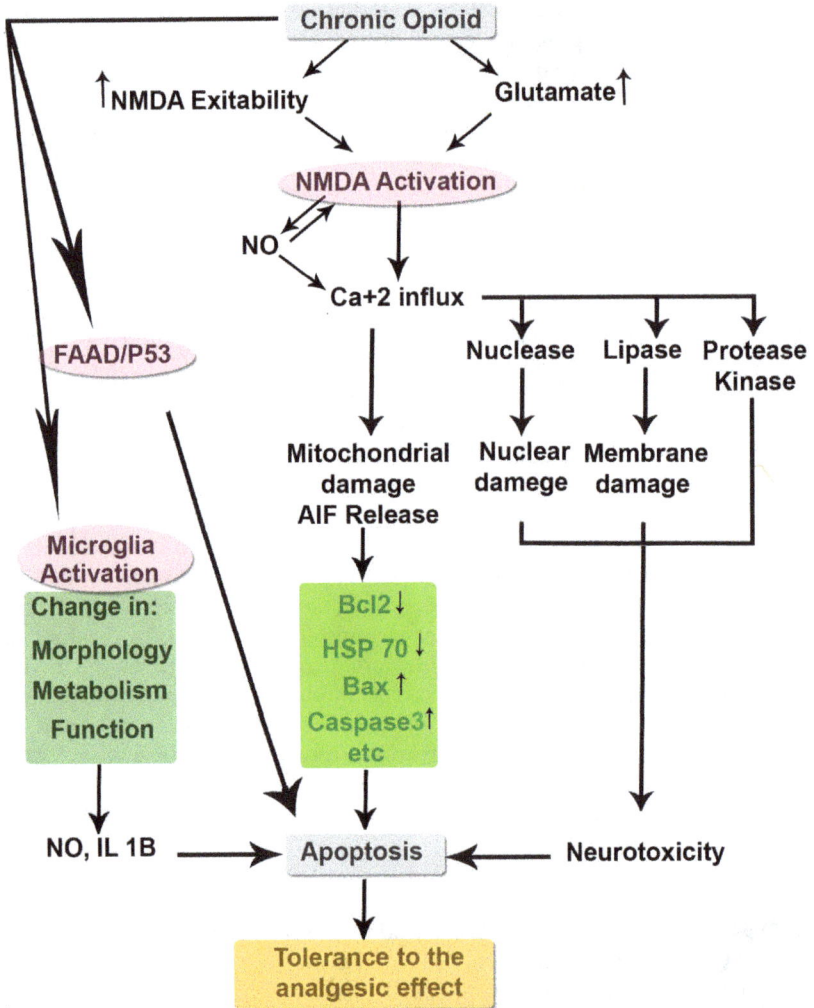

Fig. 1. Schematic diagram illustrating the possible mechanisms of opioid-induced neuronal apoptosis and tolerance. The results of before studies suggest that chronic opioid administration may induce NMDAR, microglia, FAAD/P53,... activation resulting in intracellular positive apoptosis regulators induction. The resultant apoptosis contributes to the cellular mechanism of opioid tolerance. NMDA: N-Methyl-D-Aspartate, NO: Nitric Oxide, AIF: Apoptosis-Inducing Factor, FADD: Fas-Associated Death Domain,

Opioid tolerance manifests as a loss of agonist potency and as a shift of the dose-response curve to the right. During the past decades, many studies have focused on excitatory amino acid receptors to investigate the role which they play in the development of tolerance to the antinociceptive action of opiates. This idea was suggested by Trujillo and Akil who reported that the NMDA receptor antagonist, MK801 (dizocilpine), inhibited the development of tolerance to the antinociceptive effect of morphine and morphine physical dependence (Trujillo and Akil 1991).

Using behavioral studies, we and others have shown that a variety of NMDA receptor antagonists have the ability to inhibit the development of opiate tolerance and dependence (Trujillo and Akil 1991; Trujillo 1995; Habibi-Asl and Hassanzadeh 2004; Asl et al. 2008; Habibi-Asl et al. 2009b). There are also several lines of evidence which suggest that activation of NMDARs leads to removing the magnesium blockade (Begon et al. 2001) in the calcium channel and toxic calcium influx, which activates numerous enzymes, including neuronal nitric oxide (NO) synthase (NOS). In our unpublished data we observed that nitric oxide donors such as nitroglycerin or nicorandil increased the tolerance to the analgesic effect of morphine. On the other hand the nitric oxide synthase inhibitor, N-Nitro-L-Arginine Methyl Ester (LNAME) could prevent the tolerance. It has been demonstrated that Magnesium (Mg)-deficient rats develop a mechanical hyperalgesia which is reversed by a N-Methyl-D-Aspartate (NMDA) receptor antagonist (Begon et al. 2001). Our study in agreement with those studies showed that systemic administration of magnesium sulfate could attenuate morphine tolerance to the analgesic effect (Habibi-Asl 2005; Habibi-Asl et al. 2009b). Also we showed that selenium with similar mechanism appeared to have a weaker effect than magnesium (Charkhpour M et al. 2009).

Our recently published finding, indicated that riluzole (2- amino-6-[trifluoromethoxy] benzothiazole), an antiglutamatergic agent, decreases the development of tolerance, shifting the first day of established tolerance from the 8th day in the control group to the 13th day (Habibi-Asl et al. 2009a). Riluzole interferes with responses mediated by excitatory amino acids, even though it does not interact with any known binding sites on the NMDA, kainate or AMPA glutamate receptors (Debono et al. 1993). The neuroprotective effect of riluzole, which has been shown both in vivo and in vitro, is believed to be beneficial in various neurodegenerative diseases and amelioration of trauma and stroke (Doble 1999; Albo et al. 2004).

The results indicated that there was a significant shift to the right in the dose-response curve as well as an increase in the antinociceptive 50% effective dose (ED50) of morphine for animals who received morphine also compared with those that received morphine and riluzole. On the other hand, co-administration of riluzole delayed the onset of morphine-induced apoptosis and significantly decreased the average number of TUNEL-positive cells (p < 0.01). This finding is in line with our recent results concerning the lumbar region of the spinal cord (Hassanzadeh et al.). In addition, we found that the group that received morphine and riluzole for 13 days had developed tolerance; they showed an increase in the number of apoptotic cells, as under control conditions. This result indicates that after the completion of tolerance in both the control and the treated groups, apoptosis had already developed. Previous studies have indicated that certain addictive drugs, such as morphine, could induce apoptosis in cultured neuronal cell lines as well as human cells (Singhal et al. 1998; Singhal et al. 1999). More recently, it has been shown that in vivo neuronal apoptosis occurs in the rat's spinal cord dorsal horn after chronic morphine treatment that was associated with the expression of activated caspase- 3 and the involvement of mitogen-activated protein kinase (MAPK) (Mao et al. 2002), suggesting that chronic morphine may lead to changes within the central nervous system.

Our more recent studies demonstrated that prolonged morphine administration induces up-regulation of proapoptotic elements such as caspase-3 and down regulation of the anti-apoptotic factors Bcl-2 and HSP70 in the rat cerebral cortex and spinal cord (Hassanzadeh et al.; Hassanzadeh et al.; Tikka and Koistinaho 2001; Gabra et al. 2005; Hassanzadeh K et al. 2011). Importantly, up-regulation of caspase-3 and Bax was inhibited when morphine was co-administered with the noncompetitive NMDAR antagonist MK-801, thereby supporting a link between NMDAR activation and intracellular changes in caspase-3 and Bax in response to prolonged morphine administration (Jordan et al. 2007).

Interestingly, our results demonstrated that neuroprotective agents such as serotonin$_{1A}$ receptor agonist, minocycline (Habibi-Asl 2009; Habibi-Asl et al. 2009a), selegiline,… could prevent morphine induced tolerance and apoptosis. The stimulation of serotonin$_{1A}$ (5HT1A) receptors induces a variable level of neuroprotection in different animal models of central nervous system injury such as ischemia, (Prehn et al. 1993; Semkova et al. 1998; Schaper et al. 2000; Kukley et al. 2001; Torup et al. 2000) N-methyl-D-aspartate (NMDA) excitotoxicity, (Oosterink et al. 1998; Oosterink et al. 2003) acute subdural hematoma, (Alessandri et al. 1999) and traumatic brain injury (Kline et al. 2001). Furthermore, in vitro evidence indicates that 5HT1A agonists are able to protect neurons from apoptosis induced by staurosporine (Suchanek et al. 1998), glutamate (Semkova et al. 1998), or serum deprivation (Ahlemeyer and Krieglstein 1997; Ahlemeyer et al. 1999). There are different hypotheses on the mechanisms involved in 5HT1A-mediated neuroprotection, including neuronal membrane hyperpolarization that reduces excitability,(Ahlemeyer and Krieglstein 1997; Krüger et al. 1999), reduced glutamate release, (Mauler et al. 2001) and blockade of voltage-sensitive Na channels (Melena et al. 2000).

Other neuroprotective mechanisms have also been proposed for 5HT1A agonists such as stimulation of the anti-apoptotic proto-oncogene B-cell lymphoma protein 2 (BCL-2) expression through the mitogen-activated protein kinase (MAPK/ERK) signaling pathway (Kukley et al. 2001) and suppression of the proapoptotic protein caspase-3 in a MAPK- and protein kinase C alfa-dependent manner (Adayev et al. 2003).

More recently we examined the effect of 8-OH-DPAT, a specific 5-HT1A receptor agonist, on morphine induced tolerance to an analgesic effect in rat. We found that Intra-dorsal raphe nucleus (DRN) administration of the 5-HT1A receptor agonist, 8-OH-DPAT, prevented morphine-induced apoptosis after tolerance to the analgesic effect. On the other hand, the total analgesic effect of morphine significantly increased in animals treated with morphine and 8-OH-DPAT in comparison with the control group. In addition, the results indicated that administration of both 5HT1 agonist (8-OH-DPAT) and antagonist (NAN-190) together with morphine prevent the antiapoptotic activity of the 5HT1A agonist. This means that after antagonizing the 5HT1A receptor, the apoptosis process has already developed. Another mechanism contributes to the morphine tolerance is microglial activation. Studies showed that NMDA-induced neuronal death involved proliferation and activation of microglial cells and that neuroprotective agents such as minocycline completely prevented NMDA toxicity and the preceding activation and proliferation of microglial cells. These results support the notion that microglial activation contributes to excitotoxic neuronal death, which can be inhibited by anti- inflammatory compounds, such as minocycline (Tikka and Koistinaho 2001). The mechanism underlying the role of glial cells in the effects of morphine on naive mice is unclear. It is possible that morphine acts directly on microglia, triggering alterations in their morphology, metabolism, and function (Watkins et al. 2005). Mika et al. concluded that the effect of minocycline on morphine tolerance is related to microglia. Their results provide evidence that systemic administration of minocycline in mice influences morphine's effectiveness and delays the development of morphine tolerance by attenuating microglial activation and its markers (Mika et al. 2009).

In summary, we believe that adding the neuroprotective agents to analgesic drugs specially opioids, increase the analgesic effect and prevents the hyperalgesia and tolerance to their analgesic effects.

9. References

Adams B, Moghaddam B. Corticolimbic dopamine neurotransmission is temporally dissociated from the cognitive and locomotor effects of phencyclidine. J Neurosci 1998;18(14):5545-5554.

Adams JM, Cory S. The Bcl-2 protein family: arbiters of cell survival. Science 1998;281(5381):1322-1326.

Adayev T, Ray I, Sondhi R, Sobocki T, Banerjee P. The G protein-coupled 5-HT1A receptor causes suppression of caspase-3 through MAPK and protein kinase Calpha. Biochim Biophys Acta 2003;1640(1):85-96.

Afify EA, Law PY, Riedl M, Elde R, Loh HH. Role of carboxyl terminus of mu-and delta-opioid receptor in agonist-induced down-regulation. Brain Res Mol Brain Res 1998;54(1):24-34.

Ahlemeyer B, Glaser A, Schaper C, Semkova I, Krieglstein J. The 5-HT1A receptor agonist Bay x 3702 inhibits apoptosis induced by serum deprivation in cultured neurons. Eur J Pharmacol 1999;370(2):211-216.

Ahlemeyer B, Krieglstein J. Stimulation of 5-HT1A receptor inhibits apoptosis induced by serum deprivation in cultured neurons from chick embryo. Brain Res 1997;777(1-2):179-186.

Akaike A. Preclinical evidence of neuroprotection by cholinesterase inhibitors. Alzheimer Dis Assoc Disord 2006;20(2 Suppl 1):S8-11.

Albo F, Pieri M, Zona C. Modulation of AMPA receptors in spinal motor neurons by the neuroprotective agent riluzole. J Neurosci Res 2004;78(2):200-207.

Alessandri B, Tsuchida E, Bullock RM. The neuroprotective effect of a new serotonin receptor agonist, BAY X3702, upon focal ischemic brain damage caused by acute subdural hematoma in the rat. Brain Res 1999;845(2):232-235.

Arendt-Nielsen L, Sumikura H. From pain research to pain treatment: role of human pain models. J Nihon Med Sch 2002;69(6):514-524.

Asl BH, Hassanzadeh K, Khezri E, Mohammadi S. Evaluation the effects of dextromethorphan and midazolam on morphine induced tolerance and dependence in mice. Pak J Biol Sci 2008;11(13):1690-1695.

Bahr BA, Karanian DA, Makanji SS, Makriyannis A. Targeting the endocannabinoid system in treating brain disorders. Expert Opin Investig Drugs 2006;15(4):351-365.

Begon S, Pickering G, Eschalier A, Mazur A, Rayssiguier Y, Dubray C. Role of spinal NMDA receptors, protein kinase C and nitric oxide synthase in the hyperalgesia induced by magnesium deficiency in rats. Br J Pharmacol 2001;134(6):1227-1236.

Berridge MJ. Neuronal calcium signaling. Neuron 1998;21(1):13-26.

Brodie MS, Proudfit HK. Hypoalgesia induced by the local injection of carbachol into the nucleus raphe magnus. Brain Res 1984;291(2):337-342.

Catania MV, Hollingsworth Z, Penney JB, Young AB. Phospholipase A2 modulates different subtypes of excitatory amino acid receptors: autoradiographic evidence. J Neurochem 1993;60(1):236-245.

Charkhpour M, Habibi Asl B, Yagobifard S, Hassanzadeh K. Evaluation the effect of co-administration of gabapentin and sodium selenite on the development of tolerance to morphine analgesia and dependence in mice. Pharmaceutical Sciences 2009;14(4):209-217.

Cid C, Alvarez-Cermeno JC, Regidor I, Salinas M, Alcazar A. Low concentrations of glutamate induce apoptosis in cultured neurons: implications for amyotrophic lateral sclerosis. J Neurol Sci 2003;206(1):91-95.

Craig RW. The bcl-2 gene family. Semin Cancer Biol 1995;6(1):35-43.

Dawson G, Dawson SA, Goswami R. Chronic exposure to kappa-opioids enhances the susceptibility of immortalized neurons (F-11kappa 7) to apoptosis-inducing drugs by a mechanism that may involve ceramide.

J Neurochem 1997;68(6):2363-2370.

de Fiebre NC, de Fiebre CM. alpha7 Nicotinic acetylcholine receptor knockout selectively enhances ethanol-, but not beta-amyloid-induced neurotoxicity. Neurosci Lett 2005;373(1):42-47.

Deadwyler SA, Hampson RE, Mu J, Whyte A, Childers S. Cannabinoids modulate voltage sensitive potassium A-current in hippocampal neurons via a cAMP-dependent process. J Pharmacol Exp Ther 1995;273(2):734-743.

Debono MW, Le GJ, Canton T, Doble A, Pradier L. Inhibition by riluzole of electrophysiological responses mediated by rat kainate and NMDA receptors expressed in Xenopus oocytes. Eur J Pharmacol 1993;235(2-3):283-289.

Deutsch SI, Rosse RB, Schwartz BL, Mastropaolo J. A revised excitotoxic hypothesis of schizophrenia: therapeutic implications. Clin Neuropharmacol 2001;24(1):43-49.

Doble A. The role of excitotoxicity in neurodegenerative disease: implications for therapy. Pharmacol Ther 1999;81(3):163-221.

Ferchmin PA, Perez D, Eterovic VA, de Vellis J. Nicotinic receptors differentially regulate N-methyl-D-aspartate damage in acute hippocampal slices. J Pharmacol Exp Ther 2003;305(3):1071-1078.

Finnerup NB, Otto M, McQuay HJ, Jensen TS, Sindrup SH. Algorithm for neuropathic pain treatment: an evidence based proposal. Pain 2005;118(3):289-305.

Gabra BH, Afify EA, Daabees TT, Abou Zeit-Har MS. The role of the NO/NMDA pathways in the development of morphine withdrawal induced by naloxone in vitro. Pharmacol Res 2005;51(4):319-327.

Galve-Roperh I, Aguado T, Palazuelos J, Guzman M. Mechanisms of control of neuron survival by the endocannabinoid system. Curr Pharm Des 2008;14(23):2279-2288.

Galve-Roperh I, Rueda D, Gomez del Pulgar T, Velasco G, Guzman M. Mechanism of extracellular signal-regulated kinase activation by the CB(1) cannabinoid receptor. Mol Pharmacol 2002;62(6):1385-1392.

Ghelardini C, Galeotti N, Nicolodi M, Donaldson S, Sicuteri F, Bartolini A. Involvement of central cholinergic system in antinociception induced by sumatriptan in mouse. Int J Clin Pharmacol Res 1997;17(2-3):105-109.

Ghelardini C, Galeotti N, Uslenghi C, Grazioli I, Bartolini A. Prochlorperazine induces central antinociception mediated by the muscarinic system. Pharmacol Res 2004;50(3):351-358.

Giorgetti M, Bacciottini L, Giovannini MG, Colivicchi MA, Goldfarb J, Blandina P. Local GABAergic modulation of acetylcholine release from the cortex of freely moving rats. Eur J Neurosci 2000;12(6):1941-1948.

Glantz LA, Gilmore JH, Lieberman JA, Jarskog LF. Apoptotic mechanisms and the synaptic pathology of schizophrenia. Schizophr Res 2006;81(1):47-63.

Gomez del Pulgar T, Velasco G, Guzman M. The CB1 cannabinoid receptor is coupled to the activation of protein kinase B/Akt. Biochem J 2000;347(Pt 2):369-373.

Goswami R, Dawson SA, Dawson G. Cyclic AMP protects against staurosporine and wortmannin-induced apoptosis and opioid-enhanced apoptosis in both embryonic and immortalized (F-11kappa7) neurons. J Neurochem 1998;70(4):1376-1382.

Govitrapong P, Suttitum T, Kotchabhakdi N, Uneklabh T. Alterations of immune functions in heroin addicts and heroin withdrawal subjects. J Pharmacol Exp Ther 1998;286(2):883-889.

Greenamyre JT. Glutamatergic influences on the basal ganglia. Clin Neuropharmacol 2001;24(2):65-70.

Gross A, Jockel J, Wei MC, Korsmeyer SJ. Enforced dimerization of BAX results in its translocation, mitochondrial dysfunction and apoptosis. Embo J 1998;17(14):3878-3885.

Habibi-Asl B, Alimohammadi, B., Charkhpour, M., Hassanzadeh, K. Evaluation the Effects of Systemic Administration of Minocycline and Riluzole on Tolerance to Morphine Analgesic effect in rat. . Pharmaceutical Sciences (Journal of Faculty of Pharmacy, Tabriz University of Medical Sciences) 2009;15:205-212.

Habibi-Asl B, Hassanzadeh K. Effects of ketamine and midazolam on morphine induced dependence and tolerance in mice. DARU 2004;12:101-105.

Habibi-Asl B, Hassanzadeh K, Charkhpour M. Central administration of minocycline and riluzole prevents morphine-induced tolerance in rats. Anesth Analg 2009a;109(3):936-942.

Habibi-Asl B, Hassanzadeh K, Vafai H, Mohammadi S. Development of morphine induced tolerance and withdrawal symptoms is attenuated by lamotrigine and magnesium sulfate in mice. Pak J Biol Sci 2009b;12(10):798-803.

Habibi-Asl B, Hassanzadeh, K., Moosazadeh, S. Effects of ketamine and magnesium on morphine induced tolerance and dependence in mice. DARU 2005;13:110-115.

Hajos N, Katona I, Naiem SS, MacKie K, Ledent C, Mody I, Freund TF. Cannabinoids inhibit hippocampal GABAergic transmission and network oscillations. Eur J Neurosci 2000;12(9):3239-3249.

Harada H, Ueda H, Katada T, Ui M, Satoh M. Phosphorylated mu-opioid receptor purified from rat brains lacks functional coupling with Gi1, a GTP-binding protein in reconstituted lipid vesicles. Neurosci Lett 1990;113(1):47-49.

Harris EW, Ganong AH, Cotman CW. Long-term potentiation in the hippocampus involves activation of N-methyl-D-aspartate receptors. Brain Res 1984;323(1):132-137.

Harte SE, Hoot MR, Borszcz GS. Involvement of the intralaminar parafascicular nucleus in muscarinic-induced antinociception in rats. Brain Res 2004;1019(1-2):152-161.

Hassanzadeh K, L R, Habibi-asl B, Farajnia S, Izadpanah E, Nemati M, Arasteh M, Mohammadi S. Riluzole prevents morphine-induced apoptosis in rat cerebral cortex. Pharamacol Rep 2011;63:697-707.

Hassanzadeh K, Habibi-asl B, Farajnia S, Roshangar L. Minocycline prevents morphine-induced apoptosis in rat cerebral cortex and lumbar spinal cord: a possible mechanism for attenuating morphine tolerance. Neurotox Res;19(4):649-659.

Hassanzadeh K, Habibi-asl B, Roshangar L, Nemati M, Ansarin M, Farajnia S. Intracerebroventricular administration of riluzole prevents morphine-induced apoptosis in the lumbar region of the rat spinal cord. Pharmacol Rep;62(4):664-673.

Hassouna I, Wickert H, Zimmermann M, Gillardon F. Increase in bax expression in substantia nigra following 1-methyl-4-phenyl-1,2,3,6-tetrahydropyridine (MPTP) treatment of mice. Neurosci Lett 1996;204(1-2):85-88.

Hockenbery D, Nuñez G, Milliman C, Schreiber RD, Korsmeyer SJ. Bcl-2 is an inner mitochondrial membrane protein that blocks programmed cell death. Nature 1990;348(6299):334-336.

Hwang J, Adamson C, Butler D, Janero DR, Makriyannis A, Bahr BA. Enhancement of endocannabinoid signaling by fatty acid amide hydrolase inhibition: a neuroprotective therapeutic modality. Life Sci;86(15-16):615-623.

Ivy Carroll F, Ma W, Navarro HA, Abraham P, Wolckenhauer SA, Damaj MI, Martin BR. Synthesis, nicotinic acetylcholine receptor binding, antinociceptive and seizure properties of methyllycaconitine analogs. Bioorg Med Chem 2007;15(2):678-685.

Jevtovic-Todorovic V, Covey DF, Todorovic SM. Are neuroactive steroids promising therapeutic agents in the management of acute and chronic pain? Psychoneuroendocrinology 2009;34 Suppl 1:S178-185.

Johnson EM, Jr., Greenlund LJ, Akins PT, Hsu CY. Neuronal apoptosis: current understanding of molecular mechanisms and potential role in ischemic brain injury. J Neurotrauma 1995;12(5):843-852.

Jordan J, Fernandez-Gomez FJ, Ramos M, Ikuta I, Aguirre N, Galindo MF. Minocycline and cytoprotection: shedding new light on a shadowy controversy. Curr Drug Deliv 2007;4(3):225-231.

Kaneko S, Maeda T, Kume T, Kochiyama H, Akaike A, Shimohama S, Kimura J. Nicotine protects cultured cortical neurons against glutamate-induced cytotoxicity via alpha7-neuronal receptors and neuronal CNS receptors. Brain Res 1997;765(1):135-140.

Karanian DA, Brown QB, Makriyannis A, Bahr BA. Blocking cannabinoid activation of FAK and ERK1/2 compromises synaptic integrity in hippocampus. Eur J Pharmacol 2005a;508(1-3):47-56.

Karanian DA, Brown QB, Makriyannis A, Kosten TA, Bahr BA. Dual modulation of endocannabinoid transport and fatty acid amide hydrolase protects against excitotoxicity. J Neurosci 2005b;25(34):7813-7820.

Karanian DA, Karim SL, Wood JT, Williams JS, Lin S, Makriyannis A, Bahr BA. Endocannabinoid enhancement protects against kainic acid-induced seizures and associated brain damage. J Pharmacol Exp Ther 2007;322(3):1059-1066.

Kerr JF, Wyllie AH, Currie AR. Apoptosis: a basic biological phenomenon with wide-ranging implications in tissue kinetics. Br J Cancer 1972;26(4):239-257.

Khaspekov LG, Brenz Verca MS, Frumkina LE, Hermann H, Marsicano G, Lutz B. Involvement of brain-derived neurotrophic factor in cannabinoid receptor-dependent protection against excitotoxicity. Eur J Neurosci 2004;19(7):1691-1698.

Kihara T, Shimohama S, Sawada H, Honda K, Nakamizo T, Kanki R, Yamashita H, Akaike A. Protective effect of dopamine D2 agonists in cortical neurons via the phosphatidylinositol 3 kinase cascade. J Neurosci Res 2002;70(3):274-282.

Kline AE, Yu J, Horváth E, Marion DW, Dixon CE. The selective 5-HT(1A) receptor agonist repinotan HCl attenuates histopathology and spatial learning deficits following traumatic brain injury in rats. Neuroscience 2001;106(3):547-555.

Kish T, Kivslak T, Mayer P, Wall K, Hiller S, 5iπ mutation in the rat mu opioid receptor demonstrates the involvement of calcium/calmodulin-dependent protein kinase II in agonist-mediated desensitization. J Neurochem 1997;69(4):1767-1770.

Kreitzer AC, Regehr WG. Retrograde inhibition of presynaptic calcium influx by endogenous cannabinoids at excitatory synapses onto Purkinje cells. Neuron 2001;29(3):717-727.

Krueger KM, Daaka Y, Pitcher JA, Lefkowitz RJ. The role of sequestration in G protein-coupled receptor resensitization. Regulation of beta2-adrenergic receptor dephosphorylation by vesicular acidification. J Biol Chem 1997;272(1):5-8.

Krüger H, Heinemann U, Luhmann HJ. Effects of ionotropic glutamate receptor blockade and 5-HT1A receptor activation on spreading depression in rat neocortical slices. Neuroreport 1999;10(12):2651-2656.

Kukley M, Schaper C, Becker A, Rose K, Krieglstein J. Effect of 5-hydroxytryptamine 1A receptor agonist BAY X 3702 on BCL-2 and BAX proteins level in the ipsilateral cerebral cortex of rats after transient focal ischaemia. Neuroscience 2001;107(3):405-413.

Lake JR, Hebert KM, Payza K, Deshotel KD, Hausam DD, Witherspoon WE, Arcangeli KA, Malin DH. Analog of neuropeptide FF attenuates morphine tolerance. Neurosci Lett 1992;146(2):203-206.

Laudenbach V, Medja F, Zoli M, Rossi FM, Evrard P, Changeux JP, Gressens P. Selective activation of central subtypes of the nicotinic acetylcholine receptor has opposite effects on neonatal excitotoxic brain injuries. Faseb J 2002;16(3):423-425.

Law PY, Wong YH, Loh HH. Molecular mechanisms and regulation of opioid receptor signaling. Annu Rev Pharmacol Toxicol 2000;40:389-430.

Maldonado R, Blendy JA, Tzavara E, Gass P, Roques BP, Hanoune J, Schütz G. Reduction of morphine abstinence in mice with a mutation in the gene encoding CREB. Science 1996;273(5275):657-659.

Manzanares J, Julian M, Carrascosa A. Role of the cannabinoid system in pain control and therapeutic implications for the management of acute and chronic pain episodes. Curr Neuropharmacol 2006;4(3):239-257.

Mao J. NMDA and opioid receptors: their interactions in antinociception, tolerance and neuroplasticity. Brain Res Brain Res Rev 1999;30(3):289-304.

Mao J, Mayer DJ. Spinal cord neuroplasticity following repeated opioid exposure and its relation to pathological pain. Ann N Y Acad Sci 2001;933(175-84).

Mao J, Mayer DJ, Hayes RL, Lu J, Price DD. Differential roles of NMDA and non-NMDA receptor activation in induction and maintenance of thermal hyperalgesia in rats with painful peripheral mononeuropathy Brain Res 1992;598:271–278.

Mao J, Price DD, Mayer DJ. Thermal hyperalgesia in association with the development of morphine tolerance in rats: roles of excitatory amino acid receptors and protein kinase C. J Neurosci 1994;14(4):2301-2312.

Mao J, Price DD, Zhu J, Lu J, Mayer DJ. The inhibition of nitric oxide-activated poly(ADP-ribose) synthetase attenuates transsynaptic alteration of spinal cord dorsal horn neurons and neuropathic pain in the rat. Pain 1997;72(3):355-366.

Mao J, Sung B, Ji RR, Lim G. Neuronal apoptosis associated with morphine tolerance: evidence for an opioid-induced neurotoxic mechanism. J Neurosci 2002;22(17):7650-7661.

Martin SE, de Fiebre NE, de Fiebre CM. The alpha7 nicotinic acetylcholine receptor-selective antagonist, methyllycaconitine, partially protects against beta-amyloid1-42 toxicity in primary neuron-enriched cultures. Brain Res 2004;1022(1-2):254-256.

Martinez M, Frank A, Diez-Tejedor E, Hernanz A. Amino acid concentrations in cerebrospinal fluid and serum in Alzheimer's disease and vascular dementia. J Neural Transm Park Dis Dement Sect 1993;6(1):1-9.

Marx CE, Stevens RD, Shampine LJ, Uzunova V, Trost WT, Butterfield MI, Massing MW, Hamer RM, Morrow AL, Lieberman JA. Neuroactive steroids are altered in schizophrenia and bipolar disorder: relevance to pathophysiology and therapeutics. Neuropsychopharmacology 2006;31(6):1249-1263.

Mauler F, Fahrig T, Horváth E, Jork R. Inhibition of evoked glutamate release by the neuroprotective 5-HT(1A) receptor agonist BAY x 3702 in vitro and in vivo. Brain Res 2001;888(1):150-157.

Mayer DJ, Mao J, Holt J, Price DD. Cellular mechanisms of neuropathic pain, morphine tolerance, and their interactions. Proc Natl Acad Sci U S A 1999;96(14):7731-7736.

McMahon SB, Cafferty WB, Marchand F. Immune and glial cell factors as pain mediators and modulators. Exp Neurol 2005;192(2):444-462.

McQuay H. Opioids in pain management. Lancet 1999;353:2229-2232.

Melena J, Chidlow G, Osborne NN. Blockade of voltage-sensitive Na(+) channels by the 5-HT(1A) receptor agonist 8-OH-DPAT: possible significance for neuroprotection. Eur J Pharmacol 2000;406(3):319-324.

Mika J, Wawrzczak-Bargiela A, Osikowicz M, Makuch W, Przewlocka B. Attenuation of morphine tolerance by minocycline and pentoxifylline in naive and neuropathic mice. Brain Behav Immun 2009;23(1):75-84.

Millan MJ. N-Methyl-D-aspartate receptors as a target for improved antipsychotic agents: novel insights and clinical perspectives. Psychopharmacology (Berl) 2005;179(1):30-53.

Mitchell JM, Basbaum AI, Fields HL. A locus and mechanism of action for associative morphine tolerance. Nat Neurosci 2000 3(1):47-53.

Moghaddam B, Adams B, Verma A, Daly D. Activation of glutamatergic neurotransmission by ketamine: a novel step in the pathway from NMDA receptor blockade to dopaminergic and cognitive disruptions associated with the prefrontal cortex. J Neurosci 1997;17(8):2921-2927.

Molina-Holgado F, Pinteaux E, Heenan L, Moore JD, Rothwell NJ, Gibson RM. Neuroprotective effects of the synthetic cannabinoid HU-210 in primary cortical neurons are mediated by phosphatidylinositol 3-kinase/AKT signaling. Mol Cell Neurosci 2005;28(1):189-194.

Moncada C, Lekieffre D, Arvin B, Meldrum B. Effect of NO synthase inhibition on NMDA- and ischaemia-induced hippocampal lesions. Neuroreport 1992;3(6):530-532.

Mudo G, Belluardo N, Fuxe K. Nicotinic receptor agonists as neuroprotective/neurotrophic drugs. Progress in molecular mechanisms. J Neural Transm 2007;114(1):135-147.

Nagata S. Fas ligand-induced apoptosis. Annu Rev Genet 1999;33:29-55.

Nestler EJ. Molecular mechanisms of drug addiction. Journal of Neuroscience 1992;12(7):2439-2450.

Olney JW, Newcomer JW, Farber NB. NMDA receptor hypofunction model of schizophrenia. J Psychiatr Res 1999;33(6):523-533.

Oosterink BJ, Harkany T, Luiten PG. Post-lesion administration of 5-HT1A receptor agonist 8-OH-DPAT protects cholinergic nucleus basalis neurons against NMDA excitotoxicity. Neuroreport 2003;14(1):57-60.

Oosterink BJ, Korte SM, Nyakas C, Korf J, Luiten PGM. Neuroprotection against N-methyl-D-aspartate-induced excitotoxicity in rat magnocellular nucleus basalis by the 5-HT1A receptor agonist 8-OH-DPAT. Eur J Pharmacol 1998;358(2):147-152.

Paico JA, Ferrell B. The management of cancer pain. CA Cancer J Clin.61(3).157-182.

Polakiewicz RD, Schieferl SM, Dorner LF, Kansra V, Comb MJ. A mitogen-activated protein kinase pathway is required for mu-opioid receptor desensitization. J Biol Chem 1998;273(20):12402-12406.

Prehn JH, Welsch M, Backhauss C, Nuglisch J, Ausmeier F, Karkoutly C, Krieglstein J. Effects of serotonergic drugs in experimental brain ischemia: evidence for a protective role of serotonin in cerebral ischemia. Brain Res 1993;630(1-2):10-20.

Rahn EJ, Hohmann AG. Cannabinoids as pharmacotherapies for neuropathic pain: from the bench to the bedside. Neurotherapeutics 2009;6(4):713-737.

Razoux F, Garcia R, Lena I. Ketamine, at a dose that disrupts motor behavior and latent inhibition, enhances prefrontal cortex synaptic efficacy and glutamate release in the nucleus accumbens. Neuropsychopharmacology 2007;32(3):719-727.

Rothman SM, Olney JW. Glutamate and the pathophysiology of hypoxic--ischemic brain damage. Ann Neurol 1986;19(2):105-111.

Sastry PS, Rao KS. Apoptosis and the nervous system. J Neurochem 2000;74(1):1-20.

Scascighini L, Toma V, Dober-Spielmann S, Sprott H. Multidisciplinary treatment for chronic pain: a systematic review of interventions and outcomes. Rheumatology (Oxford) 2008;47(5):670-678.

Schaper C, Zhu Y, Kouklei M, Culmsee C, Krieglstein J. Stimulation of 5-HT(1A) receptors reduces apoptosis after transient forebrain ischemia in the rat. Brain Res 2000;883(1):41-50.

Schlesinger PH, Gross A, Yin XM, Yamamoto K, Saito M, Waksman G, Korsmeyer SJ. Comparison of the ion channel characteristics of proapoptotic BAX and antiapoptotic BCL-2. Proc Natl Acad Sci U S A 1997;94(21):11357-11362.

Schulte-Hermann R, Bursch W, Kraupp-Grasl B, Oberhammer F, Wagner A. Programmed cell death and its protective role with particular reference to apoptosis. Toxicol Lett 1992;64-65 Spec No:569-574.

Scotter EL, Abood ME, Glass M. The endocannabinoid system as a target for the treatment of neurodegenerative disease. Br J Pharmacol;160(3):480-498.

Semkova I, Wolz P, Krieglstein J. Neuroprotective effect of 5-HT1A receptor agonist, Bay X 3702, demonstrated in vitro and in vivo. Eur J Pharmacol 1998;359(2-3):251-260.

Sharma SK, Klee WA, Nirenberg M. Dual regulation of adenylate cyclase accounts for narcotic dependence and tolerance. Proc Natl Acad Sci U S A 1975;72(8):3092-3096.

Shulman Y, Tibbo PG. Neuroactive steroids in schizophrenia. Can J Psychiatry 2005;50(11):695-702.

Singhal PC, Kapasi AA, Reddy K, Franki N, Gibbons N, Ding G. Morphine promotes apoptosis in Jurkat cells. J Leukoc Biol 1999;66(4):650-658.

Singhal PC, Sharma P, Kapasi AA, Reddy K, Franki N, Gibbons N. Morphine enhances macrophage apoptosis. J Immunol 1998;160(4):1886-1893.

Suchanek B, Struppeck H, Fahrig T. The 5-HT1A receptor agonist BAY x 3702 prevents staurosporine-induced apoptosis. Eur J Pharmacol 1998;355(1):95-101.

Takada-Takatori Y, Kume T, Izumi Y, Ohgi Y, Niidome T, Fujii T, Sugimoto H, Akaike A. Roles of nicotinic receptors in acetylcholinesterase inhibitor-induced neuroprotection and nicotinic receptor up-regulation. Biol Pharm Bull 2009;32(3):318-324.

Tikka TM, Koistinaho JE. Minocycline provides neuroprotection against N-methyl-D-aspartate neurotoxicity by inhibiting microglia. J Immunol 2001;166(12):7527-7533.

Torup L, Møller A, Sager TN, Diemer NH. Neuroprotective effect of 8-OH-DPAT in global cerebral ischemia assessed by stereological cell counting. Eur J Pharmacol 2000;395(2):137-141.

Trujillo KA. Effects of noncompetitive N-methyl-D-aspartate receptor antagonists on opiate tolerance and physical dependence. Neuropsychopharmacology 1995;13(4):301-307.

Trujillo KA, Akil H. Inhibition of morphine tolerance and dependence by the NMDA receptor antagonist MK-801. Science 1991;251(4989):85-87.

Ueda H, Inoue M. Peripheral morphine analgesia resistant to tolerance in chronic morphine-treated mice. Neurosci Lett 1999;266(2):105-108.

Ueda H, Inoue M, Matsumoto T. Protein kinase C-mediated inhibition of mu-opioid receptor internalization and its involvement in the development of acute tolerance to peripheral mu-agonist analgesia. J Neurosci 2001;21(9):2967-2973.

Ueda H, Inoue M, Takeshima H, Iwasawa Y. Enhanced spinal nociceptin receptor expression develops morphine tolerance and dependence. J Neurosci 2000;20(20):7640-7647.

Ueda H, Miyamae T, Hayashi C, Watanabe S, Fukushima N, Sasaki Y, Iwamura T, Misu Y. Protein kinase C involvement in homologous desensitization of delta-opioid receptor coupled to Gi1-phospholipase C activation in Xenopus oocytes. J Neurosci 1995;15(11):7485-4799.

Wallace MJ, Blair RE, Falenski KW, Martin BR, DeLorenzo RJ. The endogenous cannabinoid system regulates seizure frequency and duration in a model of temporal lobe epilepsy. J Pharmacol Exp Ther 2003;307(1):129-137.

Watkins LR, Hutchinson MR, Johnston IN, Maier SF. Glia: novel counter-regulators of opioid analgesia. Trends Neurosci 2005;28(12):661-669.

Whiteside GT, Munglani R. Cell death in the superficial dorsal horn in a model of neuropathic pain. J Neurosci Res 2001;64(2):168-173.

Wilson RI, Kunos G, Nicoll RA. Presynaptic specificity of endocannabinoid signaling in the hippocampus. Neuron 2001;31(3):453-462.

Woolf CJ. What is this thing called pain? J Clin Invest;120(11):3742-3744.

Xiao Y, He J, Gilbert RD, Zhang L. Cocaine induces apoptosis in fetal myocardial cells through a mitochondria-dependent pathway. J Pharmacol Exp Ther 2000;292(1):8-14.

Yaksh TL, Dirksen R, Harty GJ. Antinociceptive effects of intrathecally injected cholinomimetic drugs in the rat and cat. Eur J Pharmacol 1985;117(1):81-88.

Yang XF, Xiao Y, Xu MY. Both endogenous and exogenous ACh plays antinociceptive role in the hippocampus CA1 of rats. J Neural Transm 2008;115(1):1-6.

Yin D, Mufson RA, Wang R, Shi Y. Fas-mediated cell death promoted by opioids. Nature 1999;397(6716):218.

Zhang J, Barak LS, Winkler KE, Caron MG, Ferguson SS. A central role for beta-arrestins and clathrin-coated vesicle-mediated endocytosis in beta2-adrenergic receptor resensitization. Differential regulation of receptor resensitization in two distinct cell types. J Biol Chem 1997;272(43):27005-27014.

Zhang J, Ferguson SS, Barak LS, Bodduluri SR, Laporte SA, Law PY, Caron MG. Role for G protein-coupled receptor kinase in agonist-specific regulation of mu-opioid receptor responsiveness. Proc Natl Acad Sci U S A 1998;95(12):7157-7162.

Zuo DY, Zhang YH, Cao Y, Wu CF, Tanaka M, Wu YL. Effect of acute and chronic MK-801 administration on extracellular glutamate and ascorbic acid release in the prefrontal cortex of freely moving mice on line with open-field behavior. Life Sci 2006;78(19):2172-2178.

3

Polymer Based Therapies for the Treatment of Chronic Pain

Pradeep K. Dhal, Diego A. Gianolio and Robert J. Miller*

Drug and Biomaterial R&D
Genzyme Corporation – A Sanofi Company, Waltham, MA,
USA

1. Introduction

Since chronic pain manifests functional limitation, it is the leading cause of longer term disability [1, 2]. In the US alone, an estimated 75 million people suffer from chronic pain [3]. In addition to chronic pain, proper management of postoperative acute pain impacts the clinical outcome of patients undergoing surgery [4]. Opioid family of analgesics and non-steroidal anti-inflammatory drugs (NSAIDs) are the main stays of current pharmacological agents available for the management of chronic pain [5, 6]. However, current therapies for pain management show modest efficacy and are associated with significant side effects. The major adverse effects of oral NSAIDs are gastrointestinal bleeding, gastric ulcer, renal failure and cardiovascular risks (in particular with selective COX-2 inhibitors) [7, 8]. The side effects of opioid family therapies include constipation, nausea, cognitive impairment and most importantly addiction [9, 10]. Thus, development of safer and effective treatment of chronic pain is an important goal of current pharmaceutical research.

In recent years numerous efforts have been made to develop long-acting opioid analgesics and NSAIDs to modulate their pharmacokinetic profiles. Some of these include sustained release formulations and topical gels [11, 12]. Biological agents such as antibody against nerve growth factor (NGF) have also been evaluated as therapies for chronic pain. The anti-NGF antibody acts by sequestering NGF and thus inhibits its interaction with the NGF-receptor on the sensory neurons [13].

Polymeric approach offers an attractive route to develop novel therapeutic agents for effective management of chronic pain. Interesting physical and chemical characteristics of synthetic and natural polymers enable them as promising materials for biomedical applications such as therapeutic agents, drug delivery carriers, and medical devices [14, 15]. A number of polymer derived therapies have been commercialized in the marketplace [16, 17]. The present article reviews the current state of research and development efforts to discover and develop biomedical polymer as therapeutic agents for the treatment of chronic pain. While use of polymer-derived agents for the treatment of different kinds of pains will be highlighted, the primary focus of the present article pertains to management of pain arising from osteoarthritis. Furthermore, role of polymers as intrinsically pain relieving agents either alone or as chemical conjugates of low molecular weight pain modulating agents are described in this article. The research and development efforts to develop control release formulations of low molecular weight pain therapies are outside the scope of this article. There are in fact a number of interesting articles that describe this aspect of pain management therapies [18, 19].

2. Osteoarthritis pain

Osteoarthritis (OA) is one of the most prevalent musculo-skeletal degenerative diseases [20]. Although OA affects joints of the knee, hip, hand, and spine, knee is the most affected joint [21]. As a result of pain and reduced mobility, OA leads to significant loss of quality of life. Since OA is generally considered to be a result of mechanical "wear and tear" of joints, it typically affects people over the age of 60. However, its onset can be expedited at younger age due to other factors including obesity, genetic factors, and joint injury [22, 23]. Approximately 10% of the world's adult population over the age of 60 has been affected by OA [24]. Therefore, the economic burden of this disease, which includes healthcare costs and loss of productivity, is significant. These expenditures are likely to escalate with aging population. At present approximately 27 million people in the US suffer from OA and it has been estimated that by the year 2030 25% of the US adult population (a third of which of working age) will be affected by OA [25].

Although OA manifests a broad clinical syndrome, its primary cause has been attributed to the progressive breakdown of articular cartilage and chondrocytes within the synovial joints. This degeneration leads to narrowing of the joint space, suchondral sclerosis, and synovial inflammation. Breakdown of the cartilage results in alternation in joint mechanics, which further exacerbates the disease [26, 27]. In OA, concentrations of a number of mediators of inflammation such as cytokines, chemokines, and proteolytic enzymes like matrix metalloproteinases (MMPs) as well as free radicals are elevated in the synovial fluid that catalyze further degradation of cartilage [28, 29]. This process results in a self-sustaining degenerative circle that hinders the natural process of cartilage repair.

In spite of years of intensive research in tissue engineering, there has been no breakthrough to regenerate physiologically viable articular cartilage [30]. Also, no therapeutic agent has been developed that demonstrates structure modifying efficacy in OA patients [31]. The current therapies for OA are largely symptomatic in alleviating the chronic pain. These agents largely include anti-inflammatory agents, NSAIDs, and opioid family of analgesics. The relative efficacies of these therapies to relieve OA associated chronic pain have been modest at best [32, 33]. As mentioned earlier, long term use of these pharmacological agents results in major side effects (see above). In order to minimize systemic side effects associated with oral NSAIDs, topical agents containing the active agents have been developed. These delivery systems are expected to deliver the drugs in high concentrations locally and would reduce systemic side effects [34]. However, efficacy of these topical therapies is modest. In recent years, other novel therapeutic approaches for the management of OA pain has been pursued that include antibodies targeting NGF and antagonist of Transient Receptor Potential Vanilloid (TRPV) family of ion channels [35, 36]. One of the attractive therapeutic options for treating OA associated pain are polymer based viscosupplements. The following section describes the state of viscosupplement based treatments for OA pain.

3. Hyaluronic acid derived viscosupplements

3.1 Hyaluronic acid and its biology

Hyaluronic acid or hyaluronan (HA) is a polysaccharide that belongs to the glycosaminoglycan class of biological macromolecules. This highly viscous anionic biopolymer is composed of β-1, 3-D-glucuronic acid and β-1, 4-N-acetyl-D-glucosamine arranged in an alternate fashion along the polymer backbone (Fig. 1). HA is ubiquitous in nature and is produced by every tissue of higher organisms and some bacteria. The biopolymer is found in the extracellular matrices (particularly in soft connective tissues), synovial fluid, and cartilage. HA is endogenously synthesized by chondrocytes and synoviocytes [37-39]. After being released into the synovial space, HA accumulates on the surfaces of cartilage and ligament. Endogenously synthesized HA is generally of very high molecular weight (in the range of 3 -5 million Dalton) and its fully hydrated form assumes a globular shape [40]. Unique viscoelastic properties of HA enables it to maintain rheological homeostasis of the synovial fluid in the joints and plays a critical role in providing lubrication, elasticity, and shock absorption to joint tissues. Furthermore, by providing a coat on the surface of articular cartilage, HA protects the cartilage and blocks the loss of proteoglycan from the cartilage matrix into the synovial space [41]. In healthy joint of human knee, the normal concentration of HA in the synovial fluid is in the range of 2.5 - 4.0 mg/mL. However, under pathological conditions such as osteoarthritis, the concentration of HA is significantly reduced (estimated to be ~ 1 - 2 mg/mL) [42]. Furthermore, the biopolymer undergoes degradation under diseased conditions with substantial reduction in molecular weight. A combination of lowering in concentration and molecular weights leads to lowering in viscosity and elasticity of synovial fluid and consequently adverse impact on joint function. Thus, catabolic degradation of HA directly correlates with the onset OA.

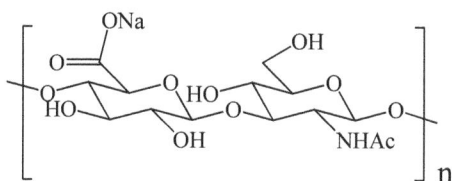

Fig. 1. Chemical structure of hyaluronic acid.

3.2 HA derivatives for the treatment of osteoarthritis

In addition to acting as a lubricant for the joint, HA has been reported to impart anti-inflammatory, anabolic, and chondroprotective effects [43, 44]. Since OA onset is attributed to degradation of high molecular weight HA and its concentration in the synovial fluid, increase in HA concentration either by increasing the rate of the proteoglycan biosynthesis or by incorporating HA exogenously to the joint space would improve joint function and relieve OA associated chronic pain. Therefore, the effect of intraarticular administration of exogenous HA to restore rheological properties of the synovial fluid have been extensively studied [45].

In order to maintain desired viscoelastic property of synovial fluid, the exogenous HA needs to have high molecular weight. It has been observed that the frequency and the amount of exogenous HA injected can be lowered by increasing the molecular weight of HA based exogenous viscosupplement. Towards that end, a variety of synthetic approaches have been undertaken to engineer high molecular weight HA derivatives [46]. In general, the desired rheological properties of HA based viscosupplements are achieved by crosslinking of naturally occurring linear HA to produce higher molecular weight compounds.

Functional group richness of HA has rendered it to be an important precursor material for the design and synthesis of numerous biomaterials with tuned physicochemical and biological properties that have found broad applications in biomedicine and biosurgery [47, 48]. HA offers three kinds of functional groups that can be used for chemical modification: carboxylic acid, primary and secondary hydroxyl, and N-acetyl (after removal of acetyl group to generate primary amine). While carboxyl groups can be modified to introduce amide and ester bonds, the hydroxyl groups can be subjected to reaction with various electrophiles such as epoxides, alkyl halides, alkyl tosylates, vinyl sulfones, etc. However, since HA is unstable at low pH, the chemical reactions employed for its modification must be selected very carefully so that they are mild and compatible to HA. This is necessary to avoid undesired degradation of HA to lower molecular weight. Furthermore, the byproducts of these reactions must be benign for both short- and long-term uses. Over the years, a great deal of research efforts have been put forth to synthesize chemically modified HA [49].

In order to synthesize HA derived viscosupplements, linear HA has been subjected to crosslinking reactions with a number of bifunctional reagents such as diepoxides, divinyl sulfone, epichlorohydrin etc [50, 51]. Some representative examples of crosslinking chemistries that were carried out to prepare HA based hydrogels are shown in Figure 2.

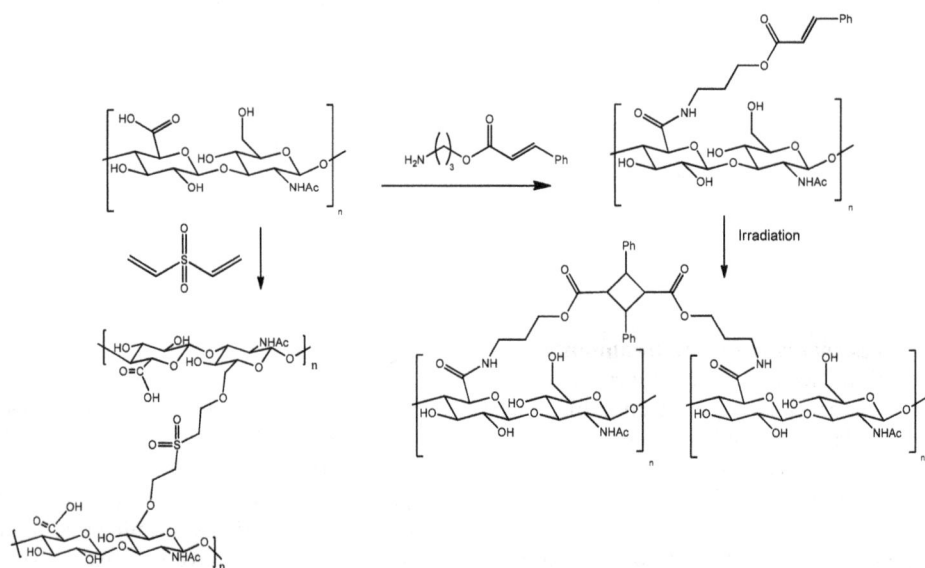

Fig. 2. Representative examples of crosslinking chemistries used to prepare HA hydrogels.

Several factors need to be taken into consideration while optimizing HA derived viscosupplementation products. For example, the rheological properties need to be tuned so that they match with those of native synovial fluid. The hydrogels must be free from any reagents that could trigger an inflammatory response associated with an exogenous material. The molecular weight of the hydrogel is critical to obtain desired clinical benefits since HA is prone to degradation and this process is accelerated in a diseased joint. A variety of HA derived crosslinked viscosupplements have been approved for human use.

The precursor HA for these preparations are obtained either from avian sources or by
biofermentation in bacteria. Table 1 summarizes some important features of
representative HA based viscosupplements that are marketed for intraarticular injection
in the knee to relieve OA pain [52]. Particularly, these products differ by their molecular
weights, which influence their rheological properties and hence residence time in the
joint.

Brand name	Generic name	HA source	Modification type	Molecular weight (kDa)
Artz®/Supartz®	Sodium hyaluronate	Avian	N/A	600 – 1,200
Euflexxa®	Sodium hyaluronate	Biofermentation	N/A	2,400 – 3,600
Hyalgan®	Sodium hyaluronate	Avian	N/A	500 - 730
Intragel®	Sodium hyaluronate	Biofermentation	N/A	800 – 1, 200
Orthovisc®	High mol. Wt. hyaluronan	Biofermentation	Chemical Modification	1,100 – 2,900
Synvisc®	Hylan G-F 20	Avian	Cross-linked	6,000

Table 1. Representative examples of clinically approved hyaluronic acid (HA) based
viscosupplementation products (reference 45).

One of the most effective viscosupplement that has been approved for clinical use is
Synvisc® (Hylan G-F 20) and its single injection formulation, Synvisc-One® [53]. The
main components of Synvisc® are HA lightly crosslinked with formaldehyde (Hylan A)
and divinyl sulfone crosslinked hylan A (Hylan B). Synvisc® contains 90% (v/v) of Hylan
A and 10% (v/v) of hylan B and its chemical structure is shown in Figure 3. Synvisc® has
been approved for the treatment of pain associated with mild to moderate OA. In
subsequent clinical studies it has been observed that intraarticular injection of Synvisc®
resulted in significant pain relief in the carpometacapal joint, temporomandibular joint
and the hip [54]. These findings suggest that pain relief from the intraarticular injections
of HA-derived viscosupplements is not limited to knee. Since, OA of the hip is the second
most common form of arthritis after OA of the knee, additional clinical investigation of
the role of viscosupplements in relieving chronic pain arising from hip arthritis is
warranted.

The biological mechanisms underlying the pharmacological action of HA derived
viscosupplements to relieve OA pain are not completely understood. It was initially
thought that since there is a reduced level of HA in OA joints, intraarticular injection of
exogenous HA restores the rheological properties of synovial fluid to the level present in
healthy joints. However, while the half-life of exogenous HA in the synovial fluid is only

few days, its clinical effect in reducing OA pain has been found to be maintained for several months [55]. This indicates that mechanism of action of HA derived viscosupplements is of multifactorial nature and is a combination of physical and biological effects. A number of *in vitro* studies have been carried out to investigate the biological activities of HA [56]. The results of these studies suggest that HA exhibits chondroprotective and anti-inflammatory effects in the synoviocytes by preventing invasion of inflammatory cells to the joint space. Biological activity of HA has also been attributed to down regulation of the gene expression of various inflammatory cytokines and catabolic enzymes like aggrecanase. Furthermore, being a natural ligand of the cell surface receptor CD44, HA has been thought to impart its effect by modulating CD44-mediated metabolism. In another *in vitro* study, when synovial fibroblasts were cultured with high molecular weight HA, newly synthesized HA molecules were found. These biological effects of exogenous HA may result in overall cartilage protection [57, 58]. Thus, well controlled clinical studies would shed further light on the chondro-protection properties of exogenous HA like Synvisc and lead to the discovery of novel therapies with disease modifying properties.

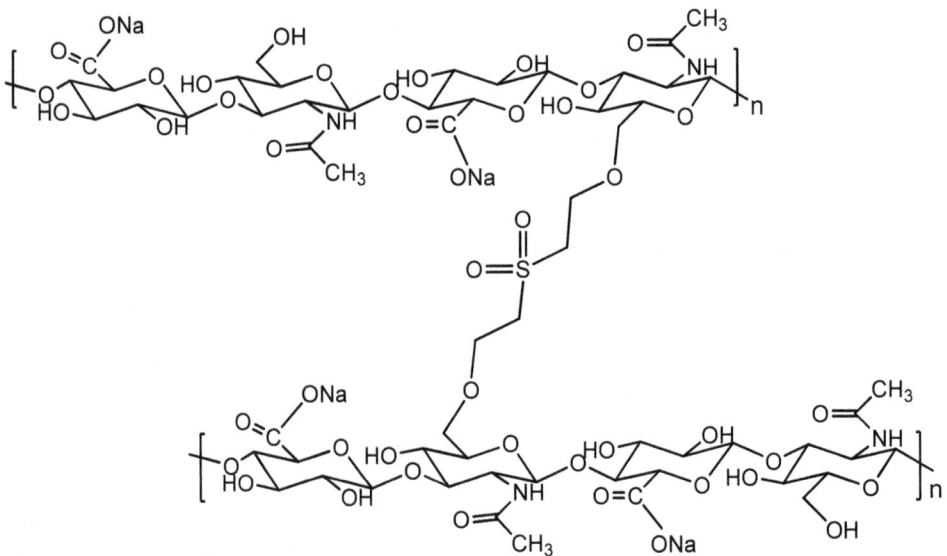

Fig. 3. Structure of Hylan B component of Synvisc®.

3.3 HA-steroid combinations for the treatment of chronic pain

One of the shortcomings of HA derived viscosupplements is their slower onset of action to reduce OA pain relative to low molecular weight drugs such as NSAIDs and steroids. Therefore, the viscosupplements are generally administered weekly over a course of three to five weeks. As described earlier, unlike traditional pain killers, pain relief from viscosupplements lasts much longer (up to several months). Although intraarticular injection of corticosteroids achieves maximum benefit within few days of injection, repeated injection of these catabolic agents can have adverse effect [59] In order to achieve fast and longer lasting pain relief while minimizing the side effects of steroids, combination therapy of HA and corticosteroids have been envisioned. Non-covalently bound admixtures of HA gel with steroids, where the steroid is dispersed within the HA hydrogel matrix have been investigated as combination therapy to treat OA pain. This approach allows sustained local delivery of the steroid at OA site and would overcome the side effects associated with steroid overdose. Figure 4 shows the structures of representative corticosteroids that have used to prepare HA derived drug-viscosupplement composites.

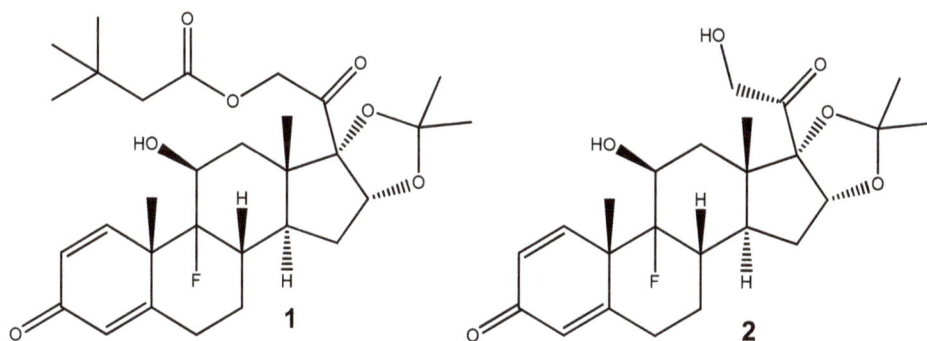

Fig. 4. Corticosteroids used to prepare HA-steroid composite hydrogel viscosupplements.

Preparation stable formulation of crosslinked HA hydrogel, Synvisc® with triamcinolone hexaacetonide (TAH) (Figure 4, 1) was investigated by dispersing Tween-80 stabilized TAH colloidal suspension within a swollen gel of Syvisc® [60]. By optimizing the ratio of Synvisc® to TAH in the formulation mixture, a stable composite was obtained. The rheological properties of Synvisc® were not adversely affected by the presence of the hydrophobic corticosteroid and the composition was found to be stable in an accelerated shelf life test.

Another steroid-viscosupplement composite was prepared by crosslinking linear HA in the presence of triamcinolone acetonide (Figure 4, 2). In this study, divinyl sulfone was allowed to react partially with HA to generate a linear HA structure with pendant vinyl sulfone group. To a solution of this vinyl sulfone functionalized HA was added a suspension of 2 and resulting reaction mixture was treated with α,ω-dithio polyethylene glycol (PEG) as the crosslinking agent. A crosslinked HA gel with relatively homogeneously distributed steroid particles within the gel matrix was obtained. The synthetic strategy adopted for the preparation of this dual-acting viscosupplement is shown in Figure 5 [61]. In a preliminary clinical study, this steroid-HA composite (Hydros-TA) showed faster pain relief compared to the corresponding native viscosupplement alone. Long term clinical study involving larger patient population needs to be carried out to demonstrate the clinical efficacy of such steroid-viscosupplement composites to treat OA associated chronic pain.

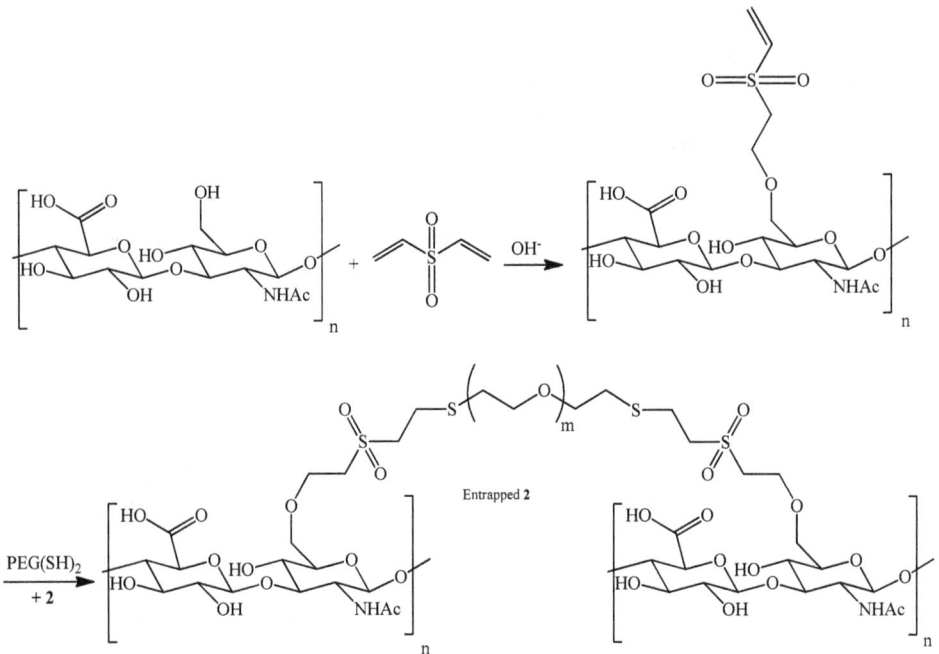

Fig. 5. Crosslinking of HA in the presence of a dispersion of triamcinolone acetonide to prepare viscosupplment-steroid composite hydrogel

3.4 Covalent conjugates of HA and low molecular pain killers

Intrinsic biocompatibility and its versatility for chemical modification make HA an attractive biomaterial to synthesize conjugated drug delivery systems. Chemical modification of HA has allowed the preparation of an array HA-drug conjugates and HA-protein conjugates as sustained-release carriers for drugs and biotherapeutics [62, 63]. Covalent conjugates of HA containing hydrogels with pain relieving agents have been explored as dual acting agents to treat chronic pain. This approach would offer a number of potential clinical benefits, that include: i) retaining viscosupplementation property of soluble HA, ii) minimizing the systemic exposure of NSAIDs and opioid family pain killers by localizing administration to the target site, iii) modulating the duration of action of these pain killers by incorporating appropriate conjugation chemistry to control the rate of cleavage of the drug from the HA gel, and iv) minimizing the frequency of administration of viscosupplement and the pain killer in the clinic. These features of the HA-drug conjugates could lead to better patient compliance and improved quality of life.

A series of HA derived functional hydrogels conjugated with local analgesics (e.g. bupivacaine) and opioid drugs (e.g. morphine) were synthesized in our laboratories as long acting treatments for chronic pain [64, 65]. Divinyl sulfone crosslinked HA hydrogel (Hylan B) was used as the polymer matrix for the synthesis of these drug conjugates. Appropriate linker arms were designed to tether these pain relieving agents to the HA matrix. Bupivacaine was conjugated to HA through a hydrolysable imide bond (Figure 6A). On the other hand, opioid drugs such as morphine, naloxone analogs were conjugated via a hydrolysable ester bonds (Figure 6B). A number of conjugates were synthesized by varying the nature of the linker arm, spacer length, and the amount of the drug loading. A systematic evaluation of the release kinetics of the drugs from the HA gel was carried out under *in vitro* conditions to identify an optimum composition. The optimum drug-HA conjugate from each class was evaluated *in vivo* for its biological activity. These drug-conjugated HA hydrogels exhibited therapeutic benefits by prolonging pain relief and were more effective than the individual agents and their admixtures. These preclinical research findings suggest that development of HA based viscosupplements conjugated with traditional pain relieving agents might lead to a promising new generation of long acting therapies for the treatment of OA associated chronic pain.

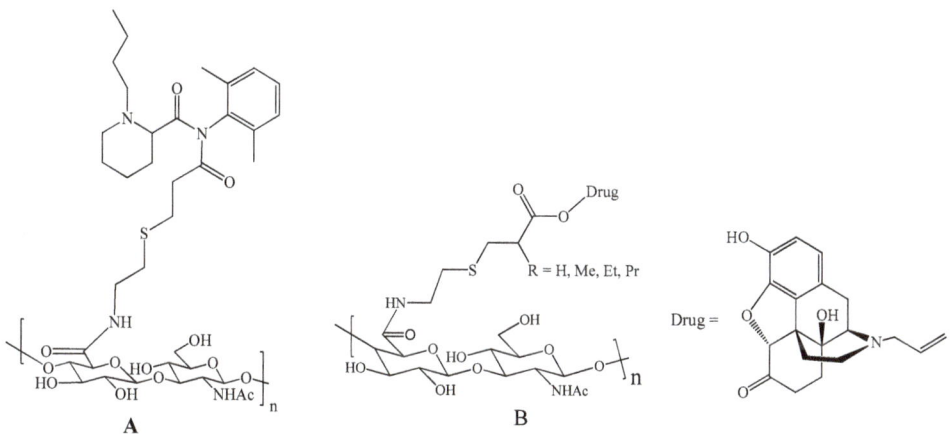

Fig. 6. HA conjugated local analgesics (A) and opioids.

In related work, conjugates of HA with methotrexate (MTX) were synthesized to achieve viscosupplementation and anti-inflammatory effect concurrently intraarticularly [66]. Increased levels of TNF-α have been found in the synovium of OA affected joints that can be mitigated by oral administration of MTX [67]. However, systemic administration of MTX is associated with certain side effects such as pneumonitis and myelosuppression [68]. Therefore, by localizing MTX to target joint by delivering it as a polymer conjugate, the systemic side effect could be minimized. After a careful structure-activity study by screening various linker arms and enzyme target groups, an optimized HA conjugate of MTX was identified (Figure 7). A peptiditic linker was chosen as target for cathepsin enzymes, which are over-expressed in OA joints. The polyethyleneglycol (PEG) linker was chosen to enable the peptide target to be accessible to the cathepsin enzyme in the joint environment. *In vitro* and *in vivo* studies revealed that the HA-MTX conjugate is capable of reducing joint pain and swelling of the knee. On the other hand, admixture of HA and MTX showed marginal efficacy.

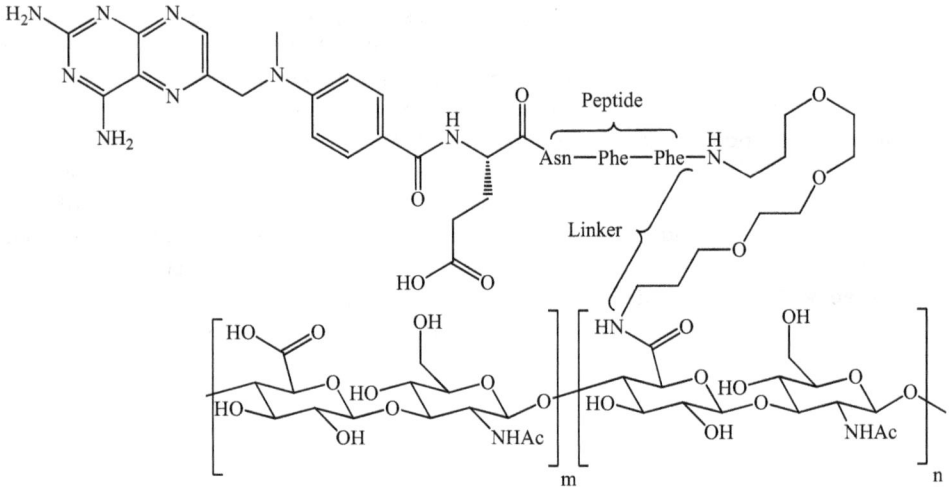

Fig. 7. HA conjugate of methotrexate as an intraarticular combination therapy for the treatment of OA pain.

4. Polymer-opioid conjugates and polymeric opioid derivatives

Besides being a first-line analgesic therapy for acute pain, opioids have been found to be useful in treating chronic pain. However, the adverse effects associated with their long term use limit the therapeutic benefits of opioid analgesics, thus leading to discontinuation of the therapy. Constipation (opioid-induced bowel dysfunction (OBD)) is one of the significant side effects associated with opioid therapies. OBD affects up to 80% of the patients undergoing opioid therapy. While other side effects associated with chronic use of opioids resolve with time, constipation continues to persist [69].

Efforts have been made to utilize polymeric approach to design and develop new generation of opioid analogs as pain killers. These polymeric compounds enable the patients to overcome OBD without losing the benefits of opioid therapy by limiting drugs' systemic absorption. Pegylation chemistry was utilized to synthesize these macromolecular opioids. The technology of pegylation has been successfully utilized to improve pharmacokinetic properties of a number of (bio)pharmaceutical agents [70]. Two representative polymer conjugated opioid derivatives are shown in Figure 8. These compounds consist of naloxol analogs linked to PEG chains through hydrolytically stable ether linkage [71, 72]. In preclinical studies, these pegylated opioid derivatives were found to maintain their centrally mediated analgesia, while antagonizing peripherally mediated constipation. One of the key conjugates, NKTR-118 (Figure 8A, n = 7) has proceeded to advanced clinical trial. In the phase II clinical trial, patients receiving NKTR-118 exhibited significant increase in bowel movement compared to patients receiving native naloxol, without compromising the analgesic property of the opioid [73]. NKTR-118 is currently undergoing phase III clinical trial.

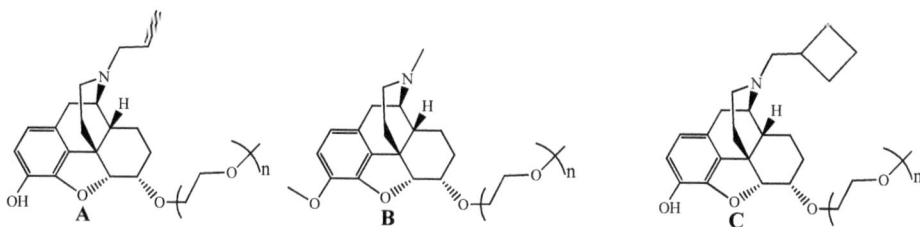

Fig. 8. Polymer modified naloxol derivatives to prevent opioid induced constipation.

Another interesting approach to develop polymeric pain relievers has been reported that utilizes a polymerization chemistry to synthesize poly(anhydride-esters), where the bioactive drug becomes part of the polymer backbone [74]. The general structure of this class of polymeric pain relievers is shown in Figure 9. Following this strategy, they were able to incorporate significant amounts (~ 62%) of the deliverable drug to the polymer chain. Hydrolytic degradation of these poly(anhydride-ester) polymers under physiological pH conditions releases the drug in a controlled manner. As a result, the side effects associated with the native drug (if released immediately) can be minimized. Some of the polymeric pain relievers reported are poly(anhydride-esters) containing the anti-inflammatory agent, salicylic acid and the opioid drug, morphine (Figure 10). Although syntheses of polymeric pain relievers based on these poly(anhydride-ester) scaffolds have been studied extensively, there is limited information about the biological activities of these polymers as treatments for chronic pain [75, 76]. Nevertheless, these polymeric opioids and anti-inflammatory agents offer a new perspective to develop novel treatments for chronic pain.

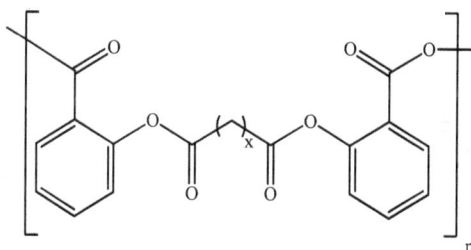

Fig. 9. Structure of salicylic acid-based poly(anhydride-esters) as polymeric anti-inflammatory agents.

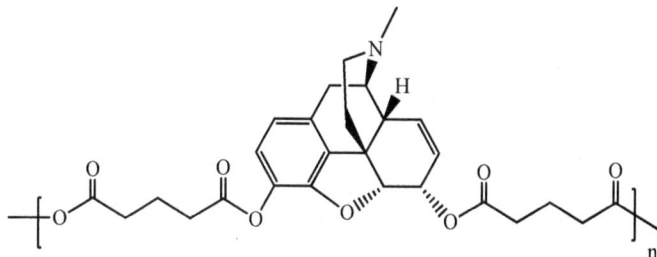

Fig. 10. Structure of morphine-based poly(ester-anhydride).

5. Conclusion

Because of its clinical relevance, development of novel pharmacologic agents for effective management of chronic pain continues to be an important goal of pharmaceutical research. Although numerous therapeutic agents with different modes of action have been developed to treat chronic pain, no single agent exhibits the most desired profile. For example, while opioids and NSAIDs remain the main stay of therapeutic options, concerns over their associated side effects have begun to limit their use. Polymeric approach offers a variety of options to develop a new generation of pain relievers, which include intrinsically bioactive polymers to different delivery systems for traditional pain killers. HA derived viscosupplements offer an attracting option to treat chronic pain due to excellent biocompatibility and various biological functions of HA. The ability to trigger various biological functions makes HA based viscosupplements as promising agents to not only relieve symptomatic effects of chronic OA pain, but also to bring about potentially disease modifying effects. Therapies comprising of polymers in combination with traditional pain killers (either as conjugates or as stable non-covalent formulations) have been found to minimize the side effects of the latter. By targeting the disease via different mechanisms of actions, these combination agents could become superior therapeutic options to treat chronic pain. With increasing understanding of the pathobiology of chronic pain and intense research in biomedical polymers, it will be possible to develop novel polymer based therapies in the near future that are safe and could act as structure modifying treatments for chronic pain.

6. References

[1] Smith B. H & Torrance N. (2011). Management of Chronic Pain in Primary Care. *Cur. Opin. Suppor. Palliat. Care*, Vol. 5, No.2, pp. 137-142
[2] Teets, R.Y.; Dahmer, S. & Scott, E. (2010). Integrative Medicine Approach to Chronic Pain. *Primary Care*, vol.37, No.2, 407-421.
[3] National Center for Health Statistics (2006), *Health, United States, 2006 with Chartbook on Trends in the Health of Americans*. Hyattsville, MD: Dept. of Health and Human Services, Centers for Disease Control and Prevention.
[4] Vadivelu, N.; Mitra, S. & Narayan, D. (2010). Recent Advances in Postoperative Pain Management. *Yale J. Biol. Med.* Vol.83, No.1, pp.11-25
[5] Turk, D. C.; Wilson, H.D. & Cahana, A. (2011). Treatment of Chronic Non-cancer Pain. *Lancet*, Vol. 377, No.9784, pp. 2226-2235
[6] Chan, B. K. B.; Tam, L. K.; Wat, C. Y.; Chung, Y. F. ; Tsui, S. L. & Cheung, C. W. (2011). Opioids in Chronic Non-cancer Pain. *Expert. Opin. Pharmacother.* , Vol. 12, No.5, pp.705-720
[7] Scanzello, C. R.; Moskowitz, N. K. & Gibofsky, A. (2010). The Post-NSAID Era: What to Use Now for the Pharmacologic Treatment of Pain and Inflammation in Osteoarthritis. *Cur. Rheomatol. Rep.*, Vol. 10, No.1, pp49-56
[8] Roth, S. H. (2011). Nonsteroidal Anti-Inflammatory Drug Gastropathy: New Avenues for Safety. *Clin. Interven. Aging.*, Vol. 6, pp 125-131
[9] Crofford, L. J. (2010). Adverse Effects of Chronic Opioid Therapy for Chronic Musculoskeletal Pain. *Nat. Rev. Rheumatol.* Vol. 6, No. 4, pp. 191-197

[10] Merza, Z. (2010). Chronic Use of Opioids and Endocrine System. *Hormone Metabol. Res.*, Vol. 42, No. 9, pp. 621-626.

[11] Weiniger, C. F.; Golovanevski, M.; Sokolsky-Papkov, M. & Domb, A. J. (2010). Review of Prolonged Local Anesthetic Action. *Expert. Opin. Drug. Deliv.*, Vol. 7, No.6, pp.737-752.

[12] Haroutiunian, S.; Drennan,D. A.; Lipman, A. G. (2010). Topical NSAID Therapy for Musculoskeletal Pain. *Pain. Med.*, Vol. 11, No. 4, pp.535-549

[13] Cattaneo, A. (2010). Tanezumab, a Recombinant Humanized mAb Against Nerve Growth Factor for the Treatment of Acute and Chronic Pain. *Cur. Opin. Mol. Ther.*, Vol. 12, No.1, pp.94-106

[14] Nair, L.S.& Laurencin, C. T. (2006). Polymers as Biomaterial for Tissue Engineering and Controlled Drug Delivery, *Adv. Biochem. Eng. Biotechnol.*, Vol. 102, No. 1, pp47-90

[15] Dhal, P. K., Huval, C. C. Holmes-Farley, S. R. & Jozefiak, T. J. Polymers as Drugs. *Adv. Polym. Sci.*, Vol. 192, No.1, pp 9-58 (2006)

[16] Duncan, R. (2003). The Dawning Era of Polymer Therapeutics. *Nat. Rev. Drug. Discov.*, Vol. 2, No. pp. 347-360

[17] Dhal, P. K. Polomoscanik, S.C.; Avila, L. Z.; Holmes-Farley, S.R. & Miller, R. J. (2009). Functional Polymers as Therapeutic Agents: Concept to Marketplace. *Adv. Drug Deliv. Rev.*, Vol. 61, No.13, pp1121-1130

[18] Manjanna, K. M.; Shivakumar, B. & Kumar, T. M. P. (2010). Microencapsulation: An Acclaimed Novel Drug-Delivery System for NSAIDs in Arthritis. *Crit. Rev. Therap. Drug Carr. Sys.*, Vol. 27, No.6, pp. 509-545

[19] Rainsfold, K. D.; Kean, W. F. & Ehrlich, G. E. (2008). Review of the Pharmaceutical Properties and Clinical Effects of the Topical NSAID Formulation, Diclofenac Epolamine. *Cur. Med. Res. Opin.*, Vol. 24, No.10, pp. 2967-2992

[20] Felson, D. T. (2004). An Update on the Pathogenesis and Epidemiology of Osteoarthritis. *Radiol. Clin. N. Am.* , Vol. 42, No. 1, pp. 1-9

[21] Kean, W. F. & Buchanan, W. F. (2004). Osteoarthritis: Symptoms, Sign, and Source of Pain. *Inflamm. Pharmacol.*, Vol. 12, No. 1, pp. 3-31

[22] Sharma, L.; Kapoor, D. & Issa, S. (2006). Epidemiology of Osteoarthritis: An Update. *Cur. Opin. Rheumatol.*, Vol. 18, No. 2, pp. 147- 156

[23] Spector, T. D. & MacGregor, A. J. (2004). Risk Factors for Osteoarthritis: Genetics. *Osteoarthr. Cartil.*, Vol. 12, pp. S39-S44

[24] WHO Scientific Group (2003). The Burden of Musculoskeletal Condition at the Start of the New Millennium. *World Health Organ. Tech. Rep. Ser.*, Vol. 919, pp 1-218

[25] Centers for Disease Control and Prevention (2010). Arthritis-related Statistics, August 2010. Available from:
http://www.cdc.gov/arthritis/data_statistics/ arthritis_related_stats.htm

[26] Wieland, H. A.; Michaelis, M.; Kirschbaum, B. J. & Rudolphi, K. A. (2010). Osteoarthritis: An Untreatable Disease. *Nat. Rev. Drug. Discov.*, Vol. 4, No. 4, pp. 331-345

[27] Felson, D. T. & Neogi, T. (2004). Osteoarthritis: Is It a Disease of Cartilage or Bone? *Arthrit Rheumatol.*, Vol. 50, pp 341-344

[28] Roach, H. I.; Aigner, T.; Soder, S.; Haag, J.; Welkerling, H. (2007). Pathobiology of Osteoarthritis: Pathomechanisms and Potential Therapeutic Targets. *Cur. Drug. Targets,* Vol.8, No. 2, pp. 271- 282

[29] Burrage, P.S.; Mix, K. S. & Brinckerhiff, C. E. (2006). Matrix Metalloproteinases : Role in Arthritis. *Front. Biosci.*, Vol. 11, No. 1, pp 529-543

[30] Becerra, J.; Andrades, J. A.; Guerado, E.; Zamora-Navas, P.; Lopez-Puertas, J. M. & Reddi, A. H. (2010). Articular Cartilage: Structure and Regeneration. *Tissue Eng. Part B.*, Vol. 16, No. 6, pp. 617- 627

[31] Altman, R. D. (2005). Structure-/Disease-modifying Agents for Osteoarthritis. *Semin. Rheumatol. Arthritis*, Vol. 34, No. 6 (suppl. 2), pp. 3 -5

[32] Kroenke, K.; Krebbs, E. E. & Bair, M. J. (2009). Pharmacotherapy of Chronic Pain: A Synthesis of Recommendation from Systematic *Reviews. Gen. Hosp. Psychiatry*, Vol. 31, 206 -219

[33] Manchikanti, L & Singh, A. (2008). Therapeutic Opioids: A Ten-year Perspective on the Complexities and Complications of the Escalating Use, Abuse, and Nonmedical Use of Opioids. *Pain Physician*, Vol.11, No.2, pp. S63-S88

[34] Schuelert, N.; Russell, F. A. & McDougall, J. J. (2011). *Ortho. Res. Rev.*, Vol. 3, No. 1, pp. 1-8

[35] Seidel, M. F.; Herguijuela, M.; Forkert, R. & Otten, U. (2010). Nerve Growth Factor in Rheumatic Diseases. Semi. *Arthritis. Rheumatol.*, Vol. 40, No.2, pp. 109- 126

[36] Wong, G. Y. & Gavva, N. R. (2009). Therapeutic Potential of Vanilloid Receptor TRPV1 Agonists and Antagonists as Analgesics: Recent Advances and Setbacks. *Brain Res. Rev.*, Vol. 60, No. 1, pp. 267- 277

[37] Laurent, T. C. & Fraser, J. R. (1992). Hyaluronan. *FASEB J.*, Vol. 6, No. &, pp. 2397- 2404

[38] Yamada, T. & Kawasaki, T. (2005). Microbial Synthesis of Hyaluronan and Chtin: New Approaches. *J. Biosci. Bioeng.*, Vol. 99, No. 6, pp. 521- 528

[39] Balazs, E. (1982). The Physical Properties of Synovial Fluid and the Specific Role of Hyaluronic Acid. In *Disorders of the Knee*, Helfert A. J. (Ed), J. B. Lippincott, Philadelphia, pp. 61-74

[40] Scott, J. E. & Heatley, F. (1999). Hyaluronan Forms Specific Stable Tertiary Structures in Aqueous Solution: A ^{13}C NMR Study. *Proc. Natl. Acad. Sci. USA*, Vol. 96, No. 9, pp. 4850-4855

[41] Shen, B.; Wei, A.; Bhargav, D., Kishen, T. & Diwan, A. D. (2010). Hyaluronan: Its Potential Application in Intervertebral Disc Regeneration. *Ortho. Res. Rev.*, Vol. 2, No. 1, pp. 17-26

[42] Watterson, J. R. & Esdaile, J. M. (2000). Viscosupplementation: Therapeutic Mechanisms and Clinical Potential in Osteoarthritis of the Knee. *J. Am. Acad. Orthop. Surg.*, Vol. 8, No. 5, pp. 277- 284

[43] Volpi, N.; Schiller, J. & Stern, R. (2009). Role, Metabolism, Chemical Modification, and Applications of Hyaluronan. *Cur. Med. Chem.*, Vol. 16, No. 14, pp. 1718- 1745

[44] Bastow, E. R., Byers, S. & Golub, S. B. (2008). Hyaluronan Synthesis and Degradation in Cartilage and Bone. *Cell Mol. Life Sci.*, Vol. 65, No. 3, pp. 395- 413

[45] Gigante, A. & Callegari, L. (2011). The Role of Intra-articular Hyaluronan in the Treatment of Osteoarthritis. *Rheumatol. Int.*, Vol. 31, pp 427 -444

[46] Burdick, J. A. & Prestwich, G. D. (2011). Hyaluronic Hydrogels for Biomedical Applications. *Adv. Mater.*, Vol. 23, No.12, pp. H41-H56

[47] Avila, L. Z.; Gianolio, D. A.; Konowicz, P. A.; Philbrook, M.; Santos, M. R. & Miller, R. J. (2008). Drug Delivery and Medical Applications of Chemically Modified

Hyaluronan. In *Carbohydrate Chemistry, Biology and Medical Applications*. Garg, H.G.; Cowman, M. K. & Hales, C. A. (Eds.), Elsevier, Amsterdam, pp. 333- 357

[48]   Leonelli, F.; La Bella, A.; Migneco, L. M.& Bettelo, R. M. (2007). Design, Synthesis and Applications of Hyaluronic acid- Paclitaxel Bioconjugates. *Molecules*, Vol. 13, pp. 360 -378

[49]   Schante, C. E.; Zuber, G.; Herlin, C. & Vandamme, T. F. (2011). Chemical Modification of Hyaluronic Acid for the Synthesis of Derivatives for a Broad Range of Biomedical Applications. *Carbohy. Polym.*, Vol. 85, No.3, pp.469- 489

[50]   Balazs, E. A. (2009). Therapeutic Use of Hyaluronan. *Struct. Chem.*, Vol. Vol.20, No. 2, pp. 341-349

[51]   Allison, D. D. & Grande-Allen, K. J. (2006). Hyaluronan: A Powerful Tissue Engineering Tool. *Tissue. Eng.*, Vol. 12, No. 8, pp. 2131- 2140

[52]   Abate, M.; Pulcini, D.; Di Iorio, A.& Schiavone, C. (2010). Viscosupplementa-tion with Intra-articular Hyaluronic Acid for the Treatment of Osteoarthritis in the Elderly. *Cur. Pharm. Des.*, Vol. 16, No. 6, pp. 331- 340.

[53]   Stitik, T. P.; Kazi, A. & Kim, J.-H. (2008). Synvisc in Knee Osteoarthritis. *Future Rheumatol.*, Vol. 3, No. 3, pp. 215- 222

[54]   Migliore, A.; Giovannangeli, F.; Granta, M. & Lagana, B. (2010). Hylan G-F 20: Review of Its Safety and Efficacy in the Management of Joint Pain in Osteoarthritis. *Clin. Med. Insights: Arthr. Musculo. Disord.*, Vol. 3, No. 1, pp 55-68

[55]   Bagga, H.; Burkhardt, D.; Sambrook, P. & March, L. (2006). Long-term Effects of Intrarticular Hyaluronan on Synovial Fluids in Osteoarthritis of the Knee. *J. Rheumatol.*, Vol. 33, No. 5, pp. 946- 950

[56]   Moreland, L. W. (2002). Intra-articular Hyaluronan and Hylans for the Treatment of Osteoarthritis: Mechanisms of Action. *Arthr. Res. Ther.*, Vol. 5, No. 2, pp. 54 – 67

[57]   Waddell, D. D. (2007). Viscosupplementation with Hyaluronan for Osteoarthritis of Knee: Clinical Efficacy and Economic Implications. *Drug & Aging,* Vol. 24, No. 8, pp. 629- 642

[58]   Altman, R. D. (2010).Non-avian-derived Hyaluronan for the Treatment of Osteoarthritis of the Knee. *Exper. Rev. Clin. Immunol.*, Vol. 6, No.1, pp. 21- 27

[59]   Gossec, L.; Dougados, M. (2006). Do Intra-articular Therapies Work and Who Will Benefit Most? *Best Pract. Res. Clin. Rheumatol.*, Vol. 20, No. 1, pp 131 – 144

[60]   Chang, G.; Voschin, E.; Yu, L.-P. & Skrabut, E. (2011). Stable Hyaluronan/Steroid Formulation. *United States Patent Application*, No.2011/00559918 A1

[61]   Gravett, D. M; Daniloff, G. Y. & He, P. (2010). Modified Hyaluronic Acid Compositions and Related Methods. *Unites States Patent*, No. 7,829, 118 B1

[62]   Varghese, O.P.; Sun, W.; Hilborn, J. & Ossipov, D. A. (2009). In-situ Crosslinkable High Molecular Weight Hyaluronan-bisphosphonate Conjugates for Localized Delivery and Cell-specific Targeting: A Hydrogel Linked Prodrug Approach. *J. Am. Chem. Soc.*, Vol. 131, No. 25, pp. 8781 – 8783

[63]   Sun, L. T.; Buchholz, K. S.; Lotze, M. T. & Washburn, N. R. (2010). Cytokine Binding by Polysaccharide-Antibody Conjugates. *Mol. Pharm.*, Vol. 7, No. 5, pp. 1769 – 1777

[64]   Gianolio, D. A.; Philbrook, M.; Avila, L. Z.; MacGreggor, H.; Duan, S. X.; Bernasconi, R.; Slavsky, M.; Dethlefsen, S.; Jarrett, P. K. & Miller, R. J. (2005). Synthesis and Evaluation of Hydrolyzable Hyaluronan-Tethered Bupivacaine Delivery Systems. *Bioconj. Chem.*, Vol. 16, No. 6, pp. 1512 - 1518

[65] Gianolio, D. A.; Philbrook, M.; Avila, L. Z.; Young, L. E.; Plate, L.; Santos, M. R.;
      Bernasconi, R.; Liu H.; Ahn, S., Sun, W. Jarrett, P. K. & Miller, R. J. (2008).
      Hyaluronan-Conjugated Opioid Depots: Synthetic Strategies and Release Kinetics
      In Vitro and *In vivo. Bioconj. Chem.*, Vol. 19, No. 9, pp. 1767 – 1774

[66] Homma, A.; Sato, H.; Okamachi, A. et. al. (2009).Novel Hyaluronic Acid- Methotrexate
      Conjugates for Osteoarthritis Treatment. *Bioorg. Med. Chem.*, Vol. 17, No. pp. 4647 –
      4656

[67] Bondeson, J. (2010). Activated Synovial Macrophages as Targets for Osteoarthritis
      Drug Therapy. *Cur. Drug. Tar.*, Vol. 11, No. 5, pp. 576 - 585

[68] Hamstra, D. A.; Page, M.; Maybuam, J. & Rehemtulla, A. (2000). Expression of
      Endogenously Activated Secreted or Cell Surface Carboxypeptidase A Sensitizes
      Tumor Cells to Methotrexate-α-Peptide Prodrugs. *Cancer Res.*, Vol. 60, No. 3, pp
      657.

[69] Asai, T. & Power, I. (1999). Naloxone Inhibits Gastric Emptying in Rats. *Anesth. Analg.*,
      Vol. 88, No. 1, pp. 204 – 208

[70] Harris, J. M. & Chess, R.B. (2003). Effect of Pegylation on Pharmaceuticals. *Nat. Rev.
      Drug. Discov.*, Vol. 2, No.3, pp. 214 - 221

[71] Jude-Fishburn, C. S.; Riley, T. A.; Zacarias, A. N. & Gursahani, H. (2011). Pegylated
      Opioids with Low Potential for Abuse and Side Effects. *PCT Int. Appl.*,
      WO 2011088140 A1

[72] Diego, L.; Atayee, R.; Helmons, P.; Hsiao, G & von Gunten, C.F. (2011). Novel Opioid
      Antagonists for Opioid-Induced Bowel Dysfunction. *Exper. Opin. Investig. Drugs*,
      Vol. 20, No. 8, pp. 1047- 1056

[73] Hipkin, R. W. & Dolle, R. E. (2010). Opioid Receptor Antagonists for Gastrointestinal
      Dysfunction. *Ann. Rep. Med. Chem.* Vol. 45, No. 1, 143 – 155

[74] Schemltzer, R. C. ; Johnson, M; Griffin, J. & Uhrich, K. (2008). Comparison of Salicylate
      Based Poly(anhydride-esters) formed via Melt Condensation versus Solution
      Polymerization. *J. Biomat. Sci. Polym. Edn.*, Vol. 19, No. 10, pp. 1295- 1306

[75] Feng, W. Yu, L. & Uhrich, K. E. (2008). Opioid-Based Poly(anhydride-esters): New
      Approach to Preventing Drug Abuse. *Polym. Prepr.*, Vol. 49, No. 2, pp. 454 – 455

[76] Rosario-Melendez, Roselin; Delgado-Rivera, Roberto; Yu, Lei & Uhrich, K. E. (2011).
      Synthesis, Characterization, and *In Vitro* Studies of a Morphine-Based
      Poly(anhydride- ester). *Polym. Mater. Sci. Eng.*, Vol. 105, No. 2, pp 833 - 835

4

Molecular Aspects of Opioid Receptors and Opioid Receptor Painkillers

Austin B. Yongye and Karina Martínez-Mayorga
Torrey Pines Institute for Molecular Studies, Port Saint Lucie, FL,
USA

1. Introduction

The unpleasant sensation of pain is experienced by all human beings at a given point in life. When pain gets severe and/or chronic it requires medical treatment. For over a thousand years, opioid agonists have been employed therapeutically to treat pain, with the first reports of such use involving the alkaloid morphine dated to the second century B.C.(Waldhoer, Bartlett et al. 2004) The term *opioid* refers to any substance with opium-like activity. Opium is extracted from the juice of the poppy plant *Papaver somniferum*. Opium contains in excess of 20 different alkaloids, and for centuries its crude form was used for pain management and for its psychological effects. In 1806 the German pharmacist Sertürner isolated a pure substance from opium, which he called morphine after the Greek god of dreams, Morpheus. Thereafter other alkaloids such as codeine (1832) and papaverine (1848) were isolated.(Reisine and Pasternak 1996) These discoveries paved the way for the use of pure alkaloids as opposed to crude opium in the medical profession. It became apparent that these alkaloids had a high potential for abuse and addiction. However, it was not until 1973 that the first descriptions of the pharmacological properties of morphine, along with other agonists and antagonists, at the level of the receptor were reported.(Pert, Pasternak et al. 1973)

Opioid receptors are of therapeutic relevance because they constitute the primary targets in the clinical treatment of both acute and chronic pain. They are members of the superfamily of seven helix transmembrane (TM) proteins known as G-protein coupled receptors (GPCRs); so-called because they are coupled in the cytoplasmic side to a group of G_i/G_o hetero-trimeric proteins called G-proteins: G_α, G_β and G_γ.(Eguchi M 2004) Currently four types of opioid receptors have been identified: μ (mu for morphine), κ (kappa for ketocyclazocine), δ (delta for deferens given that it was originally discovered in the vas deferens of mice)(Waldhoer, Bartlett et al. 2004) and orphan opioid receptor-like 1. They are in turn sub-divided into additional subtypes on the basis of their ligand binding and pharmacological profiles: μ_1-μ_2, κ_1-κ_3, and δ_1-δ_2.(Pasternak 1993; Blakeney, Reid et al. 2007) The μ, κ and δ main types are the most studied, each playing a different role in pain sedation: the μ-receptor generates the most profound analgesia, but is also associated with constipation, respiratory depression, euphoria, tolerance, dependence and addition;(Schmauss and Yaksh 1984; Cowan, Zhu et al. 1988) the δ-receptor is involved in pain relief from thermal sources,(Mansour, Khachaturian et al. 1988) but like the μ-receptor, it is also associated with respiratory depression and addiction;(Abdelhamid, Sultana et al.

1991; Maldonado, Negus et al. 1992) the κ-receptor mediates pain originating from chemical stimuli,(Leighton, Johnson et al. 1987; Wollemann, Benyhe et al. 1993) but it promotes dysphoria, diuresis and sedation.(von Voigtlander, Lahti et al. 1983; Lahti, Mickelson et al. 1985) There is also evidence that opioid receptors exist as homo- or hetero-oligomeric complexes and that their pharmacological responses may be cross-modulated.(Zhu, King et al. 1999; Rutherford, Wang et al. 2008) For instance, Waldhoer M et al. used 6'-GNTI to demonstrate the existence of a δ-κ hetero-dimer *in vivo*.(Waldhoer, Fong et al. 2005) Furthermore, δ-opioid antagonists suppress some of the side effects of μ-opioid agonists such as dependence and tolerance while retaining their analgesic properties.(Ananthan 2006) The realization of this potential for cross-modulation generated interests in developing so-called bivalent ligands of opioid receptors.(Dietis, Guerrini et al. 2009; Balboni, Salvadori et al. 2011) One therapeutic relevance of opioid receptors worth mentioning is that opioid receptors antagonists such as naloxone are utilized clinically in the treatment of morphine and heroin addiction and overdose.(Blakeney, Reid et al. 2007) In this chapter, we summarize structural aspects of opioid receptors and opioid receptor ligands, with special emphasis on the μ-opioid receptor. The importance of the combined use of experimental information and computational models is highlighted.

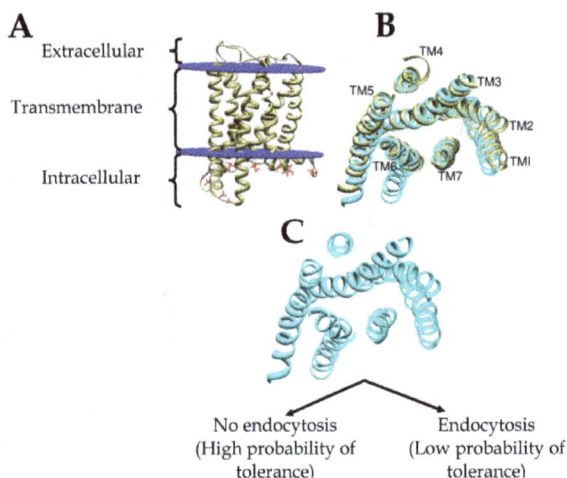

Fig. 1. (A) The three domains of the μ-opioid receptor. Intracellular serine, threonine and tyrosine residues are shown in red. (B) Extracellular perspective: the seven transmembrane helices are arranged sequentially in a counterclockwise direction. The modeled active and inactive structures are shown in cyan and tan, respectively. A substantial structural difference between the two states can be seen at TM6. (C) Hypothesized outcome of degree of ligand-induced receptor endocytosis. Homology models from Pogozheva, I. D., A. L. Lomize, et al. (1998), Fowler, C. B. et al. (2004).

2. Biochemical and biophysical characterization of the μ-opioid receptor

2.1 Structural studies of the μ-opioid receptor

The notion of preferential stabilization of distinct conformational states by agonists and non-agonists has been established experimentally and also demonstrated computationally (see Figure1). The experimental studies include: Li et al. (Li, Han et al. 2007) employing agonists and inverse-agonists of the muscarinic acetylcholine GPCR; Xu et al. (Xu, Sanz et al. 2008) identified inter-residue interaction differences between the active and inactive states for the μ-opioid receptor. From the computational side, molecular dynamics simulations studies suggest that μ-opioid receptor agonists and antagonists bind to the receptor with a set of interactions that are specific to each class.(Kolinski and Filipek 2008) In addition, MD simulations have been utilized to elucidate an increase in solvent exposure of the intracellular domains between helices 3 and 6, and different interactions between the arginine of the E/DRY motif for active and inactive GPCRs.(Fanelli and De Benedetti 2006)

2.2 Mechanism of activation of opioid receptors

To describe the mechanism of activation and action of opioid receptors it suffices to describe the cellular assembly of these receptors. Opioid receptors comprise three domains: an extracellular N-terminus, seven transmembrane α-helices and an intracellular C-terminus, Figure 1. The 7TM helices are arranged sequentially in a counter-clockwise manner when viewed from the extracellular side, and are linked by loops called EL1, EL2, EL3, IL1, IL2 and IL3. EL and IL denote extracellular loop and intracellular loop, respectively. Across the receptors the intracellular loops share the highest sequence homology (90%), followed by TM domains (70%), while the extracellular loops, the N- and C-termini show the greatest diversity.(Knapp, Malatynska et al. 1995) Coupling between the receptors and G-proteins occurs via the pertussis toxin sensitive G_α unit.

Activation and signaling from opioid receptors by different classes of ligands are regulated by a highly conserved mechanism.(Finn and Whistler 2001; Eguchi 2004) They are activated naturally by endogenous peptides, but also by exogenous opiates. Agonist-dependent opioid receptor activation induces conformational changes in the receptor, which promote exchange of G_α-bound GDP for unbound GTP, followed by dissociation of the G-proteins from the receptor. The G_α unit further dissociates from the $G_{\beta\gamma}$ units. Signal transduction occurs via GTP-bound G_α inhibiting adenylate cyclase, responsible for producing cyclic adenosine monophosphate (cAMP). Down-regulation of cAMP results in the reduction of voltage-dependent current and neurotransmitter release.(Eguchi 2004) Moreover, the threshold of voltage-dependent ion channels becomes more negative, decreasing inward flow of current responsible for spontaneous neuronal activity resulting in a drop in cellular excitability. cAMP reduction also leads to a decrease in neurotransmitter release by cAMP-dependent protein kinase. The G_β and G_γ subunits also play key roles in decreasing cell excitability by inhibiting voltage-gated Ca^{2+} channels, hyperpolarizing the membrane and up-regulating the conduction of potassium.(Eguchi 2004) These combined decreases in neurotransmitter release and excitability are manifested as analgesia. Finally, the inactive state is re-constituted when G_α-bound GTP is hydrolyzed to GDP, re-association with $G_{\beta\gamma}$ and recoupling with the receptor.

Numerous experimental approaches have been utilized to investigate GPCR structure and activation including: solution and solid-state NMR, fluorescence, IR and UV spectroscopy, spin-labeling, site-directed mutagenesis, substituted cysteine accessibility, disulphide cross-linking, engineering metal-binding sites, and identification of constitutively active mutants.(Gether 2000; Meng and Bourne 2001; Parnot, Miserey-Lenkei et al. 2002; Decaillot, Befort et al. 2003; Hubbell, Altenbach et al. 2003; Struts, Salgado et al. 2011) Experimentally and computationally, the importance of the lipid membrane should be recognized. It is well documented that membrane composition affects receptor function.(Botelho, Gibson et al. 2002; Botelho, Huber et al. 2006) From the computational side, molecular dynamics simulations showed that the modification of the original positioning of the lipids in the membrane influences the dynamics of the protein.(Lau, Grossfield et al. 2007) In addition, water flux though the transmembrane helices, has been proposed to affect rhodopsin activation. (Grossfield, Pitman et al. 2008) Lastly, the time scale involved in the activation of GPCRs is a challenging task. However, the combined use of computer power and experimental information allows for the generation of detailed structural information. For instance, 2000 ns molecular dynamics simulations and solid-state 2H-NMR data were combined to elucidate the protonation state of key residues directly involved in rhodopsin activation.(Martinez-Mayorga, Pitman et al. 2006) This exemplifies how computational models can provide detailed structural information not available otherwise.

Advances in crystallography and molecular engineering have provided the three-dimensional structures of a few GPCR's: rhodopsin,(Palczewski, Kumasaka et al. 2000; Ridge and Palczewski 2007; Choe, Kim et al. 2011) β-adrenergic receptor,(Kobilka and Schertler 2008) and adenosine receptor.(Jaakola, Griffith et al. 2008) In the absence of experimental structures of opioid receptors, the 2.6-Å resolution crystal structure of bovine rhodopsin(Palczewski, Kumasaka et al. 2000) has served as a template for generating homology models of these receptors,(Pogozheva, Lomize et al. 1998; Fowler, Pogozheva et al. 2004; Fowler, Pogozheva et al. 2004; Pogozheva, Przydzial et al. 2005) Like rhodopsin, opioid receptors belong to class A of the GPCR superfamily. The crystallographic structure of the active state of rhodopsin is now available (Choe, Kim et al. 2011) and can be contrasted with the large body of literature that suggests a common active conformation among the class-A GPCRs. (Karnik, Gogonea et al. 2003) In the activated state TM6 undergoes outward rigid-body translation toward TM5, but away from TM3 and TM7. As a result, a cavity opens up in the intracellular domain in contact with G-proteins. Similar movements have been also suggested for TM1-3 and TM7.(Lin and Sakmar 1996; Gether, Lin et al. 1997; Altenbach, Cai et al. 2001) A better understanding of these activation mechanisms at the molecular level could lead to new drugs geared towards the therapeutic regulation of their functions.

Decaillot FM et al. applied mutagenesis to study the mechanism of activation of the human δ-opioid receptor.(Decaillot, Befort et al. 2003) By analyzing 30 constitutively active mutants of this receptor, mutations hypothesized to produce distinct active conformations were grouped into four abutting areas of the receptor from the extracellular (group I) to the intracellular (group IV) domain. Details about the residues that form each group can be found in Decaillot FM. A sequential binding mechanism was proposed to activate the receptor.(Decaillot, Befort et al. 2003) Sequential binding in GPCRs is not uncommon. A similar mechanism has been postulated for the β2-adrenergic receptors.(Swaminath, Xiang et al. 2004) In the case of the δ-opioid receptor agonists bind to residues in group I comprising a hydrophobic region in EL3, weakening interactions with TM6 and TM7 in the extracellular domain thus initiating a signal. Next, the ligand enters the binding pocket disrupting interactions in groups II and III. Group II residues form a molecular switch that controls movements of TM3. Group III residues are closest to the binding site, consist of patches of hydrophilic and hydrophobic residues and form a network of interactions between residues derived from TM3, 6 and 7. The disruption of these interactions results in a receptor state that is susceptible to activation and helps propagate signals to the intracellular side. It was hypothesized that the amphiphilic nature of opiates and opioid ligands makes them complementary to residues in group III, i.e., the hydrophilic portion of the ligands disrupt the hydrogen-binding network, while the hydrophobic portion compete with the hydrophobic residues. Finally, disrupting the interactions in group 4 residues results in the separation of TM6 and TM7 in the intracellular side and possibly destabilizing interactions with Gα and exposure to other secondary protein effectors.

Insights about the conformation of the activated state of the μ-opioid receptor are based on modeling experimental distance constraints derived from site-directed mutagenesis, inter-helix H-bonds, disulphide bonds, and engineered Zn^{2+} binding sites between the μ-opioid receptor and analogues of the receptor-bound conformation of a cyclic tetra-peptidomimetic, JOM6.(Fowler, Pogozheva et al. 2004) Structural data for the active state were also derived from disulphide bonds between TM5 and TM6 in the ACM3 muscarinic receptor,(Ward SD, JBC 2002) intrinsic allosteric Zn^{2+} binding sites in TM5 and TM6 of the β_2-adrenergic receptor,(Swaminath, Lee et al. 2003) engineered activating metal-coordination center akin to those between TM3 and TM7 in the β_2-adrenergic(Elling, Thirstrup et al. 1999) and tachykinin(Holst, Elling et al. 2000) receptors, between TM2 and TM3 of the MC4 melanocortin receptor. Finally one hydrogen bond constraint from the δ-opioid receptor(Decaillot, Befort et al. 2003) was introduced. A comparison between the modeled structures of the active and inactive states of the μ-opioid receptor is shown in Figure 1. A noticeable difference is seen in TM6 highlighting the rigid-body movement described for the δ-opioid receptor.

2.3 Internalization of opioid receptors and changes in downstream signaling

Signal transduction by the μ-opioid receptor is determined by properties of the ligand such as affinity, potency, efficacy, bio-availability and half-life, collectively defined as 'relative activity' or RA.(Martini and Whistler 2007) In addition, the length of time the receptor-ligand complex remains coupled to the G-protein, is controlled by receptor desensitization, endocytosis and to an extent the pharmacokinetic properties of the ligand. It has been noted that ligand activity and endocytosis do not have a linear relationship.(Martini and Whistler 2007) Hence, an interplay of relative activity versus endocytosis (RAVE) for each ligand determines the magnitude of the signal transduced. Thus each ligand-receptor complex has an associated RAVE value. As highlighted by Martini L et al.(Martini and Whistler 2007) endogenous peptides have good RA values at the μ-opioid receptor, and also induce significant desensitization and endocytosis. Based on this reasoning, the good balance between their RA and VE values explain why they do not induce tolerance. Another example is methadone. Methadone has comparable potency with encephalin and is also an equally good receptor internalizer.(Whistler, Chuang et al. 1999) Nonetheless, it has a longer half-life compared to other opioids, and consequently a larger RA value giving rise to a moderately higher RAVE value. The extension of the RAVE analysis to morphine is more complicated and invokes secondary protein effectors and region-selective differences in receptor endocytosis.(Martini and Whistler 2007) In general, agonists such as morphine with high RAVE values are more likely to induce tolerance. It has been demonstrated that the development of μ-opioid tolerance is inversely related to the ability of an agonist to promote receptor endocytosis or internalization.(Whistler, Chuang et al. 1999; Finn and Whistler 2001) This theory distinguishes two types of agonists based on their ability to stabilize different receptor conformational states, resulting in phosphorylation by different kinases. Depending on the type of kinase the receptor can be rapidly endocytosed, resensitized and recycled to the cell surface, preventing the development of tolerance.

The formation of an opioid ligand-receptor complex results in structural changes at the extracellular and transmembrane domains, which are propagated to the intracellular domain followed by the dissociation of G-proteins; phosphorylation by G-protein coupled receptor kinases (GRK), protein kinase A (PKA) and C (PKC); and binding by other proteins such as β-arrestins.(Eguchi 2004) The phosphorylated receptor is endocytosed, whereby it is re-sensitized and recycled to the cell surface or it is marked for degradation. Unlike PKA and PKC, specific GRK-phosphorylation triggers the recruitment of β-arrestins, receptor internalization, resensitization and recycling to the cell surface. This dynamic recycling process has been suggested as crucial to circumvent development to drug tolerance. Tolerance-causing agonists impede receptor endocytosis and/or resensitization, while non-tolerance-inducing drugs promote rapid receptor desensitization-internalization-resensitization and recycling.(Martini and Whistler 2007)

The exact cause of development of tolerance is still a subject of debate. Nonetheless, it is generally accepted that chronic administration of opiates for analgesia gives rise to tolerance. The cellular mechanism of tolerance may involve downstream compensatory changes in neuronal circuits.(Eguchi 2004) The continual and sustained inhibition of adenylate cyclase activity triggers a positive feedback to compensate for the low intracellular levels of cAMP, resulting in the reversible superactivation of adenylate cyclase. This up-regulation of enzyme activity restores the cellular concentration of cAMP, resulting in cells being tolerant to the opiate and also dependent on it given that withdrawing the drug or introducing an antagonist gives rise to abnormally high levels of cAMP and also a restoration of the normal activity level of adenylate cyclase.(Sharma, Klee et al. 1975) The change is delayed but relatively stable and is known to be responsible for opiate tolerance and dependence.(Sharma, Klee et al. 1975) The combined inhibition and up-regulation of adenylyl cyclase provide a means of activating and deactivating neuronal circuits and may play a role in a memory process. It was later shown that the adenylate cyclase V and Gβγ played a role in this activation.(AvidorReiss, Nevo et al. 1996)

2.4 Point-mutation studies to identify key residue targets for phosphorylation

Mutation studies have been successful in identifying key cytosolic domains and residues of ligand-activated μ-opioid receptors, which are liable to phosphorylation, and potentially directly involved in agonist-dependent receptor internalization. (Celver, Lowe et al. 2001; El Kouhen, Burd et al. 2001; Celver, Xu et al. 2004) Truncation of the μ-opioid receptor at Ser363 produced a mutant that was not phosphorylated, and was endocytosed and recycled more slowly than the wild-type,(Qiu, Law et al. 2003) suggesting that phosphorylating residues in this segment may be important for internalization. Cleaving off the entire C-terminal resulted in increased agonist-independent internalization and recycling,(Waldhoer, Bartlett et al. 2004) indicating a greater exposure of some residues critical for the dynamic recycling machinery. Utilizing a single agonist, [D-Ala^2,MePhe^4,Gly^5-ol]enkephalin (DAMGO), the mutation of Thr180 to alanine in the second intracellular loop prevented receptor desensitization, while alanine scanning of serine or threonine in the third cytoplasmic loop did not inhibit receptor desensitization.(Celver, Lowe et al. 2001) In a DAMGO-induced receptor activation study, mutations of C-terminal serine/threonine residues identified three phosphorylation sites: Ser363, Thr370 and Ser375. The S375A mutant decreased the rate of receptor internalization, while the S363A and T370A double mutant accelerated the rate of internalization,(El Kouhen, Burd et al. 2001) which may suggest that the combined phosphorylation of Ser363 and Thr370 attenuates receptor internalization. Other studies employing etorphine and multiple mutations have also identified Ser356 and Ser363,(Burd, El-Kouhen et al. 1998) and Thr394 (using DAMGO)(Pak, Odowd et al. 1997; Wolf, Koch et al. 1999) as sites for phosphorylation that result in down-regulation of the μ-opioid receptor. Mutation of Ser330 and Ser363 simultaneously did not alter receptor phosphorylation, but the mutations prevented down-regulation of the receptor suggesting that the absence of down-regulation was not due to the removal of phosphorylation sites. Down-regulation may be occurring through a phosphorylation-independent mechanism or these two sites are not phosphorylated. This is contrary to later studies that demonstrated that Ser363 is phosphorylated.(El Kouhen, Burd et al. 2001) The T394A mutant is more rapidly internalized and resensitized relative to the wild-type μ-opioid receptor. These mutation studies show that multiple phosphorylation motifs may be needed for internalization and that not every phosphorylation site is phosphorylated.

3. Discovery and development of opioid receptor ligands

3.1 Endogenous opioid ligands

Extensive structural and pharmacological studies have been performed to understand the mechanisms of action of opioids as well as for the design of new and more efficient opioid-based painkillers. The opioid agonists propagate their analgesic effects by interacting with opioid receptors. They are both endogenously expressed peptides and exogenous opiates. The term opiate is reserved for foreign substances introduced into the body to target opioid receptors. The endogenous peptides enkephalins, dynorphins, β-endorphins and nociceptins are excised from their precursors pro-enkephalin, pro-dynorphin, pro-opiomelanocortin and pro-nociceptin/orphanin FQ, respectively. The majority of these peptides comprise a conserved N-terminal YGGF motif,(Gentilucci, Squassabia et al. 2007) except the uncharacteristically short peptides endomorphin-1 (YPWF-NH$_2$) and endomorphin-2 (YPFF-NH$_2$) that are considered analogues of the YGGF motif. A list of endogenous peptides, their precursors and receptor selectivity is presented in Table 1.

Peptide	Sequences	Precursor	Selectivity
Endomorphin-1	YPWF-NH$_2$	ND[a]	μ
Endomorphin-2	YPFF-NH$_2$		
β-endorphin	**YGGF**MTSEKSQTPLVTLFK NAIIKNAYKKGE	Pro-opiomelanocortin	μ=δ
[Leu^5]enkephalin	**YGGF**L		
[Met^5]enkephalin	**YGGF**M	Pro-enkephalin	δ
Metorphinamide	**YGGF**MRRV-NH$_2$		
Deltorphin A	YmFHLMD-NH$_2$		
Deltorphin I	YaFDVVG-NH$_2$	ND[a]	δ
Deltorphin II	YaFEVVG-NH$_2$		
Dynorphin A	**YGGF**LRRIRPKLKWDNQ		
Dynorphin A(1-8)	**YGGF**LRRI		
Dynorphin B	**YGGF**LRRQFKVVT	Pro-dynorphin	κ
α-neoendorphin	**YGGF**LRKYPK		
β-neoendorphin	**YGGF**LRKYP		
Nociceptin	FGGFTGARKSARKLANQ	Pro-nociceptin / Orphanin FQ	ORL-1[b]

[a] Not yet determined. The conserved YGGF sequence is shown in bold
[b] Orphan opioid receptor-like 1

Table 1. Endogenous opioid peptides, the precursor and receptor selectivity.

Endomorphin-1 and endomorphin-2 are highly potent, selective μ-opioid receptor endogenous peptides isolated from mammals, and elicit responses similar to that of morphine.(Zadina, Hackler et al. 1997; Horvath 2000) The endogenous peptides are advantageous in that they do not display any of the side effects of opiates (see below); however, they are not effective in clinical settings because of *in vivo* degradation by peptidases.(Witt, Gillespie et al. 2001) Notwithstanding their degradation, these peptides and their analogues have been utilized extensively as tools to probe receptor categorization and structure-activity relationships.(Hruby and Agnes 1999; Gentilucci, Squassabia et al. 2007) The exogenous opiates on the other hand are more effective in pain management, but present numerous undesirable side effects, some of which are highlighted below. As such, several efforts are being undertaken to identify beneficial analgesics with minimal to no side effects.

3.2 Potent opioid-based analgesics

Interests in identifying more effective analgesics have led to the reporting of a large number potent opioid peptide and non-peptide compounds that are generally classified as agonists or antagonists.(Pan 1998; Stevens, Jones et al. 2000; Eguchi 2004; Waldhoer, Bartlett et al. 2004; Gentilucci, Squassabia et al. 2007; Prisinzano and Rothman 2008; Volpe, Tobin et al. 2011) In spite of the multitude of known opioid compounds, only a relatively small number has been approved for clinical use. The majority of these prescribed analgesics are relatively selective for the μ-opioid receptor,(Volpe, Tobin et al. 2011) though at sufficiently higher doses interactions with the other opioid receptors will occur. While some of these compounds are selective for either the μ (morphine), κ (salvinorin A), or δ (naltrindole) opioid receptors, some are non-selective and display mixed agonist/antagonist responses, for example buprenorphine, pentazocine and butorphanol. Buprenorphine is a partial μ-agonist and partial κ-antagonist that is administered clinically for opioid detoxification and maintenance.(Blakeney, Reid et al. 2007)

Compound	Receptor	Function[a]	Compound	Receptor	Function[a]
Morphine*	M	A	Cyclazocine*	μ/κ	A/AN
Fentanyl*	"	"	Pentazocine*	"	"
Hydrocodone*	"	"	Nalbuphine*	"	"
Levorphanol*	"	"	SIOM	Δ	A
Meperidine*	"	"	SCN-80	"	"
Sufentanyl*	"	"	TAN-67	"	"
Methadone*	"	"	Ketocyclazocine	K	A
Oxycodone*	"	"	Ethyl Ketocyclazocine	"	"
Oxymorphone*	"	"	U-50,488	"	"
Codeine*	"	"	Salvinorin A	"	"
Naloxone*	"	AN	6'-GNTI[a]	"	"
Buprenorphine*	μ/κ	A/AN	5'-GNTI[a]	"	AN
Butorphanol*	"	"	Bremazocine	μ/δ/κ	A/AN

A = agonist; AN = antagonist
*Currently in clinical use. [a] GNTI: guanidino-naltrindole

Table 2. Opioid receptor ligands.

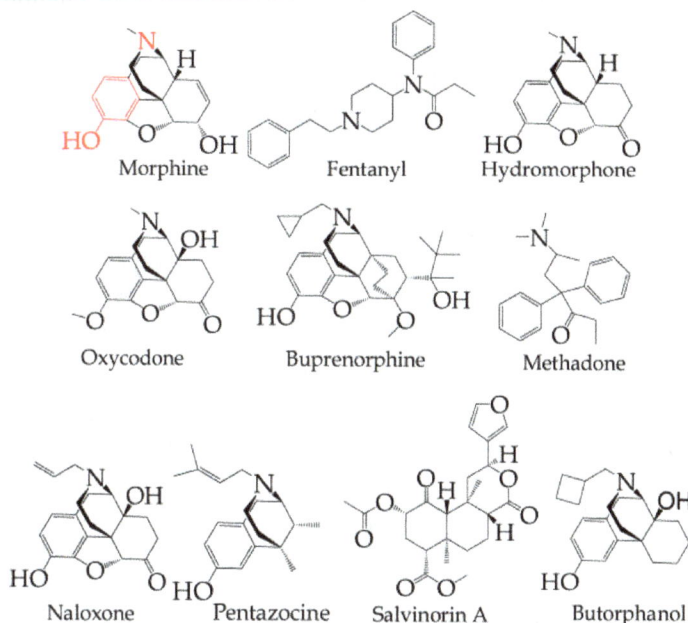

Fig. 2. The chemical structures of some exogenous opiates. The classical "message" tyramine moiety is colored in red in the structure of morphine.

The classification of some opioid compounds is given in Table 2. The chemical structures of selected compounds are shown in Figure 2. Several factors affect the potency of an analgesic, including route of administration, whether they act as full or partial agonists, ability to cross the blood-brain barrier (physico-chemical properties) and their effects on other major physiological systems.(Volpe, Tobin et al. 2011) Some potency comparisons with morphine worth mentioning include the following: fentanyl when administered intramuscularly is about 100 fold more potent; hydromorphone is 6-8 fold more potent;(Inturrisi 2002) and oral oxycodone is about 1.8 times more potent.(Curtis, Johnson et al. 1999) Though a partial agonist buprenorphine is reported to be 25-40 times more potent than morphine.(Blakeney, Reid et al. 2007)

3.3 Pharmacophoric features of opioid ligands

Numerous structure-activity relations (SAR) studies have been carried out on opioid receptor ligands to determine features that drive affinity or efficacy with the goal of generating more effective therapeutic compounds,(Eguchi 2004; Metcalf and Coop 2005; Prisinzano and Rothman 2008; Yongye, Appel et al. 2009, amongst others). SAR studies employing site-directed substitutions and constraints of endogenous peptides, as well as modifications of morphine have provided valuable insights about the pharmacophoric features, ligand selectivity and biological roles of opioid receptors.(Blakeney, Reid et al. 2007) For example it has been determined that a positively charged amine group, an aromatic moiety and a hydrophobic group result in tight binding of morphine. A salt-bridge is formed between the protonated amine and an aspartate residue in TM3, π-π stacking interactions between the aromatic group and residues in the binding pocket and hydrophobic-hydrophobic interactions. In endogenous peptides the N-terminal tyrosine contains a protonated amine and aromatic group, akin to the aromatic ring (A) and basic nitrogen (N) in morphine, Figure 3. This moiety termed tyramine is common to a majority of opioids, though there are some notable potent and selective opiates that lack this classical pharmacophore: Salvinorin A was the first highly potent, non-nitrogen opiate agonist selective towards the κ-opioid receptor;(Roth, Baner et al. 2002) one of its analogues, herkinorin became the first non-nitrogenous agonist selective towards the μ-opioid receptor.(Harding, Tidgewell et al. 2005) Furthermore, the phenylalanine side chain in endogenous peptides mimics the hydrophobic feature (B) of morphine (ring C). It should be pointed out that due to size differences between the peptides and morphine, the interactions between their respective hydrophobic features (B) and the receptor are different.

The observation of the occurrence of a common structural feature amongst opioid ligands gave rise to the "message-address" concept of ligand-receptor interactions, i.e., the same message (signal transduction) is delivered to different addresses (receptors). For the endogenous peptides the message comprises the conserved YGGF motif, with the exceptions cited in Table 1, while for the opiates the tyramine moiety represents the message. The other varied segments of the ligands make up the address and confer selectivity.

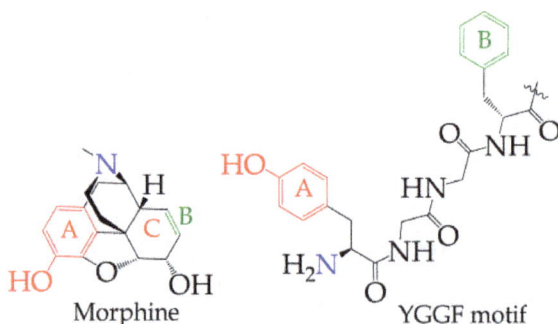

Morphine   YGGF motif

Fig. 3. Chemical structures of morphine and the truncated "message" motif of an endogenous peptide. The YGGF represents amino acids: Y, tyrosine; G, glycine and F, phenylalanine.

Generating pharmacophore models for opioid receptors have followed two traditional approaches: ligand-based or docking-based. Ligand-based methods involve identifying and superimposing common substructures of low energy conformers from which features that drive biological activity are determined. However, because of the inherent difficulties of superimposing structurally different scaffolds these efforts have typically revolved around congeneric series. See Shim J et al.(Shim, Coop et al. 2011) and references therein. In ligand-based virtual screenings via multi-conformer ensembles, the quality and coverage of the conformational ensemble are important. The production of the conformers can be computationally intensive, especially for compounds with a large number of rotatable bonds. Thus, reducing the size of multi-conformer databases and the number of query conformers, while simultaneously reproducing the bioactive conformer with good accuracy, is of crucial interest. A report protocol that takes into account these aspects has been proposed.(Yongye, Bender et al. 2010) This protocol and other important aspects of conformational coverage in ligand-based virtual screening methods have been recently revised.(Musafia and Senderowitz 2010) On the other hand, docking-based approaches are most valuable when experimental structures of receptors are available. The absence of experimental opioid receptor structures means docking-based methods must rely on homology models. Moreover, for docking-based virtual screening, one has to contend with no induced fit and the possibility of different binding modes.

The identification of enkephalins and δ-opioid receptors fueled interests in developing ligands that target this receptor. The observation that co-administration of δ-opioid receptor antagonists with μ-opioid receptor agonists produced analgesia without the side effect of μ-only agonists further served as motivation to identify δ-selective opioids. Hence, considerable efforts have been devoted to studying the SAR of δ-opioid receptor ligands using both pharmacophore and quantitative structure-activity relationship modeling. See Bernard D et al.(Bernard, Coop et al. 2007) and references therein. Employing the *conformationally sampled pharmacophore* (CSP) approach Bernard D et al. were able to differentiate between δ-opioid receptor agonists and antagonists.(Bernard, Coop et al. 2003; Bernard, Coop et al. 2005) An advantage of the CSP method is the inclusion of high energy conformers in describing pharmacophores, the justification stemming from the fact that ligands may bind in higher energy conformers stabilized by intermolecular interactions with receptors. The CSP methodology was later applied to peptide and nonpeptide agonists to derive pharmacophore models of δ-opioid receptor ligands.(Bernard, Coop et al. 2007) Three pharmacophore points were considered: aromatic (A), basic nitrogen (N) and hydrophobic group (B).

Utilizing efficacy as the activity index, CSP was extended to five peptides and twenty nonpeptides comprising μ-opioid receptor ligands, to derive an aggregate pharmacophore. By analyzing a diverse group of agonists, partial agonists and antagonists the following conclusions were derived: interactions with the B or hydrophobic site of oripavines (etorphine, buprenorphine and diprenorphine) modulated the degree of agonism; agonists with bulky B groups adopt a pose in which interactions occur with both the basic amine and the B site; agonists with large N-substituents are oriented such that the substituents occupy the position of the traditional B site. The resultant pharmacophore is an aromatic group (A), a basic amine (N), a hydrophobic group (B) and N-substituents (S). The investigators claim that such an approach would facilitate efforts to develop compounds that possess both μ-agonistic and δ-antagonistic properties even though the cell lines only expressed the μ-opioid receptor.(Shim, Coop et al. 2011) Furthermore, depending on the structural class of the ligand, N-subsituents can enhance agonism or antagonism. For example, *N*-allyl and *N*-cyclopropylmethyl substituents in etorphines give rise to better agonists compared to morphine,(Gorin and Marshall 1977) while they induce antagonism in 4,5-epoxymorphinans.(Shim, Coop et al. 2011)

The currently known κ-opioid receptor agonists have been classified into eight structural classes(Yamaotsu and Hirono 2011): peptides (dynorphins), benzomorphans (pentazocine), morphinans (butorphanol), arylacetamines (U-69593), diazabicyclononanones (HZ2), bicyclic guanidines (TPI-614-1), benzodiazepines (±tifluadom) and neocleorodane diterpenes (salvinorin A). A comprehensive review of these classes and the history of the development of κ-opioid receptor ligand pharmacophores was published recently by Yamaotsu N et al.(Yamaotsu and Hirono 2011) Evidently, the structural diversity of these classes making it difficult to construct a consensus pharmacophore model. Previous SAR and pharmacophore analyses of κ-opioid receptor ligands are typically confined to structural analogues. Yamaotsu N et al. proposed a consensus pharmacophore encompassing all eight classes using seven compounds in both the training and test sets. Superposition was based on the physico-chemical properties of groups of atoms. The consensus pharmacophore comprised three hydrophobic groups, a hydrogen bond donor and three hydrogen bond acceptors. These pharmacophoric features were employed to describe four binding orientations of the different classes of ligands for the κ-opioid receptor. It remains to be determined how this consensus pharmacophore will perform in virtual screening: for example screening a database, requiring that a given number of features match, followed by biological evaluation of the top scoring compounds. Additionally, in the search of opioid receptor ligands, structure similarity(Martinez-Mayorga, Medina-Franco et al. 2008; Yongye, Appel et al. 2009) and chemoinformatic analyses(Medina-Franco, Martínez-Mayorga et al. 2009) have been employed to develop SAR and to characterize highly dense combinatorial libraries.

3.4 Identification of opioid receptor ligands

A large and growing body of literature has reported the identification of opioid receptor ligands. In particular, improvements in high-throughput chemical synthesis have made possible the rapid and efficient generation of molecules, giving rise to thousands or millions of compounds in combinatorial libraries. Advances in molecular biology have also enabled the evaluation of millions of individual compounds against a number of different biological targets via high-throughput screening (HTS). However, some high content assays, such as *in vivo* studies, are not amenable to the high-throughput miniaturization required to screen millions of individual compounds. In such cases, screening libraries using a mixture-based format(Houghten, Pinilla et al. 1999; Pinilla, Appel et al. 2003; Houghten, Dooley et al. 2006) (also known as positional scanning-synthetic combinatorial libraries or PS-SCL) enables the evaluation of thousands to millions of molecules in approximately a hundred to a few hundred samples. PS-SCL have been used to successfully identify active molecules for a variety of biological targets. (Houghten, Pinilla et al. 1999; Pinilla, Appel et al. 2003; Houghten, Pinilla et al. 2008) In the case of opioid receptors highly active peptides (Dooley, Chung et al. 1994; Houghten, Dooley et al. 2006) and peptidomimetics have been identified. (Houghten, Dooley et al. 2006) This technique has recently found new applications in the search of conotoxins (Armishaw, Singh et al.) and *in-vivo* screening (Reilley, Giulianotti et al.). A step forward in the development of peptides with therapeutic relevance corresponds to the formation of cyclic structures. Cyclic peptides are therapeutically attractive due to their high bioavailability, potential selectivity, and scaffold novelty. In addition, the presence of D-residues induces conformational preferences not followed by peptides consisting of only naturally abundant L-residues. Therefore, the development of synthetic schemes and comprehending how amino acids induce turns in peptides is significant in peptide design. For example, a successful method for the synthesis of cyclic peptides by the intramolecular aminolysis of peptide thioesters, has been recently reported,(Li, Yongye et al. 2009) and the corresponding explicit solvent molecular dynamics simulations were produced and analyzed.(Yongye, Li et al. 2009) The cyclic tetra-peptidomimetic, JOM6, (Fowler, Pogozheva et al. 2004) is an example of a conformationally constrained peptide that retains activity against the μ-opioid receptor. It is anticipated that research will continue in this direction.

The search of opioid receptor ligands using experimental screening of combinatorial libraries has been complemented using computational methods. *In silico* methods can be incorporated at different stages of the drug discovery process, from library design to lead optimization. (Brooijmans and Kuntz 2003) Computational methods are largely applied to corporate chemical collections (Bajorath 2002) as well as combinatorial chemical libraries. (Houghten, Pinilla et al. 2008) However, limited efforts have been reported so far to explicitly integrate information from mixture-based combinatorial libraries and computational techniques (López-Vallejo, Caulfield et al. 2011; Yongye, Pinilla et al. 2011). The structural analogy contained in combinatorial libraries in general and in mixture-based libraries in particular deserves particular considerations. Virtual screening may assist in downsizing large compound libraries and the selection of a smaller set of promising hits, whereas mixture-based screening may screen out some of the false positives of virtual screening. The integration of mixture-based combinatorial library screening data and virtual screening information has been undertaken. In the particular case of opioid receptors, the predicted activity obtained from the experimental mixture-based screening of a large library of bicyclic guanidines was combined with structural similarity methods. This approach allowed categorizing the molecules as actives, activity cliffs, diverse compounds and missed hits.(Yongye, Pinilla et al. 2011)

4. Conclusions

Ever since the discovery of opioid receptors as the principal mediators of analgesia and the identification of endogenous peptides as well as opiates that elicit analgesic responses, considerable efforts have been devoted to finding compounds that target these receptors with the aim of alleviating the sensation of pain. While the endogenous peptides do not display any side effects, their use in clinical settings is hampered because of *in vivo* degradation by protein-digesting enzymes. Opiates are more effective, but adverse side effects such as tolerance, dependence and addiction limit their prolonged usage; thus the continual search for more efficient analgesics. Several compounds have been reported as opioid receptor ligands, however, only a relatively few are currently prescribed in clinical settings with morphine being the prototypical μ-opioid agonist. A high proportion of opioid-based drugs is selective toward the μ-opioid receptor, and still retains untoward side effects prompting extensive studies about the molecular origins of these undesirable properties.

This review focuses on structural aspects of opioid receptors and opioid receptor ligands, with special emphasis on the μ-opioid receptor. The information presented here can be summarized as follows:

1. Considerable evidence now point to the existence of opioid receptors as homo- or hetero-oligomeric complexes and that their pharmacological responses may be cross-modulated. For example the co-administration of a μ-opioid agonist with a δ-opioid antagonist suppressed side effects such as dependence and tolerance while retaining μ-agonist induced analgesia. The realization of this potential for cross-modulation has generated interests in the development of bivalent ligands. The ligands may be individual compounds that possess mixed agonist/antagonist properties or a separate agonist and antagonist tethered through a linker. Future directions of research in analgesia will continue to point towards agonists with acceptable side effects, designing bivalent ligands, or ligands with mixed receptor specificities and functions.

2. While the exact mechanisms of development of tolerance are still under debate, the current models suggest a combination of ligand-induced conformational changes and receptor desensitization, as well as down-stream compensatory changes of secondary effectors.
3. Promising computational methods such as consensus pharmacophore models using different structural scaffold might serve a role in identifying ligands with mixed secondary functional profiles. Understanding the cross-talk between the different signaling pathways of the opioid receptors will also be significant.
4. Production and analysis of a large number of compounds with potential affinity to opioid receptors are possible. However, considerably more work will need to be done to understand and design compounds with high analgesic effect and lower side effects. To that end, a more detailed understanding of the signaling process upon opioid receptor activation is needed.

5. Acknowledgement

This work was supported by the State of Florida, Executive Officer of the Governor's Office of Tourism, Trade and Economic Development.

6. References

Abdelhamid, E. E., M. Sultana, et al. (1991). "Selective blockage of delta-opioid receptors prevents the development of morphine-tolerance and dependence in mice." Journal of Pharmacology and Experimental Therapeutics 258(1): 299-303.

Altenbach, C., K. W. Cai, et al. (2001). "Structure and function in rhodopsin: Mapping light-dependent changes in distance between residue 65 in helix TM1 and residues in the sequence 306-319 at the cytoplasmic end of helix TM7 and in helix H8." Biochemistry 40(51): 15483-15492.

Ananthan, S. (2006). "Opioid ligands with mixed m/d opioid receptor interactions: An emerging approach to novel analgesics." AAPS J. 8(1): E118-E125.

Armishaw, C. J., N. Singh, et al. (2010). "A synthetic combinatorial strategy for developing alpha-conotoxin analogs as potent alpha7 nicotinic acetylcholine receptor antagonists." J. Biol. Chem. 285: 1809-1821.

AvidorReiss, T., I. Nevo, et al. (1996). "Chronic opioid treatment induces adenylyl cyclase V superactivation - Involvement of G beta gamma." Journal of Biological Chemistry 271(35): 21309-21315.

Bajorath, J. (2002). "Integration of virtual and high-throughput screening." Nat. Rev. Drug Discov. 1(11): 882.

Balboni, G., S. Salvadori, et al. (2011). "Opioid bifunctional ligands from morphine and the opioid pharmacophore Dmt-Tic." European Journal of Medicinal Chemistry 46(2): 799-803.

Bernard, D., A. Coop, et al. (2003). "2D conformationally sampled pharmacophore: A ligand-based pharmacophore to differentiate delta opioid agonists from antagonists." Journal of the American Chemical Society 125(10): 3101-3107.

Bernard, D., A. Coop, et al. (2005). "Conformationally sampled pharmacophore for peptidic delta opioid ligands." Journal of Medicinal Chemistry 48(24): 7773-7780.

Bernard, D., A. Coop, et al. (2007). "I quantitative conformationally sampled pharmacophore for delta opioid ligands: Reevaluation of hydrophobic moieties essential for biological activity." Journal of Medicinal Chemistry 50(8): 1799-1809.

Blakeney, J. S., R. C. Reid, et al. (2007). "Nonpeptidic ligands for peptide-activated G protein-coupled receptors." Chemical Reviews 107(7): 2960-3041.

Botelho, A. V., N. J. Gibson, et al. (2002). "Conformational energetics of rhodopsin modulated by nonlamellar-forming lipids." Biochemistry 41(20): 6354-6368.

Botelho, A. V., T. Huber, et al. (2006). "Curvature and hydrophobic forces drive oligomerization and modulate activity of rhodopsin in membranes." Biophysical journal 91(12): 4464-4477.

Brooijmans, N. and I. D. Kuntz (2003). "Molecular recognition and docking algorithms." Annu Rev Biophys Biomol Struct. 32: 335-373.

Burd, A. L., R. El-Kouhen, et al. (1998). "Identification of serine 356 and serine 363 as the amino acids involved in etorphine-induced down-regulation of the mu-opioid receptor." Journal of Biological Chemistry 273(51): 34488-34495.

Celver, J., M. Xu, et al. (2004). "Distinct domains of the mu-opioid receptor control uncoupling and internalization." Molecular Pharmacology 65(3): 528-537.

Celver, J. P., J. Lowe, et al. (2001). "Threonine 180 is required for G-protein-coupled receptor kinase 3- and beta-arrestin 2-mediated desensitization of the mu-opioid receptor in Xenopus oocytes." Journal of Biological Chemistry 276(7): 4894-4900.

Choe, H. W., Y. J. Kim, et al. (2011). "Crystal structure of metarhodopsin II." Nature 471(7340): 651-U137.

Cowan, A., X. Z. Zhu, et al. (1988). "Direct dependence studies in rats with agents selective for different types of opioid receptor." Journal of Pharmacology and Experimental Therapeutics 246(3): 950-955.

Curtis, G. B., G. H. Johnson, et al. (1999). "Relative potency of controlled-release oxycodone and controlled-release morphine in a postoperative pain model." European Journal of Clinical Pharmacology 55(6): 425-429.

Decaillot, F. M., K. Befort, et al. (2003). "Opioid receptor random mutagenesis reveals a mechanism for G protein-coupled receptor activation." Nature Structural Biology 10(8): 629-636.

Dietis, N., R. Guerrini, et al. (2009). "Simultaneous targeting of multiple opioid receptors: a strategy to improve side-effect profile." British Journal of Anaesthesia 103(1): 38-49.

Dooley, C. T., N. N. Chung, et al. (1994). "An all D-amino-acid opioid peptide with central analgesic activity from a combinatorial library." Science 266(5193): 2019-2022.

Eguchi, M. (2004). "Recent advances in selective opioid receptor agonists and antagonists." Medicinal Research Reviews 24(2): 182-212.

El Kouhen, R., A. L. Burd, et al. (2001). "Phosphorylation of Ser363, Thr370 and Ser375 residues within the carboxyl tail differentially regulates μ-opioid receptor internalization." Journal of Biological Chemistry 276(16): 12774-12780.

Elling, C. E., K. Thirstrup, et al. (1999). "Conversion of agonist site to metal-ion chelator site in the beta(2)-adrenergic receptor." Proceedings of the National Academy of Sciences of the United States of America 96(22): 12322-12327.

Fanelli, F. and P. G. De Benedetti (2006). "Inactive and active states and supramolecular organization of GPCRs: insights from computational modeling." Journal of Computer-Aided Molecular Design 20(7-8): 449-461.

Finn, A. K. and J. L. Whistler (2001). "Endocytosis of the mu opioid receptor reduces tolerance and a cellular hallmark of opiate withdrawal." Neuron 32(5): 829-839.

Fowler, C. B., I. D. Pogozheva, et al. (2004). "Refinement of a homology model of the μ-opioid receptor using distance constraints from intrinsic and engineered zinc-binding sites." Biochemistry 43: 8700-8710.

Fowler, C. B., I. D. Pogozheva, et al. (2004). "Complex of an active μ-opioid receptor with a cyclic peptide agonist modeled from experimental constraints." Biochemistry 43: 15796-15810.

Gentilucci, L., F. Squassabia, et al. (2007). "Re-discussion of the importance of ionic interactions in stabilizing ligand-opioid receptor complex and in activating signal transduction." Current Drug Targets 8(1): 185-196.

Gether, U. (2000). "Uncovering molecular mechanisms involved in activation of G protein-coupled receptors." Endocrine Reviews 21(1): 90-113.

Gether, U., S. Lin, et al. (1997). "Agonists induce conformational changes in transmembrane domains III and VI of the beta(2) adrenoceptor." Embo Journal 16(22): 6737-6747.

Gorin, F. A. and G. R. Marshall (1977). "Proposal for biologically-active conformation of opiates and enkephalin." Proceedings of the National Academy of Sciences of the United States of America 74(11): 5179-5183.

Grossfield, A., M. C. Pitman, et al. (2008). "Internal Hydration Increases during Activation of the G-Protein-Coupled Receptor Rhodopsin." J. Mol. Biol. 381(2): 478-486.

Harding, W. W., K. Tidgewell, et al. (2005). "Neoclerodane diterpenes as a novel scaffold for mu opioid receptor ligands." Journal of Medicinal Chemistry 48(15): 4765-4771.

Holst, B., C. E. Elling, et al. (2000). "Partial agonism through a zinc-ion switch constructed between transmembrane domains III and VII in the tachykinin NK1 receptor." Molecular Pharmacology 58(2): 263-270.

Horvath, G. (2000). "Endomorphin-1 and endomorphin-2: pharmacology of the selective endogenous mu-opioid receptor agonists." Pharmacology & Therapeutics 88(3): 437-463.

Houghten, R. A., C. T. Dooley, et al. (2006). "In vitro and direct in vivo testing of mixture-based combinatorial libraries for the identification of highly active and specific opiate ligands." Aaps Journal 8(2): E371-E382.

Houghten, R. A., C. Pinilla, et al. (1999). "Mixture-based synthetic combinatorial libraries." J. Med. Chem. 42(19): 3743-3778.

Houghten, R. A., C. Pinilla, et al. (2008). "Strategies for the use of mixture-based synthetic combinatorial libraries: Scaffold ranking, direct testing, in vivo, and enhanced deconvolution by computational methods." J. Comb. Chem. 10(1): 3-19.

Hruby, V. and R. S. Agnes (1999). "Conformation-activity relationships of opioid peptides with selective activities at opioid receptors." Biopolymers 51: 391-410.

Hubbell, W. L., C. Altenbach, et al. (2003). "Rhodopsin structure, dynamics, and activation: A perspective from crystallography, site-directed spin labeling, sulfhydryl reactivity, and disulfide cross-linking." Membrane Proteins 63: 243-290.

Inturrisi, C. (2002). "Clinical pharmacology of opioids for pain." Clinical Journal of Pain 18: S3-S13.

Jaakola, V. P., M. T. Griffith, et al. (2008). "The 2.6 Angstrom Crystal Structure of a Human A(2A) Adenosine Receptor Bound to an Antagonist." Science 322(5905): 1211-1217.

Karnik, C. O., C. Gueriva, et al. (2003). "Activation of G protein coupled receptors. a common molecular mechanism." Trends in Endocrinology and Metabolism 14(9): 431-437.

Knapp, R. J., E. Malatynska, et al. (1995). "Molecular-biology and pharmacology of cloned opioid receptors." Faseb Journal 9(7): 516-525.

Kobilka, B. and G. F. X. Schertler (2008). "New G-protein-coupled receptor crystal structures: insights and limitations." Trends in Pharmacological Sciences 29(2): 79-83.

Kolinski, M. and S. Filipek (2008). "Molecular dynamics of μ opioid receptor complexes with agonists and antagonists." The Open Structural Biology Journal 2: 8-20.

Lahti, R. A., M. M. Mickelson, et al. (1985). "[^{3}H]U-69593 a highly selective ligand for the opioid κ-receptor." European Journal of Pharmacology 109(2): 281-284.

Lau, P. W., A. Grossfield, et al. (2007). "Dynamic structure of retinylidene ligand of rhodopsin probed by molecular simulations." Journal of Molecular Biology 372(4): 906-917.

Leighton, G. E., M. A. Johnson, et al. (1987). "Pharmacological profile of PD-117302, a selective kappa-opioid agonist." British Journal of Pharmacology 92(4): 915-922.

Li, J. H., S. J. Han, et al. (2007). "Distinct structural changes in a g protein-coupled receptor caused by different classes of agonist ligands." Journal of Biological Chemistry 282(36): 26284-26293.

Li, Y., A. Yongye, et al. (2009). "Synthesis of Cyclic Peptides through Direct Aminolysis of Peptide Thioesters Catalyzed by Imidazole in Aqueous Organic Solutions." Journal of Combinatorial Chemistry 11(6): 1066-1072.

Lin, S. W. and T. P. Sakmar (1996). "Specific tryptophan UV-absorbance changes are probes of the transition of rhodopsin to its active state." Biochemistry 35(34): 11149-11159.

López-Vallejo, F., T. Caulfield, et al. (2011). "Integrating virtual screening and combinatorial chemistry for accelerated drug discovery." Comb. Chem. High Throughput Screening 14(6): 475-487.

Maldonado, R., S. Negus, et al. (1992). "Precipitation of morphine-withdrawal syndrome in rats by administration of mu-selective, delta-selective and kappa-selective opioid antagonists." Neuropharmacology 31(12): 1231-1241.

Mansour, A., H. Khachaturian, et al. (1988). "Anatomy of CNS opioid receptors." Trends in Neuroscience 11: 308.

Martinez-Mayorga, K., J. L. Medina-Franco, et al. (2008). "Conformation-opioid activity relationships of bicyclic guanidines from 3D similarity analysis." Bioorg. & Med. Chem. 16(11): 5932-5938.

Martinez-Mayorga, K., M. C. Pitman, et al. (2006). "Retinal counterion switch mechanism in vision evaluated by molecular simulations." J. Am. Chem. Soc. 128: 16502-16503.

Martini, L. and J. L. Whistler (2007). "The role of mu opioid receptor desensitization and endocytosis in morphine tolerance and dependence." Current Opinion in Neurobiology 17(5): 556-564.

Medina-Franco, J. L., K. Martínez-Mayorga, et al. (2009). "Characterization of Activity Landscapes Using 2D and 3D Similarity Methods: Consensus Activity Cliffs." J. Chem. Inf. Model. 49(2): 477-491.

Meng, E. C. and H. R. Bourne (2001). "Receptor activation: what does the rhodopsin structure tell us?" Trends in Pharmacological Sciences 22(11): 587-593.

Metcalf, M. D. and A. Coop (2005). "Kappa opioid antagonists: Past successes and future prospects." Aaps Journal 7(3): E704-E722.

Musafia, B. and H. Senderowitz (2010). "Biasing conformational ensembles towards bioactive-like conformers for ligand-based drug design." Expert Opinion on Drug Discovery 5(10): 943-959.

Pak, Y., B. F. Odowd, et al. (1997). "Agonist-induced desensitization of the mu opioid receptor is determined by threonine 394 preceded by acidic amino acids in the COOH-terminal tail." Journal of Biological Chemistry 272(40): 24961-24965.

Palczewski, K., T. Kumasaka, et al. (2000). "Crystal structure of rhodopsin: A G protein-coupled receptor." Science 289(5480): 739-745.

Pan, Z. Z. (1998). "mu-opposing actions of the kappa-opioid receptor." Trends in Pharmacological Sciences 19(3): 94-98.

Parnot, C., S. Miserey-Lenkei, et al. (2002). "Lessons from constitutively active mutants of G protein-coupled receptors." Trends in Endocrinology and Metabolism 13(8): 336-343.

Pasternak, G. W. (1993). "Pharmacological mechanisms of opioid analgesics." Clinical Neuropharmacology 16(1): 1-18.

Pert, C. B., G. Pasternak, et al. (1973). "Opiate agonists and antagonist discriminated by receptor binding in brain." Science 182(4119): 1359-1361.

Pinilla, C., J. R. Appel, et al. (2003). "Advances in the use of synthetic combinatorial chemistry: mixture-based libraries." Nat. Med. 9(1): 118-122.

Pogozheva, I. D., A. L. Lomize, et al. (1998). "Opioid receptor three-dimensional structures from distance geometry calculations with hydrogen bonding constraints." Biophysical Journal 75: 612-634.

Pogozheva, I. D., M. J. Przydzial, et al. (2005). "Homology modeling of opioid receptor-ligand complexes using experimental constraints." The AAAPS Journal 7(2): E434-E448.

Prisinzano, T. E. and R. B. Rothman (2008). "Salvinorin A analogs as probes in opioid pharmacology." Chemical Reviews 108(5): 1732-1743.

Qiu, Y., P. Y. Law, et al. (2003). "mu-opioid receptor desensitization - Role of receptor phosphorylation, internalization, and resensitization." Journal of Biological Chemistry 278(38): 36733-36739.

Reilley, K., M. A. Giulianotti, et al. (2010). "Identification of Two Novel, Potent, Low-Liability Antinociceptive Compounds from the Direct In Vivo Screening of a Large Mixture-Based Combinatorial Library." AAAPS J. 12: 318-329.

Reisine, T. and G. Pasternak (1996). Opioid analgesics and antagonists, In: Goodman and Gilman's The Pharmacological Basis of Therapeutics. Hardman J.G., Limbird L.E., pp 521-555, McGraw-Hill, New York.

Ridge, K. D. and K. Palczewski (2007). "Visual rhodopsin sees the light: Structure and mechanism of G protein signaling." Journal of Biological Chemistry 282(13): 9297-9301.

Roth, B. L., K. Baner, et al. (2002). "Salvinorin A: A potent naturally occurring nonnitrogenous kappa opioid selective agonist." Proceedings of the National Academy of Sciences of the United States of America 99(18): 11934-11939.

Rutherford, J. M., J. Wang, et al. (2008). "Evidence for a mu-delta opioid receptor complex in CHO cells co-expressing mu and delta opioid peptide receptors." Peptides 29(8): 1424-1431.

Schmauss, C. and T. L. Yaksh (1984). "*In vivo* studies on spinal opiate receptor systems mediating antinociception. 2. Pharmacological profiles suggesting a differential association of mu-receptor, delta-receptor and kappa-receptor with visceral chemical and cutaneous thermal stimuli in the rat." Journal of Pharmacology and Experimental Therapeutics 228(1): 1-12.

Sharma, S. K., W. A. Klee, et al. (1975). "Dual regulation of adenylate cyclase accounts for narcotic dependence and tolerance." Proceedings of the National Academy of Sciences of the United States of America 72(8): 3092-3096.

Shim, J., A. Coop, et al. (2011). "Consensus 3D Model of mu-Opioid Receptor Ligand Efficacy Based on a Quantitative Conformationally Sampled Pharmacophore." Journal of Physical Chemistry B 115(22): 7487-7496.

Stevens, W. C., R. M. Jones, et al. (2000). "Potent and Selective Indolomorphinan Antagonists of the Kappa-Opioid Receptor." J. Med. Chem. 43(14): 2759-2769.

Struts, A. V., G. F. J. Salgado, et al. (2011). "Retinal dynamics underlie its switch from inverse agonist to agonist during rhodopsin activation." Nature Structural & Molecular Biology 18(3): 392-394.

Swaminath, G., T. W. Lee, et al. (2003). "Identification of an allosteric binding site for ZN(2+) on the beta(2) adrenergic receptor." Journal of Biological Chemistry 278(1): 352-356.

Swaminath, G., Y. Xiang, et al. (2004). "Sequential binding of agonists to the beta(2) adrenoceptor - Kinetic evidence for intermediate conformational states." Journal of Biological Chemistry 279(1): 686-691.

Volpe, D. A., G. A. M. Tobin, et al. (2011). "Uniform assessment and ranking of opioid Mu receptor binding constants for selected opioid drugs." Regulatory Toxicology and Pharmacology 59(3): 385-390.

von Voigtlander, P. F., R. A. Lahti, et al. (1983). "U-50,488: a selective and structurally novel non-*mu*-(*kappa*)-opioid agonist." Journal of Pharmacology and Experimental Therapeutics 224(1): 7-12.

Waldhoer, M., S. E. Bartlett, et al. (2004). "Opioid receptors." Annual Review of Biochemistry 73: 953-990.

Waldhoer, M., J. Fong, et al. (2005). "A heterodimer-selective agonist shows in vivo relevance of G protein-coupled receptor dimers." Proceedings of the National Academy of Sciences of the United States of America 102(25): 9050-9055.

Whistler, J. L., H. H. Chuang, et al. (1999). "Functional dissociation of mu opioid receptor signaling and endocytosis: Implications for the biology of opiate tolerance and addiction." Neuron 23(4): 737-746.

Witt, K. A., T. J. Gillespie, et al. (2001). "Peptide drug modifications to enhance bioavailability and blood-brain barrier permeability." Peptides 22(12): 2329-2343.

Wolf, R., T. Koch, et al. (1999). "Replacement of threonine 394 by alanine facilitates internalization and resensitization of the rat mu opioid receptor." Molecular Pharmacology 55(2): 263-268.

Wollemann, M., S. Benyhe, et al. (1993). "The kappa-opioid receptor: evidence for the different subtypes." Life Sciences 52(7): 599-611.

Xu, W., A. Sanz, *et al.* (2008). "Activation of the mu opioid receptor involves conformational rearrangements of multiple transmembrane domains." Biochemistry 47(40): 10576-10586.

Yamaotsu, N. and S. Hirono (2011). "3D-pharmacophore identification for κ-opioid agonists using ligand-based drug-design techniques." Topics in Current Chemistry 299: 277-307.

Yongye, A. B., J. R. Appel, *et al.* (2009). "Identification, structure-activity relationships and molecular modeling of potent triamine and piperazine opioid ligands." Bioorg. & Med. Chem. 17(15): 5583-5597.

Yongye, A. B., A. Bender, *et al.* (2010). "Dynamic clustering threshold reduces conformer ensemble size while maintaining a biologically relevant ensemble." J. Comput. Aided. Mol. Des. 24: 675-686.

Yongye, A. B., Y. M. Li, *et al.* (2009). "Modeling of peptides containing D-amino acids: implications on cyclization." J. Comp.-Aid. Mol. Des. 23(9): 677-689.

Yongye, A. B., C. Pinilla, *et al.* (2011). "Integrating computational and mixture-based screening of combinatorial libraries." Journal of Molecular Modeling 17: 1473-1482.

Zadina, J. E., L. Hackler, *et al.* (1997). "A potent and selective endogenous agonist for the mu-opiate receptor." Nature 386(6624): 499-502.

Zhu, Y. X., M. A. King, *et al.* (1999). "Retention of supraspinal delta-like analgesia and loss of morphine tolerance in delta opioid receptor knockout mice." Neuron 24(1): 243-252.

5

Creation of New Local Anesthetics Based on Quinoline Derivatives and Related Heterocycles

Igor Ukrainets
National University of Pharmacy
Ukraine

1. Introduction

Pain is a widely spread symptom and one of the most common causes making people seek medical attention. Though at present, different methods of pain control such as general narcosis, acupuncture, hypnosis, electroanaesthesia, homeopathy, etc., are known, nothing is better for safety and reliability than local anaesthesia. More often it is an effective alternative to general narcosis and promotes decreasing and even eliminating the use of narcotic analgesics in surgery. Dentists, dermatologists and other medical professionals apply it in their work. Unfortunately, an "ideal" local anesthetic has not been created yet, and all current medicines of the given pharmacological group have some drawbacks. The most serious disadvantages are high neuro- and cardiotoxicity, as well as tendency to cause allergy. Thus, the search for new, more effective and safe local anesthetics is ongoing and scientists all over the world continue to work on this problem.

Quinolines are the interesting compounds for research in this area. Numerous derivatives of this azaheterocycle are widely distributed in nature. Some of them are well-known to man and used for curative purposes from ancient times. For example, alkaloids cinchonine (**1a**, R = H) and quinine (**1b**, R = OMe, Figure 1) with antimalarial properties are isolated from *Cinchona* L. The utility of the majority of other natural quinolines prospects are to be determined. However, recently there has been a noticeable progress toward a solution of this problem. Natural compounds themselves more often attract the attention of scientists working in different fields of science and engineering. The stimulating motive for their research is the widely spread conviction that the living nature does nothing without purpose and everything it synthesizes is important at all events for life and, therefore, for man (Bochkov & Smith, 1987). This conviction finds the experimental confirmation constantly, as a result, at present the spectrum of biological properties of natural quinolines has expanded significantly (Kartsev, 2007).

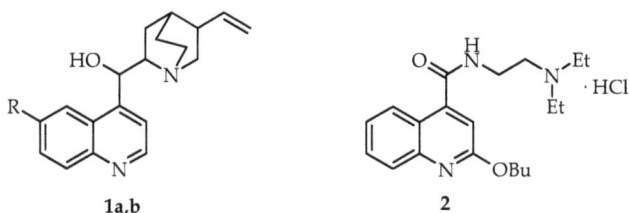

1a,b   **2**

Fig. 1. Natural antimalarial drugs and the first synthetic local anesthetic of the quinoline group

Hence the increased interest in quinolines by synthetic chemists becomes clear. Their belonging to natural metabolites, as well as practically unlimited possibilities for chemical transformations make this molecular system, especially its hydroxyanalogues, rather convenient matrices for fixing various structural elements-pharmacophores on them. It allows making systematic changes into the structure of the finished products and thus to purposefully change their physical and chemical, as well as biological properties. Finally one can succeed in obtaining new substances corresponding to high requirements for medicines. So, in particular, the first local anesthetic of the quinoline group – Cinchocaine (**2**, Figure 1) was synthesized; though it was created 85 ago (Kleemann & Engel, 2001), it has been applied successfully in medical practice nowadays (Tomoda et al., 2009; Kang & Shin, 2010; Douglas et al., 2011).

2. 1-R-4-Hydroxy-2-oxo-1,2-dihydroquinoline-3-carboxamides as a source of new privileged structures with the local anesthetics activity

When systematically studying the biological properties of 1-R-4-hydroxy-2-oxo-1,2-dihydro-quinoline-3-carboxamides we repeatedly noted the opportunity of creating new potential medicines with various effects on a living organism on their basis, including local anesthetics (Ukrainets, 1992; Ukrainets et al., 1994). After the experimental study of anaesthetic properties of a large group of compounds of this chemical range, our attention was paid to the most active of them. Hydrochlorides of (2-diethylaminoethyl)amides of 1-ethyl- (**3a**, R = Et) and, especially, 1-propyl- (**3b**, R = Pr) substituted 4-hydroxy-2-oxo-1,2-dihydroquinoline-3-carboxylic acids (Figure 2), were superior the known local anesthetic Lidocaine by the specific activity possessing at the same time the lower toxicity.

Later (Gorokhova, 1993) in the same range one more compound – hydrochloride of 1-ethyl-4-hydroxy-2-oxo-1,2-dihydroquinoline-3-carboxylic acid (2-morpholin-4-ylethyl)amide (**4**) was found. By the level of infiltration anaesthesia this amide had some more activity than its 1-N-ethyl analogue **3a**, but it was noticeably inferior to 1-N-propyl derivative **3b**. However, after the primary screening it was also included into the list of candidates for profound research as it possessed another important for future medicine property – a relatively low toxicity. By this parameter amide **4** prevailed over its acyclic analogues **3a,b** by a factor of almost 2.

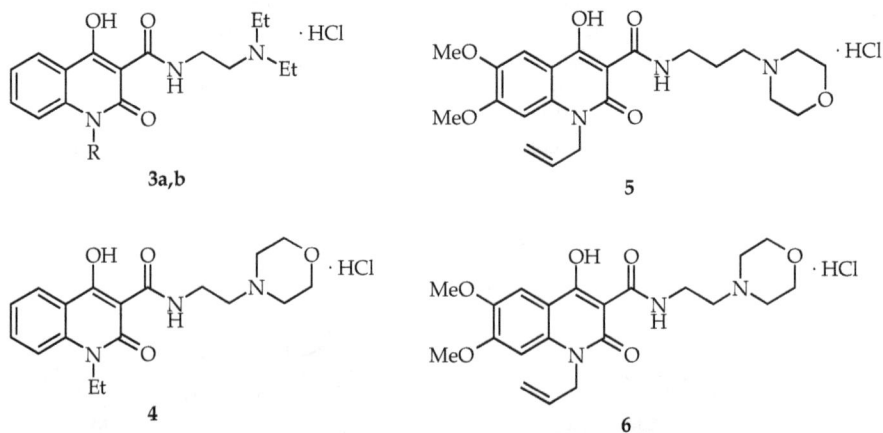

Fig. 2. Biologically active 4-hydroxy-2-oxo-1,2-dihydroquinoline-3-carboxamides

Аnd recently (Davidenko, 2010) a new pharmacological property – the ability to block opioid receptors – has been revealed in 4-hydroxy-2-oxo-1,2-dihydroquinoline-3-carboxamides. It has also been found that substances closely related in structure can reveal quite opposite biological effects. Hydrochloride of 1-allyl-4-hydroxy-6,7-dimethoxy-2-oxo-1,2-dihydro-quinoline-3-carboxylic acid (3-morpholin-4-ylpropyl)amide (5) in the dose of 1 mg/kg completely eliminates the analgesic effect of Tramadol and its homologue – (2-morpholin-4-yl-ethyl)amide 6 – prolongs the analgesic effect significantly. This fact requires further research and is doubtless of interest for researchers engaged in searching not only new opioid receptors antagonists, but highly effective pain-killers as well.

3. Chemical modification of Chinoxicaine by its transformation into pro-drugs

All compounds that passed the stage of primary pharmacological screening were subjected to more profound and thorough analysis in pre-clinical trials. To evaluate the local anaesthetic properties a greater number of parameters were taken into account; these parameters characterized the main specific manifestations of the biological effect: potency of local anaesthesia, the rate of its onset and duration. Additionally at this stage some experimental models, such as repeated infiltration and additional conduction anaesthesia, epidural and surface anaesthesia, were involved. The local irritant properties of the compounds, as well as their acute and chronic toxicity were studied.

From the experiments, only one compound emerged – hydrochloride of 4-hydroxy-2-oxo-1-propyl-1,2-dihydroquinoline-3-carboxylic acid (2-diethylaminoethyl)amide (3b), which further was studied as a privileged structure under the name of Chinoxicaine and was transferred to the next level of investigations. This amide causes a rapid, deep and long local anaesthesia on all models studied and has a low toxicity. It has been found that prolonged introduction of Chinoxicaine to the experimental animals does not produce any statistically significant changes in the activity of central nervous and cardio-vascular systems and does not cause negative reactions of the liver and gastrointestinal tract. The medicine does not produce nephrotoxic action and, thus, it can be used safely by the patients with renal pathology. While using Chinoxicaine, there were no cases of blood pressure decrease, which is its beneficial advantage over many known anesthetics. Additional advantages of Chinoxicaine are that together with the high specific activity it shows clear antiarrhythmic, antimicrobial, antioxidant, and fungicidal effects.

Simultaneously with the pharmacological studies, diversified synthetic research to find the most available method for obtaining Chinoxicaine substance was carried out. As the result, principally different synthetic schemes providing a high quality of the final product have been suggested (Ukrainets et al., 1998; Ukrayinecz & Bezuhliy, 2002; Romanov & Ukrainets, 2006).

Unfortunately, the "Chinoxicaine" project faced some problems. For example, possessing a unique set of pharmacological properties Chinoxicaine appeared to be surprisingly poorly soluble in water. Its solubility is only 13.85 g in 100 ml of water at 20°C, and this caused great difficulty when preparing a stable medicinal form for injections. We solved this problem rather rapidly, though water had to be replaced by the combined solvent.

At the later stages of introduction of a new local anesthetic into medical practice, namely at the stage of clinical trials, one more serious drawback was revealed. In some patients, Chinoxicaine solution in the site of injection caused a transient feeling of burning. Though this undesirable effect lasted less than one minute, further work with the medicine practically lost any progress without its removal. Theoretically a rather simple and effective solution of the problem has been found. The irritant action of Chinoxicaine is completely eliminated by addition such substances as adrenaline in insignificant concentrations in its solution.

However, we tried to solve the problem by structure modification well known in the art to modern researchers (Kubinyi, 2006).

For example, on the basis of structural biological regularities previously revealed a quite new analogue of Chinoxicaine with the improved properties can be synthesized. But is should be taken into account that in such case all complex of biological and pharmaceutical trials have to be carried out in a full volume. Besides to achieve the aim is quite unreal as a result of synthesis of only one new substance. Most likely, to solve the task successfully is possible only after the study of the series of new compounds.

Taking this into account we began to improve pharmaceutical properties of Chinoxicaine from the most rational variant – creation of pro-drugs on its basis. Biologically active source in this approach remains the same, that is why both the terms of development and costs for its implementation are greatly reduced.

However, the practical realization of the method is linked with certain difficulties. In particular, to increase the water solubility, as a rule, it is necessary to introduce additional ionizing groups into the structure of the modified compounds, while to eliminate the irritant action the same ionizing groups in the molecule should be masked (Kuznetsov et al., 1991). In other words, theoretically possible methods of elimination of the revealed drawbacks of Chinoxicaine mutually exclude each other.

Most likely the irritant action of Chinoxicaine is related to the presence of 4-OH-group in its structure, which accounts for the marked acid properties in 1-R-4-hydroxy-2-oxo-1,2-dihydroquinoline-3-carboxamides (Ukrainets, 1988). However, it has been noted (Gorokhova, 1993) that the potency of the given side effect to a great extent depends on the structure of the amide fragment as well. For example, hydrochloride of 4-hydroxy-2-oxo-1-propyl-1,2-dihydroquinoline-3-carboxylic acid (2-morpholin-4-ylethyl)amide (7, Figure 3) and its 1-N-ethyl analogue 4 mentioned above do not yield to Chinoxicaine in the specific activity, but they do not practically render the irritant action. This fact was the foundation for performing bioreversible chemical modification of Chinoxicaine by the tertiary amino group (Ukrainets et al., 2009).

One of the obvious solutions of the target trasformation of the Chinoxicaine molecule is trasformation into quaternary ammonium salts, which is simple in its performance. It should be noted here that common alkyl halides are not suitable for such transformation since they form with the medicine – tertiary amine – the stable compounds, which are almost not subjected to metabolism and are excreted from the organism unchanged (Kuznetsov et al., 1991). Carboxylic acid haloalkyl esters are more interesting. They allow to transform tertiary amines in quaternary ammonium salts with labile grouping N^+-C-O, which is capable of relatively easily to be splitted by hydrolysis and release the initial medicine in the form of the corresponding hydrohalide (Kuznetsov et al., 1991; Vinogradova et al., 1980). One of this reagents is commercially available bromomethylacetate, by its interaction with (2-diethylaminoethyl)amide of 4-hydroxy-2-oxo-1-propyl-1,2-dihydro-quinoline-3-carboxylic acid (8) in the anhydrous acetonitrile medium the target bromo-acetoxymethylate 9 was obtained (Figure 3).

The biological screening has demonstrated that quaternization conducted eliminated the irritant action of Chinoxicaine almost completely, unlike it bromoacetoxy-methylate 9 in the form of 2% aqueous solution which causes only insignificant hyperemia of conjunctiva of the rabbit's eye. At the same time in spite of expectations, dissolution in water decreased significantly (up to 8.86 g per 100 ml), but usually it increases sharply in pro-drugs of this type in 1-2 thresholds comparing to hydrohalides (Vinogradova et al., 1980). Significantly there is almost a threefold shortening of the duration of the surface anesthesia by the bromoacetoxymethylate 9 and this is evidently due to the low rate of liberation of the starting tertiary amine.

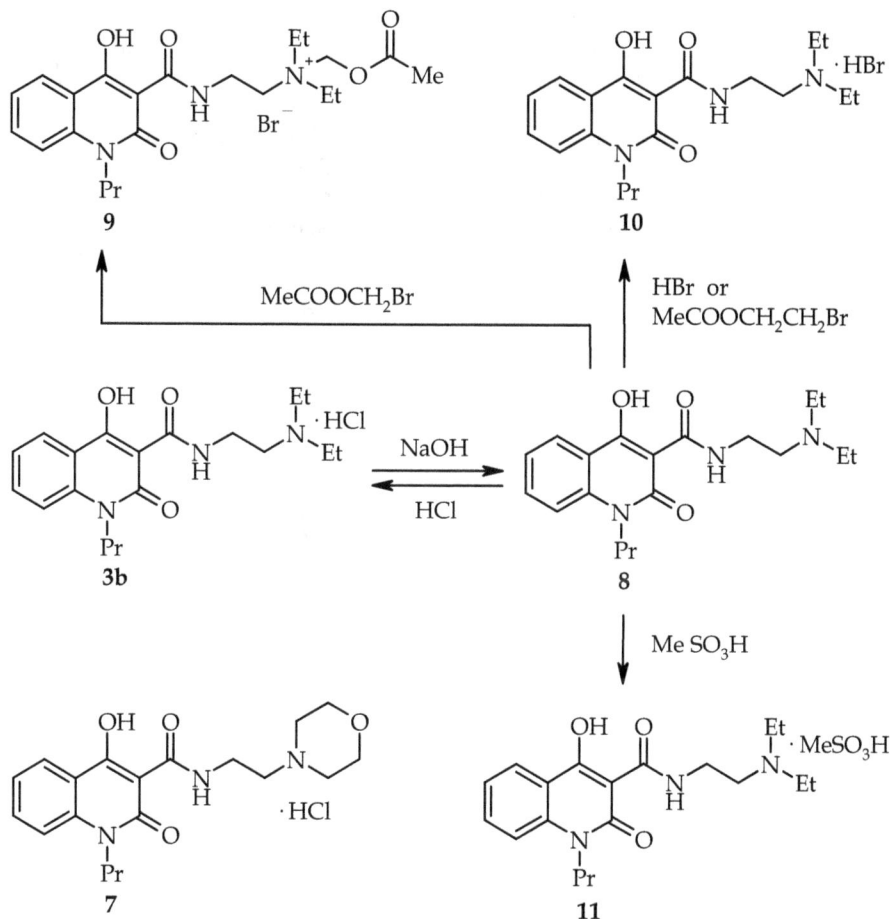

Fig. 3. Modification of Chinoxicaine into pro-drugs

The attempt to optimize the value by substitution of 2-bromomethyl acetate with 2-bromo-ethyl failed. Under the action of amide 8 the reagent is dehydrobrominated, as a result, instead of bromoacetoxyethylate hydrobromide 10 was isolated, it could be also obtained by neutralization of the tertiary amino group of amide 8 by hydrobromic acid. Though salt formation is not accompanied with the change of number, character and location of covalent bonds, it is widely used as an individual type of chemical modification of medicinal substances in medical chemistry. Hence, hydrobromide **10** can be considered as an original pro-drug of Chinoxicaine. However, there was no positive results due to transfer of hydrochloride to hydrobromide. Absolutely all the parameters worsened: solubility decreased to 3.40 g in 100 ml of water, the irritant action increased considerably, and the local anaesthetic activity decreased.

The substitution of hydrogen chloride as a salt-forming reagent of methanesulfonic acid, which forms methanesulfonate **11** practically with the quantitative yield reacting with amide **8** in the anhydrous diethyl ester medium, was more successful.

According to the X-ray structural data, in the symmetrically independent part of the unit cell of the methanesulfonate **11** there is a molecule of the 4-hydroxy-2-oxo-1-propyl-1,2-dihydroquinoline-3-carboxylic acid (2-diethylaminoethyl)amide protonated at atom $N_{(19)}$ and the methanesulfonic acid anion (see Figure 4).

The dihydroquinolone fragment is planar within 0.02 Å. The deviations of atoms $C_{(11)}$ and $C_{(15)}$ from the mean square plane of the dihydropyridine ring are 0.067 and 0.022 Å respectively. A marked deviation of atom $C_{(11)}$ from the ring plane is explained by the presence of a shortened intramolecular contact $H_{(9)} \cdots H_{(11B)}$ of 1.986 Å. The amide fragment is virtually coplanar with the dihydroquinolone (torsional angle $C_{(4)}-C_{(3)}-C_{(15)}-O_{(15)}$ = 4°). Such an orientation is stabilized by two intramolecular hydrogen bonds: $O_{(4)}-H_{(4)} \cdots O_{(15)}$ ($H \cdots O$ 1.74 Å, $O-H \cdots O$ 155°) and $N_{(16)}-H_{(16)} \cdots O_{(2)}$ ($H \cdots N$ 1.91 Å, $N \cdots H-O$ 140°).

The $O_{(4)}-C_{(4)}$ 1.319(3), $N_{(16)}-C_{(15)}$ 1.313(3), and $C_{(2)}-C_{(3)}$ 1.451(3) Å bonds in the compound studied are shortened (mean values 1.331, 1.334, and 1.464 Å respectively) but the $O_{(15)}-C_{(15)}$ 1.264(3) and $C_{(3)}-C_{(4)}$ 1.379(3) Å bonds are lengthened (mean values 1.231 and 1.363 Å respectively).

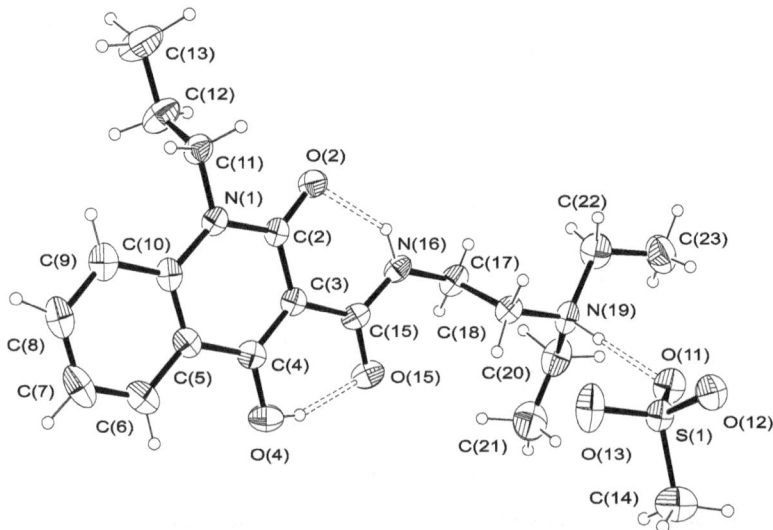

Fig. 4. The structure of the methanesulfonate **11** molecule with atomic numbering. The dotted lines indicate the intra- and intermolecular hydrogen bonds

Atom $N_{(1)}$ has a planar trigonal configuration. The substituents at atoms $N_{(1)}$ and $N_{(16)}$ have an *anti*-periplanar conformation (torsional angles $N_{(1)}-C_{(11)}-C_{(12)}-C_{(13)}$ and $N_{(16)}-C_{(17)}-C_{(18)}-$

$N_{(19)}$ 176.2 and 176.0° respectively. The plane of the carbon atoms of the propyl group on the $N_{(1)}$ atom is virtually perpendicular to the mean-square plane of the dihydropyridine ring, the angle between them being 89.1°.

In the crystal the molecules of the methanesulfonate **11** form dimers *via* stacking interactions between the dihydroquinolone fragments, the benzene rings being situated over the dihydropyridines. The distance between the ring centroids is 3.54 Å and the mean-square planes of the dihydropyridine and benzene fragments form a dihedral angle of 2.2°.

The cation and anion are mutually bonded by an intermolecular hydrogen bond $N_{(19)}$– $H_{(19)} \cdots O_{(11)}$ (H $\cdots$ O 1.88 Å, N–H $\cdots$ O 176°).

The biological screening has shown that methanesulfonate **11** demonstrates a significant improvement of all pharmaceutical properties comparing to the initial hydrochloride **3b** (Chinoxicaine). In particular, the local irritant action was successfully decreased to the level of bromoacetoxymethylate **9**. Dissolution in water increased in more than six times – up to 85.72 g per 100 ml, and it has eliminated the problem of choosing a solvent for preparation of a stable medicinal form for injections. Finally, there are also some positive aspects of revealing the specific activity: the rate of anaesthesia onset remains the same, but the total duration of the surface anaesthesia and the deep anaesthetization phase increased.

4. Synthesis of conformation stable forms of quinolones as an attempt to improve pharmaceutical properties of Chinoxicaine

In modern medical chemistry several standard methods are successfully applied for improving the privileged structures chosen according to the results of preliminary pharmacological trials. Recently with accumulation of information about the spatial structure of active binding sites for many types of receptors a greater attention has been paid to methodology of conformation restrictions (Chen et al., 2010; Watanabe et al., 2010; Nirogia et al., 2011). In general, this method of the structural transformation of a molecule suggests the preservation of all functional groups contacting with a biological target in their original form and at the same time it is directed to fixing of some of them in "active" conformation.

One of the most wide-spread ways of practical realization of the method is cyclization, which allows transformation of the open side chains of the initial molecule in endo- or exo-cyclic fragments, making possible the change of the pharmaceutical and (or) pharmacokinetic properties. Taking into account the given data it is quite logical to study N-R-amides of 1-hydroxy-3-oxo-5,6-dihydro-3H-pyrrolo- (**12a-m**) and 1-hydroxy-3-oxo-6,7-dihydro-3H,5H-pyrido- (**13a-m**) [3,2,1-*ij*]quinoline-2-carboxylic acids as potential local anesthetics (Figure 5).

The interest of these compounds is caused by the fact that they are very similar to Chinoxicaine (**3b**) and its 1-N-ethyl analogue **3a** by their structure. At the same time amides **12-13a-m** have a principally important structural difference: though their 1-N-alkyl substituents contain the same two-three carbon atoms, they are situated not in the open alkyl chains, but are included in the composition of pyrrole or tetrahydropyridine cycles annelation with the quinolone nucleus. Such modification is known to lead to the essential spatial trasformation of the molecule. In particular, in 1-propylsubstituted 4-hydroxy-quinolones-2 the ethyl fragment is placed perpendicular the plane of the quinolone nucleus, as a result the terminal methyl group is far from the bicycle more than 3 Å (Ukrainets et al., 2009). And on the contrary, the tricyclic pyrido[3,2,1-*ij*]quinoline system is much compact – in spite of the *sofa* conformation of the tetrahydropyridine ring, $C_{(6)}$ atom deviates from its relative plane only in 0.56 Å (Ukrainets et al., 2008). Unlike 1-N-ethylsubstituted 4-hydroxyquinolones-2, in which the methyl group of ethyl substituent is never located in the quinolone cycle plane (Baumer et al., 2004; Ukrainets et al., 2007), tricyclic pyrrolo[3,2,1-*ij*]- quinoline system is practically flat (Ukrainets et al., 2006a). It is clear that transfer from 1-N-ethyl- and 1-N-propylsubtituted **3a,b** to conformation limited pyrrolo- and pyridoquinolines **12-13** should be obligatory reflected to the biological properties. The answer to the question about this influence has been found in one of the recent investigations (Kravtsova, 2011).

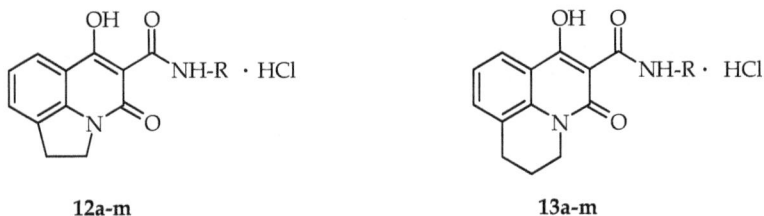

12a-m	**13a-m**

12-13: **a** R = 2-aminoethyl; **b** R = 3-aminopropyl; **c** R = 4-aminobutyl; **d** R = 6-aminohexyl;
e R = 2-ethylaminoethyl; **f** R = 2-(2-hydroxyethylamino)ethyl; **g** R = 2-dimetylaminoethyl;
h R = 2-diethylaminoethyl; **i** R = 3-dimethylaminopropyl; **j** R = 3-diethylaminopropyl;
k R = 2-piperazin-1-ylethyl; **l** R = 2-morpholin-4-ylethyl; **m** R = 3-morpholin-4-ylpropyl

Fig. 5. Tricyclic analogues of Chinoxicaine

Testing of the samples synthesized has been carried out on the infiltration anaesthesia model by Buelbring-Yueid method (Table 1).

Analysis of the experimental data obtained demonstrates that compounds with the primary amino groups, i.e. amides **12-13a-d**, do not practically show the anesthetic properties. The weak activity (the anaesthesia lasts for not more 5 min, and the phase of complete sensitivity loss has not come) has appeared in monoalkylaminoalkylamides **12-13e,f**. And only when the second alkyl residue is introduced into the terminal amino group (amides **12-13g-m**), the local anaesthetic action increases noticeably, but though in this case its duration remains rather short. For example, for the most active diethylaminoethyl derivative **13h** this index is approximately 40 min, though the infiltration anaesthesia index reaches the maximum possible value. As compared, Chinoxicaine in the similar conditions causes total anaesthesia lasting for approximately 75 min (with the general duration of anaesthesia of 4 hours), and its 1-N-ethyl analogue **3a** – approximately 60 min (with the general duration of anaesthesia of 2 hours).

It is interesting to note that the irritant action of 2% aqueous solutions of tricyclic amides **12-13,** determined by the rabbit's eye cornea according to the simplified modification of Setnikar method, is absent in most examples at all or decreases significantly comparing to its bicyclic prototypes **3a,b**. And it is in spite of the fact that acidity of enolic OH-groups in 1-hydroxy-3-oxo-5,6-dihydro-3H-pyrrolo[3,2,1-*ij*]quinoline-2-carboxylic acid and its 1-N-ethyl analogue is practically the same, and in 1-hydroxy-3-oxo-6,7-dihydro-3H,5H-pyrido[3,2,1-*ij*]-quinoline-2-carboxylic acid is similar with its 1-N-propyl analogue (pKa^{OH} = 13,44-13,48).

In general, based on the biological trials conducted, it can be stated that the structural transformation of the molecule, which accompanies the transfer from 1-alkylsubstitued 4-hydroxyquinolin-2-ones to conformation limited tricyclic pyrrolo- or tetrahydropyrido-quinolones, allows to decrease the irritant action of compounds of this class, but at the same time it has a strong negative effect on the local anesthetic properties and that is why it can be considered as unperspective.

| Compound | Infiltration anaesthesia | | | Irritative effect, points |
	The start of anaesthesia, min	Index	Duration of total anaesthesia, min	
12a	4.32 ± 0.28	1.1	Undetermined	0
12b	3.81 ± 0.21	2.7	Undetermined	0
12c	4.60 ± 0.33	2.0	Undetermined	0
12d	4.93 ± 0.39	1.2	Undetermined	0
12e	3.27 ± 0.30	5.1	Undetermined	0
12f	3.66 ± 0.27	3.5	Undetermined	0
12g	2.82 ± 0.31	12.2	10.64 ± 1.20	2
12h	2.05 ± 0.17	36.0	39.82 ± 2.37	1
12i	3.09 ± 0.28	9.8	9.27 ± 1.33	2
12j	2.91 ± 0.32	14.2	15.92 ± 1.24	1
12k	3.87 ± 0.45	6.4	5.30 ± 1.45	1
12l	2.24 ± 0.26	27.0	25.56 ± 1.62	0
12m	3.04 ± 0.34	16.2	14.75 ± 1.18	0
13a	5.26 ± 0.44	2.8	Undetermined	0
13b	4.32 ± 0.35	3.9	Undetermined	0
13c	4.63 ± 0.41	4.2	Undetermined	0
13d	5.65 ± 0.48	2.3	Undetermined	0
13e	3.72 ± 0.33	7.6	Undetermined	0
13f	4.08 ± 0.29	5.4	Undetermined	0
13g	3.26 ± 0.30	16.7	13.51 ± 1.81	1
13h	2.23 ± 0.23	36.0	40.24 ± 3.06	1
13i	3.92 ± 0.22	14.1	8.83 ± 1.26	1
13j	3.10 ± 0.25	17.3	11.48 ± 2.55	1
13k	4.05 ± 0.36	9.7	6.63 ± 1.14	0
13l	2.64 ± 0.23	21.4	28.96 ± 3.73	0
13m	3.22 ± 0.31	15.8	15.37 ± 2.02	0
3a	1.84 ± 0.10	36.0	58.92 ± 4.11	2
Chinoxicaine	1.61 ± 0.13	36.0	74.79 ± 4.71	2

Table 1. Biological properties of tricyclic compounds **12-13**

5. Application of the bioisosteric replacements methodology for optimization of the Chinoxicaine molecule

The term „isosters" was introduced by Irwing Langmuir at the beginning of the 20th century. By his definition, isosters are molecules or ions containing the same number of atoms, as well as the same number and arrangement of electrons. Therefore, "isosteric replacements" in the created drugs are replacement of an atom or the group to the similar one by size or valency. If the physiological activity remains at the same time, then such replacement is called "bioisosteric". After a while the term "bioisoster" has been referred to compounds obtained by replacement of quite "unsimilar" groupings, but with preserving their biological properties (King, 2002). As a result, the concept of bioisosteric replacements at present has become one of the most powerful means for creating effective and safe medicines (Devereux & Popelier, 2010; Wassermann & Bajorath, 2011; Large et al., 2011). Its application allows not only to optimise the known biologically active substances, but to reveal new structures with the similar or related properties and, thus, to increase the patent protection of a future medicine.

5.1 Hydrochlorides of 4-hydroxy-2-oxo-1,2,5,6,7,8-hexahydroquinoline-3-carboxylic acids N-R-amides

The first attempt to optimize the Chinoxicaine molecule by the method of bioisosteric replacements was replacement of its 1,2-dihydroquinoline nucleus by 1,2,5,6,7,8-hexahydroquinoline. We did it expecting that such transformation may appear to be bioisosteric. With this aim a large group of hydrochlorides of 4-hydroxy-2-oxo-1,2,5,6,7,8-hexahydroquinoline-3-carboxylic acids N-R-amides **14a-y** has been synthesized by the method developed earlier (Kolisnyk, 2009) (Figure 6).

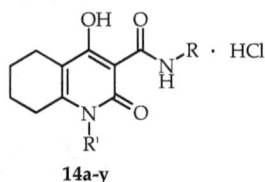

14a-y

14: R' = H: **a** R = 2-aminoethyl; **b** R = 3-aminopropyl; **c** R = 4-aminobutyl; **d** R = 6-aminohexyl; **e** R = 2-ethylaminoethyl; **f** R = 2-(2-hydroxyethylamino)ethyl; **g** R = 2-dimetylaminoethyl; **h** R = 2-diethylaminoethyl; **i** R = 3-dimethylaminopropyl; **j** R = 3-diethylaminopropyl; **k** R = 1-ethylpyrrolidin-2-ylmethyl; **l** R = 2-morpholin-4-ylethyl; **m** R = 3-morpholin-4-ylpropyl; **o** R = 3-piperidin-1-ylpropyl; **p** R = 3-(4-methylpiperazin-1-yl)propyl; **q** R = 4-diethylamino-1-methylbutyl

R' = Pr: **r** R = 2-diethylaminoethyl; **s** R = 3-diethylaminopropyl

R' = *cyclo*-Pr: **t** R = 2-ethylaminoethyl; **u** R = 2-(2-hydroxyethylamino)ethyl; **v** R = 2-dimetylaminoethyl; **w** R = 2-diethylaminoethyl; **x** R = 3-dimethylaminopropyl; **y** R = 3-diethylaminopropyl

Fig. 6. Hydrogenated analogues of Chinoxicaine

The biological screening conducted allow to state that reduction of the benzene part of the quinolone ring, unfortunately, leads to practically complete loss of local anaesthetic properties and that is why such modification should be considered unsuccessful. In other words, there is no reason to declare 4-hydroxy-2-oxo-1,2-dihydroquinoline and 4-hydroxy-2-oxo-1,2,5,6,7,8-hexahydroquinoline molecular systems to be bioisosteric (at least, in relation to local anaesthesia).

5.2 1-R-3-(2-Diethylaminoethyl)-1H-quinazoline-2,4-diones hydrochlorides

All ways of modification of Chinoxicaine molecule considered by us previously could not remove the local irritant action completely, therefore, it can be assumed that this drawback had been stipulated mainly by the presence of a OH group. Thus, the next step of potentially bioisosteric transformation of Chinoxicaine was the synthesis of compounds known to be without groupings with acid properties. One of the examples of such substances were 1-R-3-(2-diethylaminoethyl)-1H-quinazoline-2,4-diones hydrochlorides **15a-f** (Figure 7). We considered various variants of obtaining compounds of this class allowing to choose the most suitable of them depending on the structure of the target product (Ukrainets et al., 2010)

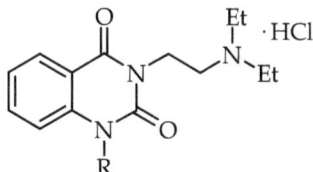

15: a R = H; **b** R = Me; **c** R = Et; **d** R = Pr; **e** R = Bu; **f** R = *i*-Bu

Fig. 7. Derivatives of 1H-quinazoline-2,4-dione

The study of the local irritant action of 1-R-3-(2-diethylaminoethyl)-1H-quinazoline-2,4-diones hydrochlorides **15** conducted in rabbits by the method of Lebo and Camage, has shown that the substances under research in the form of aqueous solutions with 2% concentration do not cause any reactive changes on the surface of the skin of the experimental animals. It should be worth mentioning that in similar conditions Chinoxicaine also does not reveal the irritating effect. That is why other, more sensitive, models should be involved in further research.

The ability of 2% aqueous solutions of the compounds synthesized to cause infiltration anaesthesia of the skin and subcutaneous cellulose has been studied in guinea pigs (Buelbring-Yueid method). Simultaneously several parameters characterizing the basic specific manifestations of the pharmacological effect such as the rate of anaesthesia onset, its depth (potency) and duration were taken into account. The data given in Table 2 shows that all 1-R-3-(2-diethylaminoethyl)-1H-quinazoline-2,4-diones hydrochlorides **15**, without exception, possess the local anaesthetic properties in some degree. In most cases anaesthesia occurs rather quickly and in some minutes after injection, the phase of deep anaesthesia begins. However, in spite of high values of the infiltration anaesthesia index, sometimes reaching the duration of the total anaesthesia caused by quinazolones **15** remains comparatively short and they yield to Chinoxicaine and Lidocaine greatly by this parameter. However, unlike the reference drugs the most active of the compounds synthesized – hydrochlorides **15a,e,f** – reveal a number of new properties, which can be considered as useful in the complex of the short, but powerful local anaesthetic action. They are sedation as well as movement disorder or motor block on the site of introduction of the substance examined. The motor block was estimated on the "peak" of the local anesthesia by 5 point scale: 0 points - the tail root tone preserved, movements preserved in full; 1 point - weakening of the tail root tone; 2 points - the weak tail root tone, sluggish movement, the animal sitting more; 3 points - lowering of the tail root tone and possible slight movement of the animal during stimulation of the skin section not occurring in the anesthetized zone, slight inhibition of the animal; 4 points - general atonia of the tail root, appearance of some inhibition of movement in response to stimulation, overall inhibition of the animal; 5 points

- the state of general atonia of the tail root without movement upon pain or electrical stimulation of the skin outside the area of anesthesia, the animal lying on side.

Compound	Infiltration anaesthesia			Motor block, points	Sedative effect, points
	The start of anaesthesia, min	Index	Duration of total anaesthesia, min		
15a	1.14 ± 0.16	36.0	32.35 ± 1.38	4	1
15b	1.53 ± 0.19	35.8	30.19 ± 0.75	0	0
15c	4.46 ± 0.29	18.5	15.74 ± 1.05	0	1
15d	2.97 ± 0.32	35.7	29.82 ± 0.59	0	0
15e	2.82 ± 0.43	36.0	36.46 ± 2.53	5	1
15f	1.59 ± 0.25	34.2	29.20 ± 1.43	5	3
Chinoxicaine	1.50 ± 0.04	36.0	75.61 ± 4.54	0	0
Lidocaine	2.12 ± 0.19	36.0	52.80 ± 3.76	0	0

Table 2. Biological properties of the quinazoline-2,4-diones hydrochlorides 15

The sedative effect was estimated in the following way: 0 points - absent, the animal moving independently in cage; 1 point - the animal calm, sitting more, moving around the cage only when disturbed by the researcher; 2 points - the animal slowed down, sitting in the corner of the cage, anxiety with the researcher significantly set aside and again sitting, often closing eyelids, sleep onset; 3 points - the animal sleeping, lying on side, not responsive to stimulation by the researcher or to needle stick.

In general, the combination of analgesic, sedative and immobile extremities effects rendering by hydrochlorides 15a,e,f can be used in creating medicines on their basis that are available for practical application in tiny surgical interventions, for example, in veterinary medicine. Thus, it can be stated confidently that 1-R-quinazoline-2,4-dionic cycle is bioisoster of 4-hydroxy-2-oxo-1,2-dihydroquinoline nucleus.

5.3 The irreversible chemical modification of Chinoxicaine at position 4 of the quinolone nucleus

The complex research described by us above has shown convincingly that 4-OH-group is the main cause of the local irritant properties of Chinoxicaine. Therefore, after its blocking one can expect the elimination of the undesired side effect. Meanwhile, we have not even considered alkylation or acylation of 4-OH-group as the most obvious variant of another bioreversible modification of Chinoxicaine. The reason is quite simple. Within a rather limited choice of pharmacologically available protective groups, neither 4-O-alkyl, nor 4-O-acyl derivatives of 4-hydroxyquinolin-2-ones have a high chemical stability. It is the tendency to hydrolysis that is a serious obstacle when synthesizing such compounds, as well as when further preparing sterile solutions for injections on their basis.

Taking it into account we tried to modify 4-OH-group of Chinoxicaine not by means of forming pro-drugs, but by using the same method of bioisosteric replacements, i.e. by its irreversible replacement with the groupings similar not by sizes or volume, but having the same physical and chemical properties and that is why inducing the similar pharmacological effect (King, 2002).

The first example of such transformation was 4-chloro-2-oxo-1-propyl-1,2-dihydroquinoline-3-carboxylic acid (2-diethylaminoethyl)amide hydrochloride 16 (Figure 8).
A high reactivity of the chlorine atom in 1-R-4-chloro-3-ethoxycarbonyl-2-oxo-1,2-dihydro-quinolines in relation to nucleophilic reagents allows to transform them easily into 4-methyl-2-oxo-1,2-dihydroquinoline-3-carboxylic acids, one being the basis for synthesis of one more bioisoster of Chinoxicaine – 4-methyl substituted analogue 17.
N-R-Amides of 2-oxo-1,2-dihydroquinoline-3-carboxylic acid with a primary amino group in position 4 of the quinolone ring exist in the 2-hydroxy-4-imino form rapidly hydrolyzed by mineral acids to 4-hydroxy-2-quinolones (Ukrainets et al., 2006b). Proceeding from it as the next object for pharmacological screening we deliberately obtained hydrochloride of 4-diethylamino-2-oxo-1-propyl-1,2-dihydroquinoline-3-carboxylic acid (2-diethylaminoethyl)-amide 18 as chemically more stable product. Amides 19a-d containing no substituents at position 4 are of particular interest, in spite of the fact that due to the absence of these substituents they cannot be considered to be classical bioisosters of Chinoxicaine.
The study of local irritant action of the compounds synthesized, the ability to cause infiltration anaesthesia of the skin and subcutaneous cellulose, as well as the evaluation of the motor block and the sedative effect were carried out by standard methods previously described in detail by us (Ukrainets et al., 2010). It has been determined that all substances tested in the form of aqueous solutions with 2% concentration do not cause any reactive changes on the skin surface of the experimental animals.
From the data presented in Table 3 it follows that bioisosteric replacement of 4-OH-group to the chlorine atom – amide 16 – leads to significant decrease of all pharmacological indexes and, therefore, it is unsuccessful.

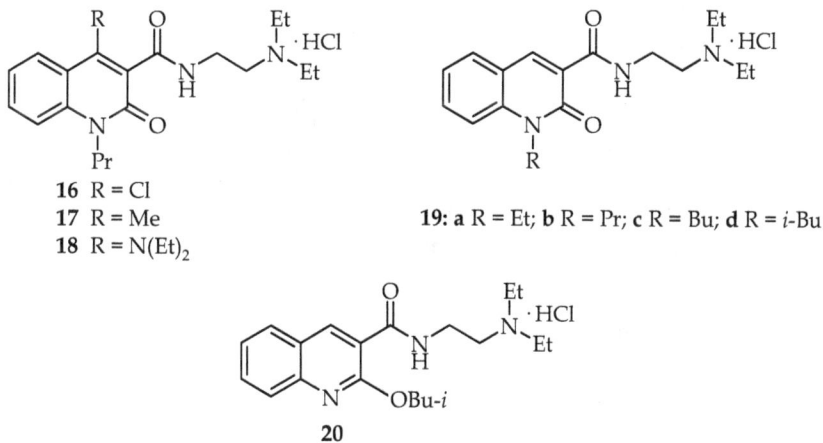

16 R = Cl
17 R = Me
18 R = N(Et)$_2$

19: a R = Et; b R = Pr; c R = Bu; d R = i-Bu

20

Fig. 8. Modification of 4-OH-group of Chinoxicaine

More interesting was the replacement of the hydroxyl group to the methyl one. From all substances of the last series 4-methyl-substituted amide 17 possesses the most rapid development of the biological effect (less than 2 min after injection). The infiltration anaesthesia index reaches the maximum possible value, and the total anaesthesia or the time of absence of pain and all types of sensitivity (tactile, temperature, etc.), during which the surgical intervention can be made (the section of tissues, wound suture, etc.), last approximately 55 min. These data prove the sufficient high activity of amide **17**, which are comparable to the reference drugs - Chinoxicaine and Lidocaine. However, amide **17** yields them significantly in the total duration of anaesthesia, i.e. time when the sensitivity increases gradually and then restores completely.

Compound	Infiltration anaesthesia				Motor block, points	Sedative effect, points
	The start of anaesthesia, min	Index	The total anaesthesia, min	The general duration of anaesthesia, min		
16	3.96 ± 0.42	26.3	14.25 ± 1.11	24.72 ± 2.18	0	0
17	1.94 ± 0.21	36.0	55.33 ± 2.74	68.38 ± 2.68	0	0
18	2.28 ± 0.31	36.0	37.51 ± 2.83	67.85 ± 2.37	0	0
19a	4.52 ± 0.32	19.3	13.20 ± 1.00	21.01 ± 1.67	0	0
19b	4.50 ± 0.36	35.5	27.89 ± 1.89	32.34 ± 2.92	0	0
19c	3.03 ± 0.28	36.0	39.04 ± 2.12	58.26 ± 2.81	5	2
19d	2.71 ± 0.37	36.0	53.77 ± 1.93	83.28 ± 2.05	5	3
20	2.82 ± 0.44	35.6	47.56 ± 1.74	85.48 ± 2.33	5	3
Chinoxicaine	1.62 ± 0.13	36.0	74.74 ± 4.71	236.89 ± 9.34	0	0
Lidocaine	2.34 ± 0.20	36.0	51.26 ± 3.45	140.27 ± 6.20	0	0

Table 3. Biological properties of 4-OH-modified derivatives of Chinoxicaine

A special attention should be paid to 4-diethylamine derivative **18**, not only for its high anaesthetic properties, but for the perspective to perform further modifications of such type easily and practically in unlimited quantity as well and to reach the result required.

From the series of non-substituted amides **19** at position 4 it is worth mentioning only compounds with butyl and *iso*-butyl substituents at the cyclic nitrogen atom (amides **19c** and **19d** respectively). Both are characterized by a rather rapid onset of action and high values of infiltration anaesthesia indexes. The distinctive feature of the first one is the signs of drowsiness, inertia in animals in 10-15 min after the injection and complete sleepiness can occur at 15-20 min. The motor block with the strength of 5 points lasts for approximately 20 min on the site of introduction of the substance examined. In the case of amide **19d** already by 7-10 min after injection the animals had the state of deep sleep: they slept on their side without the reaction to the active stimulation by the needle (tactile, pain and temperature sensitivity is absent). In 15-20 min the animals awoke, but they were drowsy and motionless for approximately 20 min and then began to move their paws. Therefore, one can speak about the deep and prolonged motor block and the marked sedative effect, which can be very useful properties of local anesthetic while conducting a number of short-termed surgical interventions, especially when rendering aid to patients with the increased excitability and possible fear before any surgical manipulations.

The study of hydrochloride of 2-isobutoxyquinoline-3-carboxylic acid (2-diethylamino-ethyl)amide **20** is of particular interest. This compound has been specially synthesized by us as an aromatic analogue of the most active of 1,2-dihydro derivatives, i.e. amide **19d**. A comparative analysis of biological properties of these isomers demonstrates that with transfer to the aromatic structure some parameters decrease, and others, vice versa, intensify. For example, amide **20** differs with the later start of anaesthesia, decrease of the indon and reduction of duration of the deep anaesthesia phase. At the same time the general duration of anaesthesia increases a little, as well as duration of the sedative effect. Unfortunately, transfer of the isobutyl substituent from the nitrogen atom to the oxygen atom is accompanied by appearance of undesirable properties – unlike amide **19d** its aromatic isomer **20** has been found to have the irritant action, though a transient one.

6. Conclusion

The research carried out by us gives reason to suppose that 4-hydroxy-2-oxo-1,2-dihydro-quinoline-3-carboxylic acids are of great interest as a base in creating new effective medicines to eliminate pain. Such medicines can be not only local anesthetics possessing the unique complex of pharmacological properties, but, as it has been found quite recently, non-narcotic analgesics with high activity and low toxicity as well. The rich arsenal of structural and biological regularities accumulated, as well as practically unlimited synthetic potential of 4-hydroxyquinolin-2-ones allow to change the character of impact of such compounds on a living organism easily and in the required direction, and thus, to provide their direct practical value and a great perspective.

7. Acknowledgment

We appreciate the assistance of professor V.I. Mamchur (Dnepropetrovsk State Medical Academy, Ukraine) in studying biological properties of the compounds synthesized and useful comments while discussing the results obtained.

8. References

Bochkov, A.F. & Smit, V.A. (1987). *Organic Synthesis. Purposes, Methods, Tactics, Strategy* [in Russian], Nauka, Moscow, Russia

Kartsev, V.G. (Ed.). (2007). *Selected Methods for Synthesis and Modification of Heterocycles. Vol. 6. Quinolines: Chemistry and Biological Activity* [in Russian], International charitable foundation "Scientific Partnership Foundation" (ICSPF), ISBN 978-5-903078-10-3, Moscow, Russia

Kleemann, A. & Engel J. (2001). *Pharmaceutical Substances: Syntheses, Patents, Applications*, Thieme Medical Publishers, ISBN 1588900312, Stuttgart, Germany

Tomoda, K.; Asahiyama, M.; Ohtsuki, E.; Nakajima, T.; Terada, H.; Kanebako, M.; Inagi, T. & Makino, K. (2009). Preparation and Properties of Carrageenan Microspheres Containing Allopurinol and Local Anesthetic Agents for the Treatment of Oral Mucositis. *Colloids and Surfaces. B, Biointerfaces*, Vol.71, No.1, pp. 27-35, ISSN 0927-7765

Kang, C. & Shin, S.C. (2010). Preparation and Evaluation of Bioadhesive Dibucaine Gels for Enhanced Local Anesthetic Action. *Archives of Pharmacal Research*, Vol.33, No.8, pp. 1277-1283, ISSN 0253-6269

Douglas, H.A.; Callaway, J.K.; Sword, J.; Kirov, S.A. & Andrew, R.D. (2011). Potent Inhibition of Anoxic Depolarization by the Sodium Channel Blocker Dibucaine. *Journal of Neurophysiology*, Vol.105, No.4, pp. 1482-1494, ISSN 0022-3077

Ukrainets, I.V. (1992). Synthesis, Chemical Transformation and Biological Properties of Alkyl(aryl)amides of Malonic Acid Derivatives [in Russian]. *Thesis for Doctor Degree in Chemistry in speciality 15.00.02 – Pharmaceutical Chemistry and Pharmacognosy,* Manuscript, Kharkov, Ukraine

Ukrainets, I.V.; Gorokhova, O.V.; Taran, S.G.; Bezugly, P.A.; Filimonova, N.I. & Turov, A.V. (1994). 4-Hydroxy-2-Quinolones. 24. Improved Synthesis and Biological Properties of 1-Alkyl-4-Hydroxy-2-Quinoline-3-Carboxylic Acid β-Dialkylaminoalkylamide Hydrochlorides. *Chemistry of Heterocyclic Compounds,* Vol.30, No.10, pp. 1214-1219, ISSN 0009-3122

Gorokhova, O.V. (1993). Synthesis, Chemical and Biological Properties of Alkyl- and Arylamides of Malonic Acid Derivatives [in Russian]. *Thesis for Candidate Degree in Chemistry in speciality 15.00.02 – Pharmaceutical Chemistry and Pharmacognosy,* Manuscript, Kharkov, Ukraine

Davidenko, O.O. (2011). Synthesis, Physical, Chemical Properties and Biological Activity of Substituted 4-Hydroxy-2-Oxo-1,2-Dihydroquinoline-3-Carboxylic Acids and Their Derivatives [in Ukrainian]. *Thesis for Candidate Degree in Pharmacy in speciality 15.00.02 – Pharmaceutical Chemistry and Pharmacognosy,* Manuscript, Kharkov, Ukraine

Ukrainets, I.V.; Bezugly, P.A.; Gorokhova, O.V.; Taran, S.G. & Treskach, V.I. (1998). Method for Preparing 1-Propyl-2-Oxo-4-Hydroxyquinoline-3-Carboxylic Acid Diethylami-noethylamide Hydrochloride (Chinoxycaine). *Patent Ukraine 24967,* Available from http://base.ukrpatent.org/searchINV/

Ukrayinecz, I.V. & Bezuhliy, P.A. (2002). Injectable Anesthetic. *Patent USA 6340692,* Available from
http://worldwide.espacenet.com/searchResults?NUM=US6340692&DB=EPODOC&locale=en_EP&ST=number&compact=false

Romanov, I.V. & Ukrainets, I.V. (2006). Method for Preparing 1-Propyl-2-Oxo-4-Hydroxy-quinoline-3-Carboxylic Acid Diethylaminoethylamide Hydrochloride (Chinoxy-caine). *Patent Russia 2285692,* Available from
http://worldwide.espacenet.com/searchResults?NUM=RU2285692&DB=EPODOC&locale=en_EP&ST=number&compact=false

Kubinyi, H. (2006). In Looking ups of the New Compounds-leaders for Creation of Drugs [in Russian]. *Russian Chemical Journal,* Vol.L, No.2, pp. 5-17, ISSN 0373-0247, Available from http://www.chem.msu.su/rus/journals/jvho/2006-2/5.pdf

Kuznetsov, S.G.; Chigareva, S.M. & Ramsh, S.M. (1991). Pro-drugs. Chemical Aspect. *Summaries in Science and Technology. Organic Chemistry* [in Russian], VINITI, ISSN 0137-0251, Moscow, Russia

Ukrainets, I.V. (1988). Synthesis and Research of New Biological Active Derivatives of Malonic Acid 2-Carboxyphenylamide [in Russian]. *Thesis for Candidate Degree in Pharmacy in speciality 15.00.02 – Pharmaceutical Chemistry and Pharmacognosy,* Manuscript, Kharkov, Ukraine

Ukrainets, I.V.; Kravtzova, V.V.; Tkach, A.A. & Rybakov, V.B. (2009). 4-Hydroxy-2-Quino-lones. 155. Bioreversible Chemical Modification of Chinoxycaine at the Tertiary Amino Group as a Method of Improving its Pharmaceutical Activity. *Chemistry of Heterocyclic Compounds,* Vol.45, No.6, pp. 698-704, ISSN 0009-3122

Vinogradova, N.D.; Kuznetsov, S.G. & Chigareva, S.M. (1980). Quaternary Ammonium Salts with Labile N+-C Bonds as Drug Precursors. *Pharmaceutical Chemistry Journal,* Vol.14, No.9, pp. 604-609, ISSN 0091-150X

Chan, H.; Gong, Y.; Giles, K.M. & Pletther, E. (2010). Synthesis and Biological Activity of Conformationally Restricted Gypsy Moth Pheromone Mimics. Bioorganic and Medicinal Chemistry, Vol.18, No.8, pp. 2920-2929, ISSN 0968-0896

Watanabe, M.; Hirokawa, T.; Kobayashi, T.; Yoshida, A.; Ito, Y.; Yamada, S.; Orimoto, N.; Yamasaki, Y.; Arisawa, M. & Shuto, S. (2010). Investigation of the Bioactive Conformation of Histamine H3 Receptor Antagonists by the Cyclopropylic Strain-based Conformational Restriction Strategy. Journal of Medicinal Chemistry, Vol.53, No.9, pp. 3585-93, ISSN 0022-2623

Nirogia, R.V.; Kambhampati, R.; Daulatabad, A.V.; Gudla, P.; Shaikh, M.; Achanta, P.K.; Shinde, A.K. & Dubey, P.K. (2011). Design, Synthesis and Pharmacological Evaluation of Conformationally Restricted N-Arylsulfonyl-3-Aminoalkoxy Indoles as a Potential 5-HT(6) Receptor Ligands. Journal of Enzyme Inhibition and Medicinal Chemistry, Vol.26, No.3, pp. 341-349, ISSN 1475-6366

Ukrainets, I.V.; Tkach, A.A. & Grinevich, L.A. (2008). 4-Hydroxy-2-Quinolones. 148. Synthesis and Anti-tubercular Activity of 1-Hydroxy-3-Oxo-6,7-Dihydro-3H,5H-Pyrido-[3,2,1-ij]quinoline-2-Carboxylic Acid N-R-Amides. Chemistry of Heterocyclic Compounds, Vol.44, No.8, pp. 956-966, ISSN 0009-3122

Baumer, V.N.; Shishkin, O.V.; Ukrainets, I.V.; Sidorenko, L.V. & El Kayal, S.A. (2004). 1-Ethyl-4-Hydroxyquinolin-2(1H)-one. Acta Crystallographica Section E, Vol.60, No.12, pp. o2356-o2358, ISSN 1600-5368

Ukrainets, I.V.; Gorokhova, O.V.; Sidorenko, L.V. & Bereznyakova, N.L. (2007). 4-Hydroxy-2-Quinolones. 111. Simple Synthesis of 1-Substituted 4-Methyl-2-Oxo-1,2-Dihydroquino-line-3-Carboxylic Acids. Chemistry of Heterocyclic Compounds, Vol.43, No.1, pp. 58-62, ISSN 0009-3122

Ukrainets, I.V.; Sidorenko, L.V.; Gorokhova, O.V.; Mospanova, E.V. & Shishkin, O.V. (2006a). 4-Hydroxy-2-Quinolones. 94. Improved Synthesis and Structure of 1-Hydroxy-3-Oxo-5,6-Dihydro-3H-Pyrrolo[3,2,1-i,j]quinoline-2-Carboxylic Acid Ethyl Ester. Chemistry of Heterocyclic Compounds, Vol.42, No.5, pp. 631-635, ISSN 0009-3122

Kravtsova, V.V. (2011). The Search of New Local Anesthetics in the Range of Amide Derivatives of Oxoquinoline-3-Carboxylic Acids [in Ukrainian]. Thesis for Candidate Degree in Pharmacy in speciality 15.00.02 – Pharmaceutical Chemistry and Pharmacognosy, Manuscript, Kharkov, Ukraine

King, F.D. (Ed.). (2002). Medicinal Chemistry: Principles and Practice, Royal Society of Chemistry, ISBN 0854046313, Cambridge, UK

Devereux, M. & Popelier, P.L. (2010). In Silico Techniques for the Identification of Bioisosteric Replacements for Drug Design. Current Topics in Medicinal Chemistry, Vol.10, No.6, pp. 657-668, ISSN 1568-0266

Wassermann, A.M. & Bajorath, J. (2011). Large-scale Exploration of Bioisosteric Replacements on the Basis of Matched Molecular Pairs. Future Medicinal Chemistry, Vol.3, No.4, pp. 425-36, ISSN 1756-8919

Large, J.M.; Torr, J.E.; Raynaud, F.I.; Clarke, P.A.; Hayes, A.; Stefano, F.; Urban, F.; Shuttleworth, S.J.; Saghir, N.; Sheldrake, P.; Workman, P. & McDonald, E. (2011). Preparation and Evaluation of Trisubstituted Pyrimidines as Phosphatidylinositol 3-Kinase Inhibitors. 3-Hydroxyphenol Analogues and Bioisosteric Replacements. Bioorganic and Medicinal Chemistry, Vol.19, No.2, pp. 836-851, ISSN 0968-0896

Kolisnyk, O.V. (2009). Synthesis, Physical, Chemical and Biological Properties of 4-Hydroxy-2-Oxo-1,2,5,6,7,8-Hexahydroquinoline-3-Carboxylic Acids Amidation Derivatives. [in Ukrainian]. *Thesis for Candidate Degree in Pharmacy in speciality 15.00.02 – Pharmaceutical Chemistry and Pharmacognosy*, Manuscript, Kharkov, Ukraine

Ukrainets, I.V., Kravtsova, V.V., Tkach, A.A., Mamchur, V.I. & Kovalenko, E.Yu. (2010). 4-Hydroxy-2-Quinolones. 173. 1-R-3-(2-Diethylaminoethyl)-1H-Quinazoline-2,4-Dione Hydrochlorides as Potential Local Anesthetic Agents. *Chemistry of Heterocyclic Compounds*, Vol.46, No.1, pp. 96-105, ISSN 0009-3122

Ukrainets, I.V.; Sidorenko, L.V.; Gorokhova, O.V. & Jaradat, N.A. (2006b). 4-Hydroxy-2-Quinolones. 93. Synthesis and Biological Properties of 2-Hydroxy-4-Imino-1,4-Dihydroquinoline-3-Carboxylic Acid N-R-Amides. *Chemistry of Heterocyclic Compounds*, Vol.42, No.4, pp. 475-487, ISSN 0009-3122

6

Reduced Antinociceptive Effect of Repeated Treatment with a Cannabinoid Receptor Type 2 Agonist in Cannabinoid-Tolerant Rats Following Spinal Nerve Transection

Matthew S. Alkaitis[1,2], Christian Ndong[1,3], Russell P. Landry III[1,3],
Joyce A. DeLeo[1,3,4] and E. Alfonso Romero-Sandoval[1,3,4]
[1]Neuroscience Center at Dartmouth, Dartmouth Medical School,
[2]Nuffield Department of Clinical Laboratory Sciences, John Radcliffe Hospital,
[3]Department of Anesthesiology, Dartmouth-Hitchcock Medical Center,
[4]Department of Pharmacology and Toxicology, Dartmouth-Hitchcock Medical Center,
[1,3,4]USA
[2]UK

1. Introduction

In both preclinical and clinical studies, agents that activate cannabinoid receptors type 1 (CB1) and 2 (CB2) have shown promise in the treatment of pain (Wade et al., 2004; Romero-Sandoval and Eisenach, 2007). Cannabinoids are licensed for the clinical treatment of cancer chemotherapy-associated nausea and vomiting (USA and Canada), immunodeficiency syndrome-associated loss of appetite and weight loss (USA and Canada), multiple sclerosis-associated spasticity (United Kingdom and Canada) and neuropathic pain (Canada). However, clinical use of cannabinoid compounds is limited both by undesirable neurological side effects and by induction of tolerance. In animal models, neurological side effects have been shown to be dependent on CB1 receptor but not CB2 receptor activation (Romero-Sandoval and Eisenach, 2007). Furthermore, sustained spinal or subcutaneous administration of the CB1 receptor agonist, WIN 55,212-2 has been shown to induce hypersensitivity and antinociceptive tolerance in naive mice and rats. In contrast, we (Romero-Sandoval and Eisenach, 2007; Romero-Sandoval et al., 2008a) and others (Yao et al., 2009) have shown that spinal CB2 receptor agonists (such as JWH015) relieve postoperative and neuropathic pain in rodent models without inducing neurological side effects or antinociceptive tolerance. Despite advancements in the molecular mechanisms involved in cannabinoid tolerance (Martini et al., 2010), a better understanding of the respective roles of CB1 and CB2 receptors is required to design effective therapies that do not induce tolerance. Further advances in this area may also guide clinical treatment of patients who have already developed tolerance through prior exposure to non-selective cannabinoid agonists for recreational or medical purposes.

Using the L5 nerve transection (L5NT) rodent model of chronic neuropathic pain, this study was designed to test: 1) whether a non-selective cannabinoid agonist (CP55940) induces tolerance following repeated intrathecal (i.t.) administration in a model of neuropathic pain; 2) whether this antinociceptive tolerance could be reversed by the cessation of drug exposure; and 3) whether sustained spinal administration of the non-selective cannabinoid CP55940 affects antinociception induced by a CB2 receptor agonist (JWH015). To determine the site of action of these agonists we additionally examined expression levels and cellular localization of CB1 and CB2 receptors in the spinal cord of rats receiving either L5NT or sham surgery.

2. Materials and methods

2.1 Animals and surgical procedures

These studies were performed in accordance with the Guidelines for Animal Experimentation of the International Association for the Study of Pain (IASP) and after approval by the Institutional Animal Care and Use Committee at Dartmouth College (Dartmouth Medical School, Hanover, New Hampshire). Male Sprague-Dawley rats weighing 200–250 g (Harlan, Indianapolis, IN) at the start of surgery underwent L5NT surgery as previous described (Tanga et al., 2005). Briefly, rats were anesthetized with 2% isoflurane in oxygen and a small incision to the skin overlying L5-S1 was made followed by retraction of the paravertebral musculature from the vertebral transverse processes. The L6 transverse process was then partially removed to expose the L4 and L5 spinal nerves. The L5 spinal nerve was identified, lifted slightly, and transected. The wound was irrigated with saline and sutured in two layers. Sham surgeries were performed in other group of rats following the same procedure but without manipulating or injuring the nerves. The surgeries and anesthesia exposure lasted 15 – 20 minutes. Animals were housed individually and maintained in a 12:12 hr light/dark cycle with *ad libitum* access to food and water. Efforts were made to limit animal distress and to use the minimum number of animals necessary to achieve statistical significance.

2.2 Tissue preparation, immunohistochemistry, imaging and image analysis

After being anesthetized with 2-4% isoflurane in oxygen, rats were perfused transcardially with phosphate buffered saline (0.01 M, 150 ml) followed by 4% formaldehyde (350 ml) at room temperature. The L5 spinal cord section was collected and placed in 30% sucrose for 48-72 hr at 4 °C. The tissue was then frozen in O.C.T. Compound (Sakura Finetek, Torrance, CA) and stored at -80 °C. To determine the expression of spinal CB2 receptor immunohistochemistry was performed on transverse 20-μm L5 spinal cord free-floating sections by using the Vector ELITE ABC (Vector Labs, Burlingame, CA), avidin-biotin complex technique and a goat polyclonal antibody against the C-terminus of CB2 receptor (1:150, Santa Cruz biotechnology, Santa Cruz, CA, sc10076) as we have previously described (Romero-Sandoval et al., 2008a). Immunofluorescence was performed to determine the spinal CB1 receptor expression level using a rabbit polyclonal antibody (1:200, Cayman, Ann Arbor, MI) and a Alexa-Fluor™ 488 Goat anti-Rabbit IgG1 secondary antibody (Molecular Probes, Eugene, Oregon). For CB1 receptor and CB2 receptor expression quantification, the sections were examined with an Olympus microscope, and images were captured with a Q-Fire cooled camera (Olympus, Melville, NY). We quantified the CB1 receptor or CB2 receptor expression, blinded to experimental conditions, as the number of

pixels above a preset intensity threshold using SigmaScan Pro 5 as previously described
(Romero-Sandoval and Eisenach, 2007; Romero-Sandoval et al., 2008b). For both CB1
receptor and CB2 receptor expression, the staining intensity was examined in a standardized
area of superficial laminae (I-II) and deep laminae (III-V) of the L5 dorsal horn in 3–4 slices
examined per animal.

Immunofluorescence was also used for dual labeling with specific cell markers and CB1
receptor or CB2 receptor. All sections were blocked in 5% Normal Goat Serum (NGS) and
0.01% Triton-X-100 for 1 hour at 4 °C. Sections were incubated in the appropriate primary
antibody or antibodies diluted in a buffer composed of 1% NGS and 1% Triton-X-100 in PBS
overnight at 4 °C. To determine the cellular localization of CB1 receptor or CB2 receptor we
co-labeled antibodies for CB1 receptor and CB2 receptor with the following cellular markers
(antibodies): rabbit polyclonal anti-Iba-1 for microglia (1:1000, Wako Pure Chemical
Industries, Richmond, VA), mouse polyclonal anti-GFAP for astrocytes (1:400, Sigma, Saint
Louis, Missouri), mouse polyclonal antibody anti- ED2/CD163 for perivascular cells (1:150,
Serotec, Raleigh, NC), mouse polyclonal anti-Neuronal Nuclei, NeuN for neurons (1:10,000,
Chemicon, Billerica, Massachusetts).

The following secondary antibodies were used as indicated in table 1: Alexa-Fluor™ 488
Goat anti-Rabbit IgG1 (Molecular Probes, Eugene, Oregon), Alexa-Fluor™ 488 Goat anti-
Mouse IgG1 (Molecular Probes, Eugene, Oregon), Alexa-Fluor™ 555 Goat anti-Mouse IgG
(Molecular Probes, Eugene, Oregon) and Alexa-Fluor™ 555 Donkey anti-Goat IgG
(Molecular Probes, Eugene, Oregon).

To avoid cross-reactivity between the secondary antibodies in the CB_2 receptor colocalization experiments, sections were first incubated in Alexa-Fluor™ 555 Donkey anti-
Goat IgG (Molecular Probes, Eugene, Oregon) as described above, washed 2 times in PBS
and then incubated in the appropriate Alexa-Fluor™ 488 secondary antibody as described
above. This protocol modification prevented binding of the Alexa-Fluor™ 555 Donkey
anti-Goat IgG to the goat-derived Alexa-Fluor™ 488. The specificity of each antibody was
tested by omitting the primary antibody on 1-3 additional sections. To avoid cross-
reactivity when co-staining with primary antibodies against Iba-1 and CB_1 receptors that
are both rabbit-derived, a TSA Signal Amplification Kit was used following the
manufacturer instructions (PerkinElmer LifeSciences Inc, Boston, MA). On the first day,
normal immunofluorescence protocol was followed except that sections were incubated
only in anti-CB_1 receptor antibody at a concentration of 1:10,000. On the second day
sections were washed 2 times for 5 minutes in PBS then incubated in a biotinylated Goat α
Rabbit secondary antibody for 1 hour at 4 °C. Sections were then subjected to another
wash, incubated in SA-HRP (1:100) for 1 hour at 4 °C, washed again and incubated in the
TSA fluorophore (1:250) for 10 minutes at 4 °C. Sections were then washed again and
incubated overnight in the Iba-1 primary antibody (1:1000). The next day sections were
subjected to normal day 2 immunofluorescence protocol to visualize Iba-1 (described
above). One control was included with only the anti-CB_1 receptor primary antibody
(1:10,000) and the Alexa 555 Goat α Rabbit secondary antibody to control for any cross-
reactivity that might cause CB_1 receptor expression to appear in red. A second control
included only the anti-CB_1 receptor primary antibody and the TSA kit in order to
visualize the staining achieved in the absence of the co-stain. Finally, a third control
included the TSA kit, Iba-1 primary and the Alexa 555 Goat α Rabbit secondary antibody
but excluded the anti-CB_1 receptor primary antibody. This third control provided

visualization of the non-specific background staining produced by the kit alone. All controls confirmed the specificity of the co-stain.

Antigen (Co-stain)	Primary	Secondary	Fluorophore optimal excitation (nm)
CB1	Rabbit	Goat α Rabbit	488
Iba1 (CB1)	Rabbit (Rabbit)	Goat α Rabbit (TSA Signal Amplification Kit)	488 (555)
GFAP (CB1)	Mouse (Rabbit)	Goat α Mouse (Goat α Rabbit)	488 (555)
ED2 (CB1)	Mouse (Rabbit)	Goat α Mouse (Goat α Rabbit)	488 (555)
Iba1 (CB2)	Rabbit (Goat)	Goat α Rabbit (Donkey α Goat)	488 (555)
GFAP (CB2)	Rabbit (Goat)	Goat α Rabbit (Donkey α Goat)	488 (555)
ED2 (CB2)	Mouse (Goat)	Goat α Mouse (Donkey α Goat)	488 (555)
NeuN (CB2)	Mouse (Goat)	Goat α Mouse (Donkey α Goat)	488 (555)

Table 1. Details of antibody selections for all immunofluorescense experiments, CB1: Cannabinoid receptor type 1, CB2: Cannabinoid receptor type 2, ED2: Perivascular cell marker, GFAP: Glial Fibrillary Acidic Protein, Iba-1: Ionized Calcium–Binding Adapter Molecule 1, NeuN: Neuronal Nuclei.

Stained sections were examined with an Olympus fluorescence microscope, and images were captured with a Q-Fire cooled camera (Olympus, Melville, NY). Confocal microscopy was also performed using a Zeiss LSM 510 Meta confocal microscope (Carl Zeiss AG, Oberkochen, Germany; Englert Cell Analysis Laboratory, Dartmouth). Merged color images were processed using Adobe Photoshop 7.0 (Adobe Systems, San Jose, CA).

2.3 Behavioral testing
Mechanical allodynia was evaluated by measuring the 50% withdrawal threshold using an up–down statistical method (Chaplan et al., 1994) and calibrated von Frey filaments (1 – 60 g, Stoelting, Wood Dale, IL). At each time point, two measurements were made on the paw ipsilateral to surgery in 5-10 min intervals, and the average of these values was used for data analyses. As an internal control, withdrawal thresholds were also measured in the paw contralateral to surgery (uninjured side). The withdrawal threshold was determined for each animal before surgery, 4 days after surgery (immediately before any pharmacological treatment), and after drug administration (different time points for different paradigms, see below). The investigator was blinded to drug treatment in all behavioral tests.

2.4 Drugs and treatments
Drugs were administered by intrathecal (i.t.) injection by means of lumbar puncture under brief inhalational anesthesia (2-4% isoflurane in oxygen) using a Hamilton syringe and a 28-

gauge 5/0-Inch Hypodermic needle The needle was inserted intrathecally) on the midline
between the fourth and fifth lumbar vertebrae. The correct injection site was confirmed with
the stimulation of nerves in the cauda equina when the lumbar needle penetrated the dura and
produced a brief but obvious movement of the tail and/or the hind paws. The animals
regained consciousness 2–3 min after the discontinuation of anesthesia. Drugs were diluted in
dimethylsulfoxide and saline in a ratio of 1:1 and administered in a volume of 15 µl as
previously described (Romero-Sandoval et al., 2008a). The drugs used were: the dual (CB1
receptor and CB2 receptor) cannabinoid receptor agonist CP55940 (5-(1,1-Dimethylheptyl)-2-
[5-hydroxy-2-(3-hydroxypropyl) cyclohexyl]phenol; Sigma Chemical Co., St. Louis, MO); the
CB2 receptor agonist JWH015 ((2-Methyl-1-propyl-1H-indol-3-yl)-1-naphthalenylmethanone),
the CB1 receptor antagonist AM281 (1-(2,4-Dichlorophenyl)-5-(4-iodophenyl)-4-methyl-N-4-
morpholinyl-1H-pyrazole-3-carboxamide) and the CB2 receptor antagonist AM630 (6-Iodo-2-
methyl-1-[2-(4-morpholinyl)ethyl]-1H-indol-3-yl](4-methoxyphenyl)methanone),   purchased
from Tocris, Ellisville, MI.

2.5 Repeated CP55940 administration and monitoring of behavioral effects

Beginning four days after surgery, CP55940 (100 µg/injection, n=18) or vehicle (n=17) was
administered in single daily injections (8:00-9:00 AM) for five days. This dose and i.t.
administration method were chosen based on our previous study using CP55940 in the same
model of neuropathic pain (Romero-Sandoval and Eisenach, 2007), and on a previous study
that demonstrated induction of antinociceptive tolerance with another non-selective
cannabinoid agonist WIN 55,212-2 (Gardell et al., 2002) at a dose of 100 µg twice daily.
Drugs and vehicle were administered i.t. based on previous evidence that spinal cord
mechanisms drive induction of cannabinoid tolerance (Gardell et al., 2002). Two hours after
each injection, mechanical withdrawal thresholds in both ipsilateral and contralateral hind-
paws were evaluated as described above.

2.6 Evaluation of response to acute CP55940 dose escalation in tolerant and
non-tolerant animals

CP55940 was acutely administered i.t. in 30-min interval escalating doses: 0.4, 2, 10 and 50
µg in L5NT animals 24 hr before and 24 hr after the repeated (5 day) treatment with
CP55940 (n=5) or vehicle (n=6). As a control, vehicle was administered i.t. using the same
dose escalation paradigm in animals that had previously received L5NT followed by
repeated (5 days) treatment with CP55940 (n=8). The antinociceptive effect of escalating
doses of CP55940 was evaluated 15 min after every injection. The effectiveness and potency
of CP55940 were calculated using these dose responses and were compared in both repeated
CP55940 and repeated vehicle treatment groups. To determine whether cannabinoid-
mediated tolerance was reversed following the discontinuation of sustained CP55940
administration, the antinociceptive response to escalating doses of CP55940 were also
measured two weeks after the last day of repeated CP55940 treatment (washout period). In
summary, responses to acute CP55940 dose escalation (or vehicle) was evaluated in the
following cases: 1) prior to any additional treatment, 2) 24 hours after repeated (5-day)
treatment with CP55940, 3) 24 hours after repeated (5-day) treatment with vehicle, and 4) 2
weeks (washout period) after repeated (5-day) treatment with CP55940. To confirm that
CP55940 induced its effects via CB1 receptor and CB2 receptor as we have previously
demonstrated (Romero-Sandoval and Eisenach, 2007; Romero-Sandoval et al., 2008a), we

administered CP55940 at a dose of 50 μg in combination with vehicle, the CB1 receptor antagonist AM281 at a dose of 50 μg or the CB2 receptor antagonist AM630 at a dose of 50 μg in a separate group of rats. Mechanical withdrawal threshold was determined 2 hr after treatments.

2.7 Evaluation of response to acute JWH015 dose escalation in tolerant and non-tolerant animals

JWH015, a CB2 receptor agonist, was acutely administered i.t. in 30-min interval escalating doses: 0.4, 2, 10 and 50 μg in L5NT animals that had previously received repeated (5 days) treatment with CP55940 (n=8) or vehicle (n=8). Vehicle was acutely administered i.t. using the same dose escalation paradigm in animals that had previously received L5NT followed by repeated (5 days) treatment with CP55940 (n=8). The antinociceptive effect of escalating doses of JWH015 was evaluated 15 min after every injection and its efficacy and potency were quantified. The first set of experiments was performed 24 hr after the last day of repeated CP55940 administration to test whether the cannabinoid-mediated tolerance influenced the antinociceptive effects of a CB2 receptor agonist administered acutely. The second set of experiments was performed two weeks after the last day of repeated CP55940 treatment (washout period) to test whether the potency and/or efficacy of the CB2 receptor agonist, JWH015 improves following the discontinuation of sustained CP55940 treatment. In summary, responses to acute JWH015 dose escalation (or vehicle) were evaluated in the following cases: 1) 24 hours after repeated (5-day) treatment with CP55940 or vehicle and 2) 2 weeks (washout period) after repeated (5-day) treatment with CP55940 or vehicle.

To confirm that JWH015 induced its effects via CB2 receptors as we have previously demonstrated (Romero-Sandoval and Eisenach, 2007; Romero-Sandoval et al., 2008a), we administered JWH015 at a dose of 50 μg in combination with the CB2 receptor antagonist AM630 at a dose of 50 μg or vehicle in a separate group of animals. Mechanical withdrawal threshold was determined 2 hr after treatments.

2.8 Evaluation of response to repeated JWH015 administration in tolerant and non-tolerant animals

Following the washout period (two weeks after repeated administration of CP55940 or vehicle), JWH015 (50 μg/injection, n=9) or vehicle (n=8) was administered in single daily injections (8:00-9:00 AM) for four days. Behavioral testing were performed before and 2 hr after each injection. Antinociceptive tolerance was evaluated by testing mechanical withdrawal thresholds in the paw ipsilateral or contralateral to surgery.

2.9 Assessment of neurological side effects

Based on our previous studies (Romero-Sandoval and Eisenach, 2007; Romero-Sandoval et al., 2008a) righting and placing-stepping tests were used to evaluate motor reflexes; the bar test was used to evaluate catalepsy; vocalization was used as a sign of irritability or discomfort to manipulation and exploratory activity was used as a measure of awareness. These parameters were evaluated before, 20 minutes and 2.5 hr after each injection (following behavioral mechanical hypersensitivity testing). The placing-stepping reflex was tested by placing the rostral aspect of the hind paws on the edge of a table and was quantified as the seconds in which the animals put the paws up and forward into a position to walk. A cut-off of 60 s was used. The bar test consists of placing the forelimbs on a bar of

~1 cm of diameter and 10 cm above and parallel to a table, leaving the hind paws resting on the table. A cataleptic animal will stay in that position longer than a normal animal. The time in which the animal puts its forelimb on the table was recorded, using a cut off time of 60 s. The righting test consists of placing the animal supine and recording the ability to right itself. Righting was scored on a scale of 0-3, 0 indicating normal righting reflex (an immediate and coordinated twisting of the body to an upright position), 1 indicating mild impairment (ability to completely right, but slowly), 2 indicating moderate impairment (ability to right the forelimbs slowly followed by the hind limbs with more difficulty) and 3 indicating severe impairment (inability to right in 20 sec). Vocalization was rated on a scale of 0-3, 0 indicating absent vocalization, 1 indicating some vocalization when manipulated, 2 indicating consistent vocalization when manipulated and 3 indicating vocalization even light touch. Exploratory activity was rated on a scale of 0-3 with 0 indicating normal activity, 1 indicating only head movements without vertical and/or horizontal exploration, 2 indicating no spontaneous movements and 3 indicating splayed posture with no spontaneous movements. All behavioral measures were performed twice and the average used for analyses.

2.10 Statistical analyses

The effects of L5NT surgery and drug injections on bar test, placing-stepping test and withdrawal thresholds were examined using the repetitive measurements one-way analysis of variance. If significant effects were found, Tukey's multiple comparison or Dunnett's test was conducted. Differences between groups were examined using two-way analysis of variance. If differences were found, the Bonferroni post test was used. In the acute antinociceptive effect studies, acute i.t. JWH015 50% of maximum efficacy (ED50) and its 95% confidence limits were calculated and compared between repeated CP55940 and repeated vehicle groups using Student's t test. ED50s were calculated using the baseline and after-surgery withdrawal thresholds as maximum and minimum effect values respectively. Vocalization, righting test and exploratory activity data following treatment were compared using the Friedman Repeated Measures Analysis of Variance on Rank test. If significant effects were found, non-parametric Wilcoxon signed ranks tests were conducted comparing each time point to the baseline value (before surgery). Between group differences were compared at each time period using the Kruskal-Wallis test. Significant effects were further evaluated using the Mann-Whitney U test comparing only the novel treatment to control or agonist group. The effects of CP55940 in acute antinociception vs. CP55940 in the presence of CB1 receptor or CB2 receptor antagonist was evaluated by one-way ANOVA followed by Dunnett's post-test. The effects of JWH015 in acute antinociception in the presence of the CB2 receptor antagonist was evaluated by unpaired Student's t-test. Data are presented as mean ± SEM. In all cases a P value less than 0.05 was considered significant. SigmaStat and GraphPad inStat software were used for statistical analyses.

3. Results

3.1 Spinal cord CB1 and CB2 receptor expression and cellular localization

Compared to rats receiving sham surgery, rats receiving L5NT surgery demonstrated significantly higher CB1 receptor expression in the L5 dorsal horn on postoperative days 4 and 7 (Figure 1). The changes in CB1 receptor expression were primarily apparent in the deeper laminae (III-V) of the dorsal horn in rats that had received L5NT surgery. CB1 receptor expression on day 1 after surgery was not significantly different between groups.

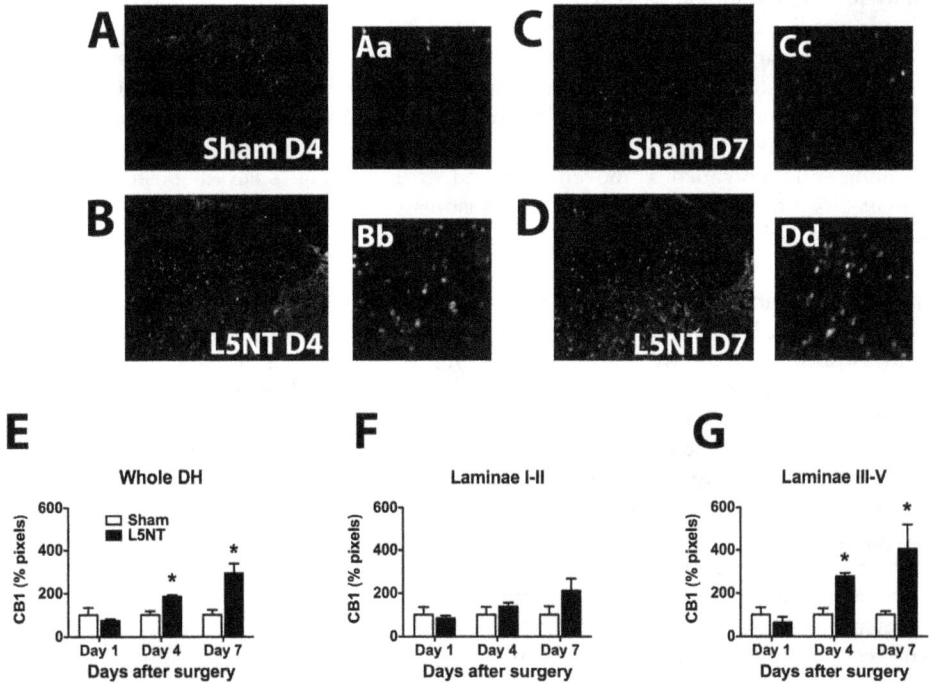

Fig. 1. CB1 receptor expression is increased on days 4 and 7 after L5 nerve transection. Representative images (A-D) show CB1 receptor expression at postoperative days 4 (D4) and 7 (D7) in the L5 dorsal horn of rats receiving sham surgery or L5 nerve transection. Details of the deep laminae (III-IV) of the dorsal horn of these spinal cord tissues are shown next to each original image (Aa-Dd). CB1 expression was quantified in the ipsilateral whole dorsal horn (E), laminae I-II (F) and laminae III-IV (G) of rats receiving sham surgery or L5 nerve transection at postoperative days 1, 4 and 7. Receptor expression was quantified as the number of pixels above a set threshold per total pixels in the selected area and normalized to percent of each control, sham group. *p<0.05 vs. respective sham group by t test. N=3 for all groups.

Compared to the sham surgery group, rats receiving L5NT also demonstrated significantly higher spinal CB2 receptor expression on postoperative day 4 (Figure 2). This increased CB2 receptor expression was mainly observed in the superficial laminae (I-II) of the dorsal horn in animals with L5NT surgery. No significant changes in CB2 receptor expression were observed on postoperative days 1 to 7 following nerve injury compared to the sham surgery group.

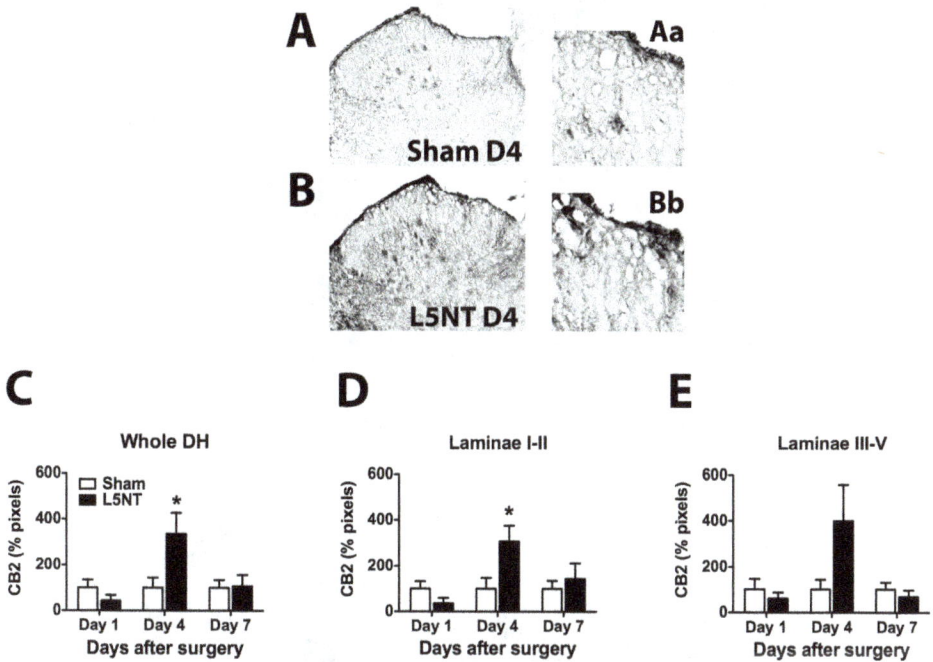

Fig. 2. CB2 receptor expression is increased on day 4 following L5 nerve transection. Representative images (A-B) show CB2 receptor expression at postoperative day 4 (D4) in the L5 dorsal horn of rats receiving sham surgery or L5 nerve transection. Details of the superficial laminae (II-III) of the dorsal horn of these spinal cord tissues are shown next to each original image (Aa and Bb). CB2 expression was quantified in the ipsilateral whole dorsal horn (C), laminae I-II (D) and laminae III-IV (E) of rats receiving sham surgery or L5 nerve transection at postoperative days 1, 4 and 7. Receptor expression was quantified as the number of pixels above a set threshold per total pixels in the selected area and normalized to percent of each control, sham group. *p<0.05 vs. respective sham group by t test. N=3 for all groups.

Using confocal microscopy, we observed that spinal CB1 receptors were primarily expressed on NeuN-positive neurons in the dorsal horns of animals receiving L5NT surgery (Figure 3). Occasionally, CB1 receptors expression co-localized with the astrocyte marker GFAP (Figure 3). CB1 receptor expression did not co-localize with Iba-1-positive microglia or ED2/CD163-positive perivascular cells at any observed time point following L5NT (Figure 3). However, cells expressing CB1 receptor were in close proximity to Iba-1-positive microglia and perivascular cells.

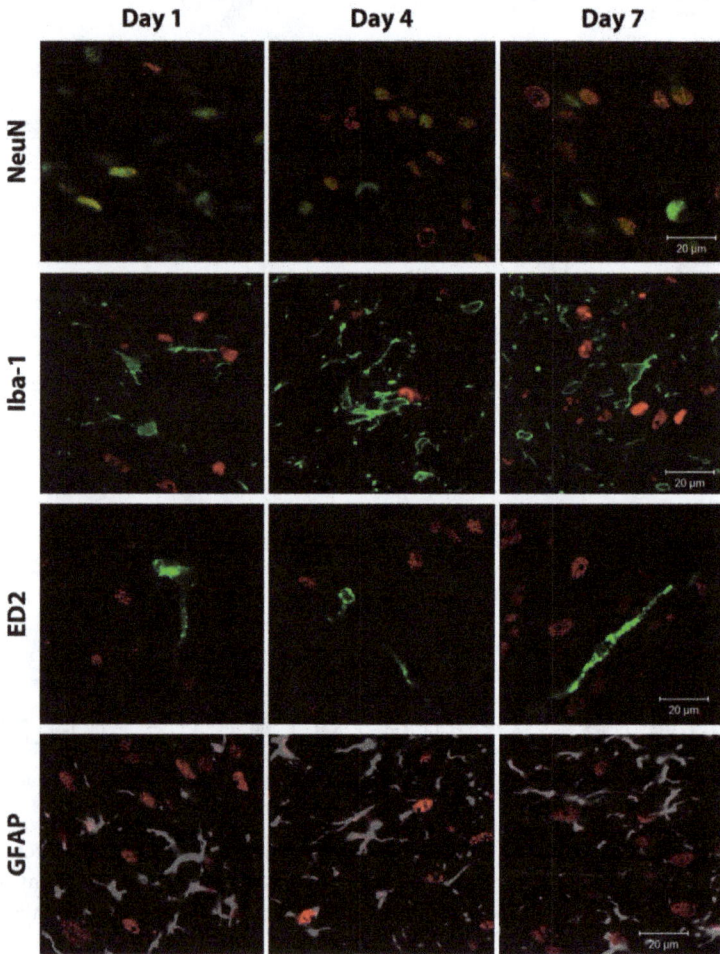

Fig. 3. CB1 receptor is expressed primarily in neurons. Representative confocal images show CB1 receptor cell localization in the ipsilateral L5 dorsal horn of rats at days 1, 4 and 7 after L5 nerve transection. CB1 receptor staining appears in red. NeuN (marker for neurons), Iba-1 (marker for microglia) and ED2/CD163 (ED2, marker for perivascular microglia) appear in green, and GFAP (marker for astrocytes) appears in grey. In the images of CB1 receptors and Iba-1, Iba-1 (originally in red) was changed to green, and CB1 receptor (originally in green) was changed to red to consistently show CB1 receptors in red in all images. GFAP color (originally in green) was changed to grey to obtain a better visualization of occasional expression of CB1 receptors on GFAP-positive cells. The colocalization of CB1 receptors with NeuN appears in yellow.

Microglia (Iba-1 positive cells) and perivascular cells (ED2/CD163 positive cells) displayed localized areas of CB2 receptor expression (Figure 4). Diffuse, punctate CB2 receptor expression was constitutionally observed in NeuN positive neuronal somata (Figure 4). Even though GFAP-positive spinal cord astrocytes did not demonstrate CB2 receptor expression, these cells were in close proximity to cells that expressed CB2 receptor (Figure 4).

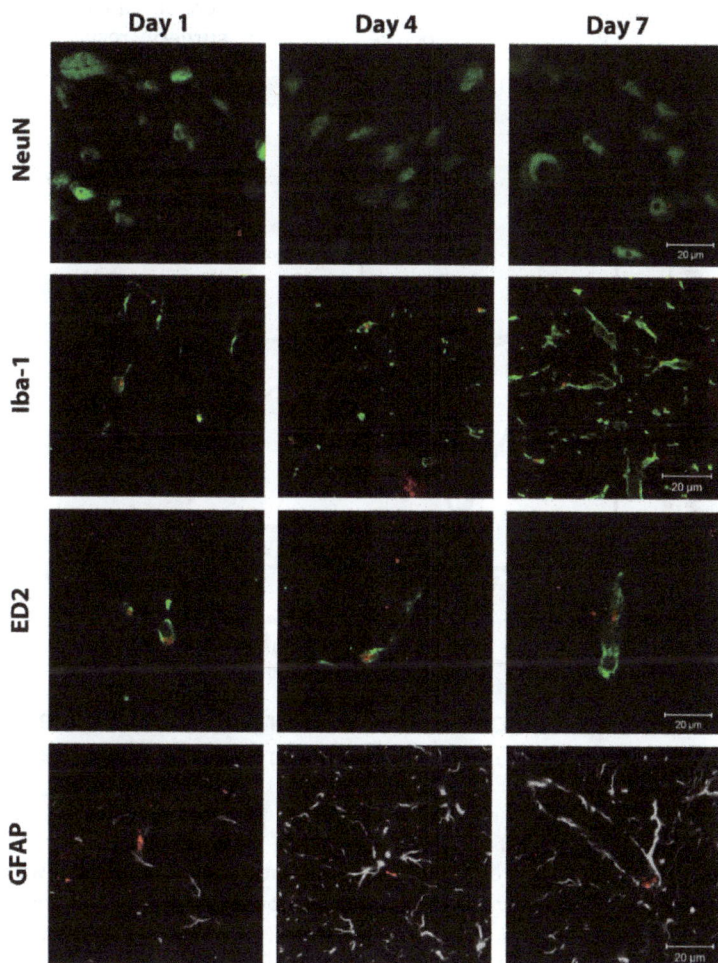

Fig. 4. CB2 receptors are mainly expressed in microglial cells. Representative confocal images show CB2 receptor cell localization in the ipsilateral L5 dorsal horn of rats at days 1, 4 and 7 after L5 nerve transection. CB2 receptor appears in red. NeuN (marker for neurons), Iba-1 (marker for microglia) and ED2/CD163 (ED2, marker for perivascular microglia) appear in green, and GFAP (marker for astrocytes) appears in grey. GFAP color (originally in green) was changed to grey to obtain a better visualization of this specific marker and any potential expression of CB2 receptors. The colocalization of CB2 receptors with the other cellular markers is visualized in yellow.

3.2 CP55940 antinociceptive tolerance

Mechanical withdrawal thresholds on the uninjured side (paw contralateral to L5NT) were not affected by surgery (26.7±1.4 g vs. 23.1±1.1 g, before and after surgery respectively), nor were they significantly different at any observed time point during the five subsequent days of intrathecal vehicle or CP55940 administration (Figure 5). In the paw ipsilateral to L5NT surgery, withdrawal thresholds were significantly reduced after surgery (26.6±1.3 g vs. 5.4±0.5 g, before and after surgery respectively, p<0.05).

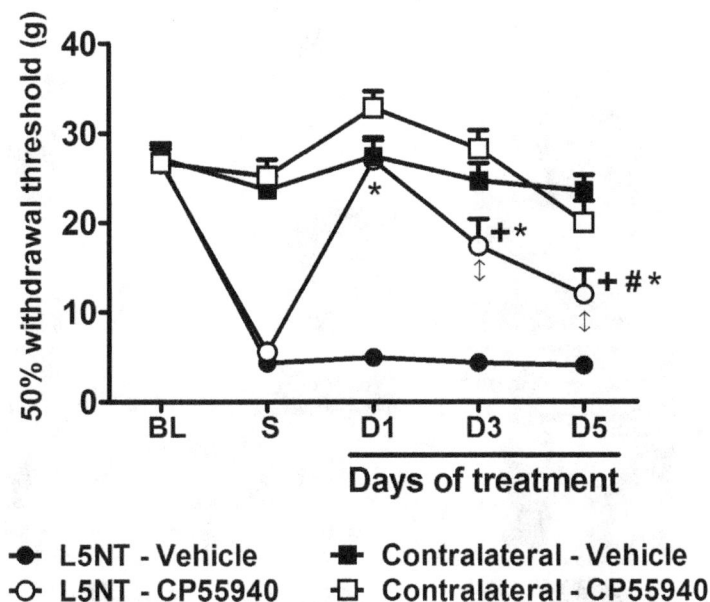

Fig. 5. Antinociceptive effects of repeated i.t. administration of CP55940. Paw withdrawal thresholds indicate responses to von Frey stimulation ipsilateral to L5NT or contralateral to surgery (uninjured side) before surgery (base line = BL), four days after surgery (S), and 2 hr after i.t. injections of vehicle (n=17) or CP55940 (n=18) on days 1, 3 and 5. Withdrawal thresholds on day 1 (D1), day 3 (D3) and day 5 (D5) vs. after surgery data significantly differ by repeated measures one way ANOVA; *p<0.05 vs. after surgery, +p<0.05 vs. D1 L5NT-CP55940, # p<0.05 vs. D3 L5NT-CP55940 by repeated measures one way ANOVA followed by Tukey's multiple comparison test. Groups significantly differ by two way ANOVA; ‡p<0.05 compared to vehicle and both contralateral groups by two way ANOVA followed by Bonferroni post tests.

Administration of vehicle (i.t.) on each of the subsequent 5 days did not significantly alter this L5NT-induced hypersensitivity at any time point observed (Figure 5). In contrast,

Reduced Antinociceptive Effect of Repeated Treatment with a Cannabinoid Receptor Type 2 Agonist in
Cannabinoid-Tolerant Rats Following Spinal Nerve Transection

113

administration of the non-selective cannabinoid agonist CP55940 (100 µg, i.t.) resulted in significantly higher withdrawal thresholds (measured 2 hours following injection) compared to vehicle-treated controls on each day observations were made (Figure 1). However, ipsilateral withdrawal thresholds in animals treated with CP55940 were significantly lower at 2 hr after injection on days 3 - 5 compared to day 1 values (Figure 1). Additionally, the anti-allodynic effect of CP55940 was significantly lower at 2 hr after injection on day 5 compared to day 3 (Figure 5).

In order to test the efficacy and potency of CP55940 before and after its repeated administration, we performed an acute dose escalation with i.t. CP55940. CP55940 reduced L5NT-induced hypersensitivity in a significant and dose-dependent manner before and 24 hr after the 5-day course of daily CP55940 administration (Figure 6). Compared to acute i.t. vehicle treatment, the minimum effective dose of CP55940 was 10 µg, and its maximum effective dose (dose that induced a return to base line values) was 50 µg (the maximum dose tested) before and after its repeated administration. However, CP55940 displayed an approximately 2-fold higher efficacy ($p<0.05$, Table 2) and an approximately 7-fold higher potency ($p<0.05$, Table 2) in untreated animals (Figure 6A) than in animals previously treated with CP55940 for five days (repeated CP55940 group, Figure 6B). The higher efficacy and potency of CP55940 observed in untreated animals were similar to the ones observed in animals previously treated for five days with vehicle (repeated vehicle group, Figure 6C, Table 2). We then evaluated the effects of acute CP55940 two weeks after repeated treatment with CP55940 was discontinued (washout period). Even though acute CP55940 was still effective (at 10 and 50 µg doses vs. vehicle) following 2 weeks of washout period, its efficacy and potency were significantly lower than in animals that had not received repeated CP55940 treatment (Figure 6D, Table 2). The acute antinociception induced by CP55940 50 µg (plus vehicle, 32.9 ± 2.1 g, n=6) in the L5NT group was blocked by either the CB1 receptor antagonist AM281 50 µg (14.5 ± 4.3 g, n=4, $P<0.05$) or the CB2 receptor antagonist AM630 50 µg (15.2 ± 4.3 g, n=4, $P<0.05$), confirming that the activity of this compound depends on activation of both CB1 and CB2 receptors.

	50% w.t. for the 50 µg dose (efficacy in g)		ED50 (95% confidence limits)	
	CP55940	JWH015	CP55940	JWH015
L5NT no previous treatment	32.9±1.94		14.7 (10.91-19.9)	
24 hr after repeated vehicle	29.7±2.85	17.0±2.7	11.9 (7.6-18.6)	26.4 (13.8-50.5)
24 hr after repeated CP55940	14.9±1.12 *	16.3±3.9	112.6 (21.2-596.6) *	37.4 (26.7-52.5)
2 weeks after repeated CP55940	15.7±4.8 *	14.2±2.5	162.6 (5.7-4567) *	32.5 (1.2-872)

Table 2. Effect of the highest dose (50 µg) and ED50 (95% confidence limits) of acute i.t. administration of CP55940 and JWH015 in L5NT, *$P<0.05$ vs. L5NT no previous treatment and 24 hr after repeated vehicle groups. Withdrawal threshold = w.t.

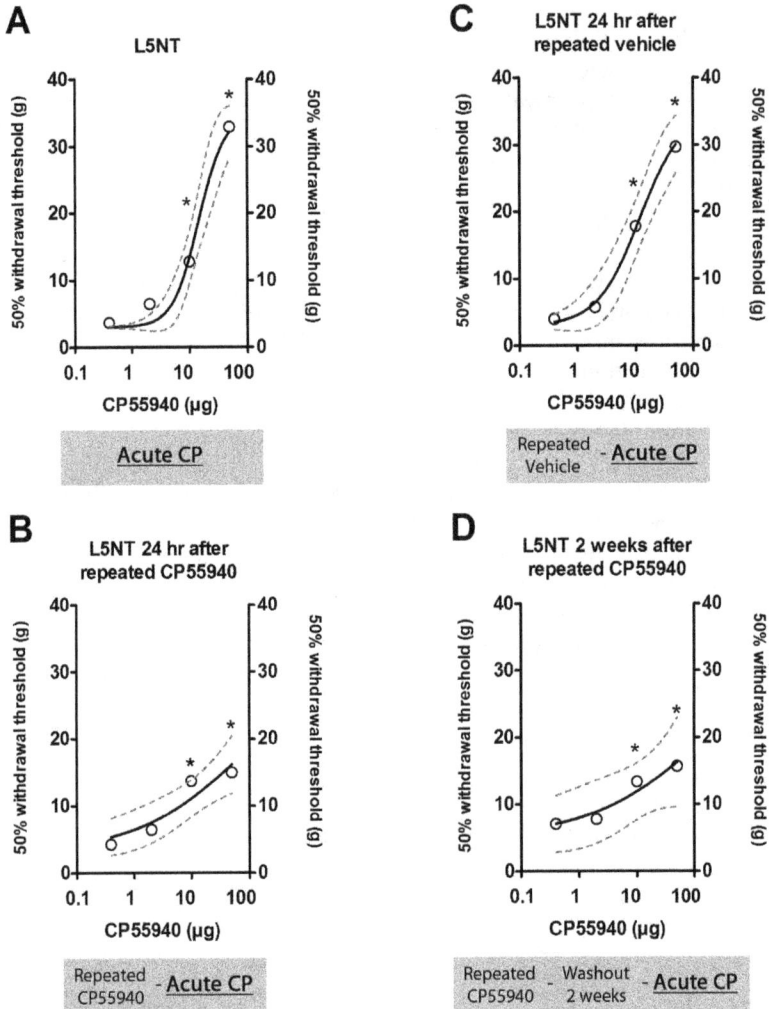

Fig. 6. Antinociceptive effects of acute i.t. administration of CP55940. Withdrawal thresholds (95% confidence limits, doted lines) indicate responses to von Frey stimulation ipsilateral to L5NT surgery 15 min after escalating doses (0.4, 2, 10 and 50 µg) of i.t. CP55940 in animals receiving no additional treatment (A, n=5), 24 hr after the discontinuation of repeated treatment (5 days) with CP55940 i.t., 100 µg (B, n=6) or vehicle (C, n=6) and 2 weeks (washout period) after the discontinuation of repeated treatment (5 days) with CP55940 100 µg (D, n=5). Withdrawal thresholds in response to dose escalation of CP55940 significantly differ from after-surgery values by repeated measures one way ANOVA, *p<0.05 vs. after surgery by repeated measures one way ANOVA followed by Tukey's multiple comparison test. Groups significantly differ by two way ANOVA; p<0.05 L5NT or L5NT 24 hr after repeated vehicle groups vs. L5NT 24 hr after repeated CP55940 or L5NT 2 weeks after repeated CP55940 groups for 50 µg by two way ANOVA followed by Bonferroni post tests.

In order to investigate the neurological side effects of CP55940 administration, we evaluated the place-stepping reflex, vocalization, exploratory activity and the bar test. Repeated vehicle injection did not significantly affect any of these behaviors at any time point observed. CP55940 significantly impaired the placing-stepping reflex (Figure 7A), induced vocalization (Figure 7B) and reduced exploratory activity (Figure 7C) on days 1, 2 and 3 compared to vehicle group, and induced catalepsy (Figure 7D) on days 1, 2, 3 and 4

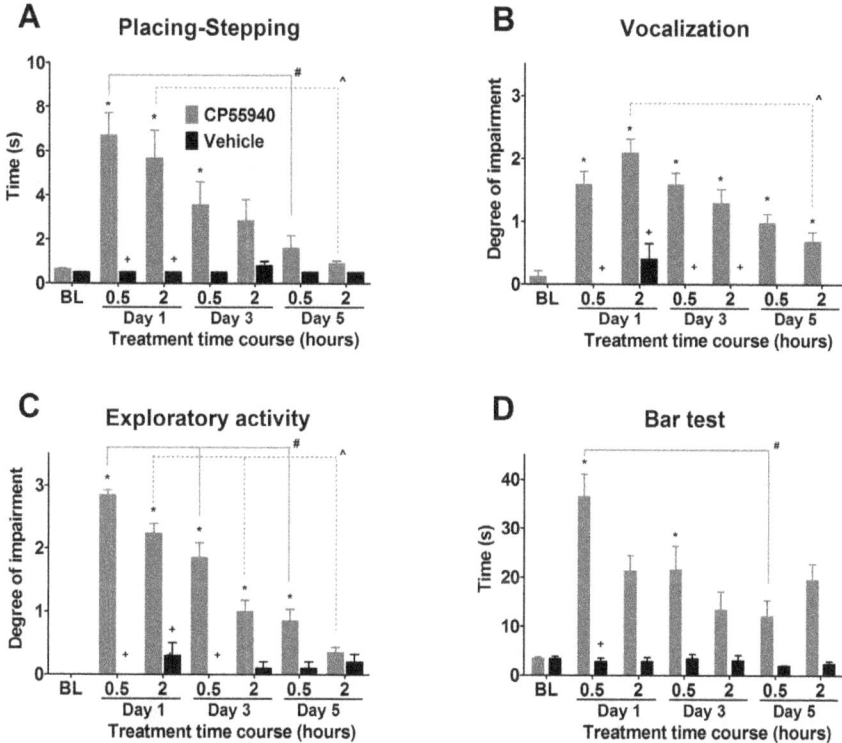

Fig. 7. Neurological side effects in response to repeated treatment with CP55940. Placing-stepping (A), vocalization (B), exploratory activity (C) and bar test (C) scores are shown from before the first injection (base line = BL), and 0.5, 2 and 24 hr after each i.t. injection (days 1 - 5) of vehicle (n=8) or CP55940 (n=13) during five consecutive days. Withdrawal thresholds on days 1, 3 and 5 in placing-stepping and bar test vs. base line data significantly differ by repeated measures one way ANOVA, *p<0.05 vs. base line, #p<0.05 vs. 0.5 hr, ^p<0.05 vs. 2 hr by repeated measures one way ANOVA followed by Tukey's multiple comparison test. Groups differ in placing-stepping and bar test by repetitive measurements two-way ANOVA, +p<0.05 vs. CP55940 group by two way ANOVA followed by Bonferroni post tests. Days 1, 3 and 5 values in vocalization and exploratory activity vs. base line significantly differ by Friedman test, *p<0.05 vs. base line, #p<0.05 vs. 0.5 hr, ^p<0.05 vs. 2 hr by Friedman test followed by Wilcoxon test. Groups in vocalization and exploratory activity significantly differ by Kruskal-Wallis test; +p<0.05 vs. CP55940 by Kruskal-Wallis test followed by Mann-Whitney U test.

compared to vehicle group. The magnitude of these neurological side effects decreased over the 5-day course of daily CP55940 injections until they were not significantly different compared to vehicle group on days 4 and 5 (except for catalepsy, 2 hr after CP55940 injection on day 4 vs. vehicle group, p<0.05). The righting reflex was significantly impaired by CP55940 compared to base line on days 1 and 3 (30 min and 2 hr after injections, data not shown). The effects of CP55940 on placing-stepping reflex, vocalization and bar test on day 1 were significantly higher compared to its effects on days 4 and 5. The effects of CP55940 on exploratory activity on day 1 were significantly higher compared to its effects on days 3, 4 and 5. For clarity, only the data obtained on days 1, 3 and 5 of treatment are shown.

3.4 Acute antinociceptive effect of JWH015 in CP55940-tolerant animals

JWH015, a selective CB2 receptor agonist, reduced mechanical hypersensitivity ipsilateral to surgery in a dose-dependent fashion when administered i.t. in cumulative, escalating doses in animals previously exposed to CP55940 or vehicle (Figure 8A). The minimum and

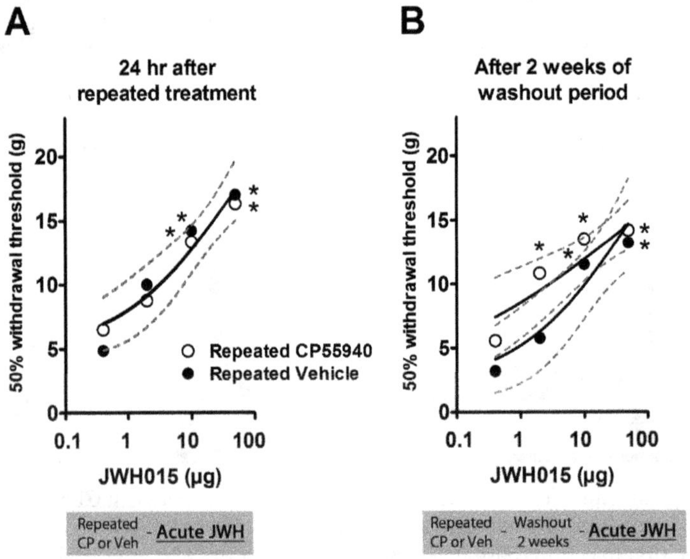

Fig. 8. Antinociceptive effects of acute i.t. administration of JWH015 in CP55940-mediated tolerant animals. Withdrawal thresholds (95% confidence limits, doted lines) indicate responses to von Frey stimulation ipsilateral to L5NT surgery 15 min after escalating doses (0.4, 2, 10 and 50 µg) of i.t. JWH015 administered 24 hr (A) or two weeks (washout period, B) after the discontinuation of repeated treatment with CP55940 100 µg (Repeated CP55940) or vehicle (Repeated Vehicle). Groups did not differ by two-way ANOVA. Withdrawal thresholds after each dose vs. after surgery values significantly differ by repeated measures one way ANOVA, *p<0.05 vs. after surgery by repeated measures one way ANOVA followed by Tukey's multiple comparison test. Twenty-four hr after repeated treatment cessation: Repeated CP55940 n=8, Repeated Vehicle n=8, Repeated CP55940-washout period n=6 and Repeated Vehicle-washout period n=5.

ımaxlıınını ptıpı tiya ʌʌϭʌϭ ʌt Jᴡ/Hᴜᵗ1ʙ in the repeated CP55940 group were 10 and 50 µg respectively (50 µg was the highest dose used). JWH015 was equally effective in both repeated CP55940 and vehicle groups since no significant difference in withdrawal thresholds was observed between groups in any dose tested. As a result, the ED50 value [95% confidence limits] of JWH015 was not significantly different in animals previously treated with repeated CP55940 compared to animals previously treated with vehicle (Table 1 and Figure 8A). Vehicle (same paradigm as cumulative JWH015) did not modify the withdrawal thresholds ipsilateral to surgery (3.5±0.6 vs. 5.3±1.4 g before and 15 min after the last injection respectively, n=6) 24 hr after repeated treatment with vehicle.

JWH015 was also effective in reversing the L5NT-induced hypersensitivity when it was administered in a cumulative manner two weeks after the cessation of CP5940 treatment (washout period). In this case, the minimum and maximum effective dose of JWH015 were 2 and 50 µg respectively in animals previously exposed to CP55940 (repeated CP55940 group), and 10 and 50 µg respectively in animals previously treated with vehicle (repeated vehicle group). Similar efficacy and potency of JWH015 were observed in both repeated CP55940 and vehicle groups (Table 2). No significant difference in withdrawal thresholds was observed between groups in any dose tested (Figure 8B). Vehicle (same paradigm as cumulative JWH015) did not modify the withdrawal thresholds ipsilateral to surgery in the repeated vehicle group after the two-week washout period (3.5±0.6 vs. 3.6±0.7 g before and 15 min after the last injection respectively, n=6). The acute antinociception induced by JWH015 50 µg (plus vehicle, 17 ± 2.7 g, n=8) in the L5NT group was completely blocked by the CB2 receptor antagonist AM630 50 µg (2.4 ± 0.4 g, n=4, P<0.05).

3.5 Antinociceptive effect of a CB2 receptor agonist administered repeatedly in CP55940 tolerant animals studies

JWH015 injected i.t. for four consecutive days induced similar antinociceptive effects on all days tested in animals previously exposed to repeated i.t. vehicle treatment (for 5 days) and a washout period of two weeks. However, JWH015 injected i.t. for four consecutive days induced antinociception only on days 1 and 4 in animals previously exposed to sustained spinal CP55940 administration (for 5 days) and a washout period of two weeks. Repeated i.t. JWH015 was significantly less effective on the last three days of treatment in animals previously exposed to repeated CP55940 when compared to those previously exposed to repeated vehicle (Figure 9A). The JWH015 repeated treatment did not modify the mechanical withdrawal threshold in the contralateral paw in the repeated vehicle or CP55940 group, and the effects of repeated JWH015 did not differ between groups, except on day 3 when the withdrawal threshold was significantly higher in the repeated vehicle group than the CP55940 one (Figure 9B). Vehicle (same paradigm as repeated JWH015) did not modify the withdrawal thresholds ipsilateral (n=6) or contralateral (n=6) to surgery in the repeated CP55940 group after the two-week washout period (data not shown).

4. Discussion

The main findings of our study are: 1) the repeated administration of a non-selective cannabinoid agonist (CP55940) induces antinociceptive tolerance and tolerance to cannabinoid-induced neurological side effects in a rat model of neuropathic pain; 2) CP55940 tolerance persists two weeks after the discontinuation of cannabinoid administration; 3) prior induction of CP55940 tolerance reduced the antinociceptive effect of repeated administration of a CB2 receptor agonist (JWH015), but did not alter the antinociceptive response to acute JWH015 dose escalation.

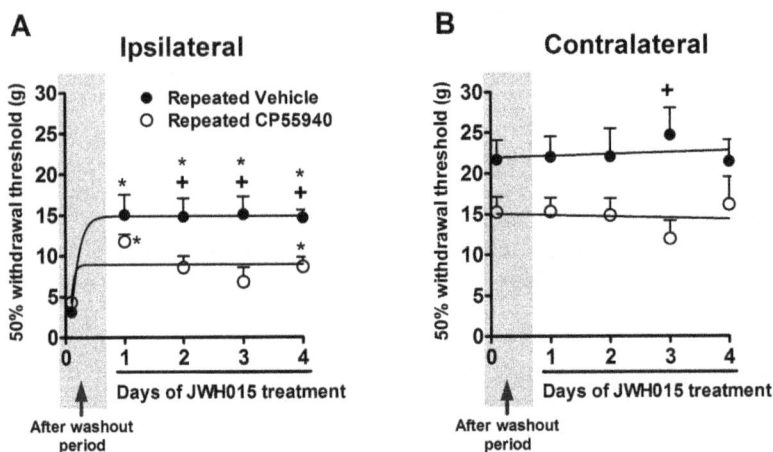

Fig. 9. Antinociceptive effects of repeated i.t. administration of JWH015 in CP55940-mediated tolerant animals. Paw withdrawal thresholds indicate responses to von Frey stimulation ipsilateral to L5NT (A) or contralateral to surgery (uninjured side, B) two weeks after the cessation of repeated CP55940 or vehicle administration (After washout period), and 2 hr after each i.t. injection of JWH015 during four consecutive days. Withdrawal thresholds on days 1-4 vs. after washout period data significantly differ by repeated measures one way ANOVA, *$p<0.05$ after washout period by repeated measures one way ANOVA followed by Tukey's multiple comparison test. Groups significantly differ by two way ANOVA; +$p<0.05$ compared to vehicle group by two way ANOVA followed by Bonferroni post tests.

We demonstrate that a non-selective cannabinoid agonist administered repeatedly at a concentration that induces neurological side effects (such as the effects that regular cannabis users seek for recreational purposes) is sufficient to produce a long lasting antinociceptive tolerance that persists weeks after the cessation of drug exposure. In agreement with these findings, diminished psychotropic effects (D'Souza et al., 2008) and analgesic tolerance to delta-9-tetrahydrocannabinol (Clark et al., 1981) have been demonstrated in frequent users of cannabis. This hypothesis has been further supported by a double-blind, placebo-controlled study demonstrating evidence of dronabinol tolerance in regular marijuana users (Bedi et al., 2010). It has also been shown that repeated administration of CB1 receptor agonists results in antinociceptive tolerance in naïve mice and rats (Gardell et al., 2002; Hama and Sagen, 2009), and that this tolerance is dependent on spinal cord mechanisms (Gardell et al., 2002). In contrast, we have previously shown that i.t. administration of the CB2 receptor agonist JWH015 effectively reverses L5 nerve transection-induced behavioral hypersensitivity without antinociceptive tolerance through at least five days of treatment (Romero-Sandoval and Eisenach, 2007). Similar findings have been described with another CB2 receptor agonist, A-836339 (Yao et al., 2009). Taken together, these previous findings suggest that CB1 rather than CB2 receptor agonism is responsible for the antinociceptive tolerance observed in response to CP55940 administration in the current study. Repeated administration of CP55940 also induced tolerance to a range of neurological side effects. We have previously observed that CP55940-induced neurological side effects are dependent on CB1 receptor activation, but not on CB2 receptor activation in rat postoperative and neuropathic pain models (Romero-Sandoval and Eisenach, 2007; Romero-Sandoval et al., 2008a). While these findings support the potential role of CB1 receptors in cannabinoid induced tolerance in our neuropathic pain model, CB1 receptor agonism does not induce antinociceptive tolerance in a spinal cord injury model (Hama and Sagen, 2009). Therefore, agonism of both CB1 and CB2 receptors may be required to induce antinociceptive tolerance to cannabinoid therapies in animals or patients with peripheral or central nerve injury.

CB1 receptor-dependent cross-tolerance among cannabinoids has recently been described between delta-tetrahydrocannabinol (the active ingredient of cannabis) and anandamide (one of the major endocannabinoids) (Falenski et al., 2010), and between 2-arachidonylglycerol (another major endocannabinoid) and the CB1 receptor agonist WIN55,212-2 (Schlosburg et al., 2010). This cross-tolerance is thought to be CB1-dependent (Falenski et al., 2010). However, we demonstrate in our current study that repeated administration of JWH015 exhibited reduced efficacy in rats with peripheral nerve injury that have been previously exposed to a non-selective cannabinoid agonist. This finding directly contrasts with our previous observation that repeated JWH015 reduces L5NT-induced hypersensitivity without signs of tolerance in the same rat model of neuropathic pain (Romero-Sandoval et al., 2008a). Taken together, these findings indicate that cannabinoid antinociceptive tolerance to non-selective cannabinoid agonists affects subsequent responsiveness of both CB1 and CB2 receptors. We also observed that CB1 receptors are predominantly expressed in neurons and that CB2 receptors are predominantly expressed in microglia in the spinal cord of both sham surgery and L5NT groups. Therefore, neuronal and glial interactions may contribute to the effects of CP55940-induced tolerance on JWH015's antinociceptive effectiveness.

Cannabinoid tolerance depends on CB receptor availability (Tappe-Theodor et al., 2007; Martini et al., 2010) and/or sensitivity (Jin et al., 1999; Selley et al., 2004). These receptor properties may change following peripheral insults such as paw incision (Alkaitis et al., 2010), peripheral nerve injury (Lim et al., 2003) or sustained activation by endogenous (Falenski et al., 2010; Schlosburg et al., 2010) or exogenous cannabinoids (Gardell et al., 2002; Hama and Sagen, 2009). In accordance with our findings, others have shown that a single intracerebroventricular dose of CB1 receptor agonists (WIN55,212-2 or ACEA) induces antinociceptive tolerance that lasts for more than 14 days through actions on the pertussis toxin-insensitive G proteins, Gz (Garzon et al., 2009). The mechanisms involved in long lasting CB1 receptor-mediated tolerance may also include the persistent cellular internalization or degradation of CB1 receptor (Sim-Selley et al., 2006). These data suggest that cannabinoid responsiveness and tolerance are shaped by a number of factors including type of pain or injury, exposure to endogenous or exogenous cannabinoids and receptor expression and sensitivity.

5. Conclusion

We demonstrate that a non-selective cannabinoid drug induces tolerance under neuropathic pain conditions, that this tolerance persists several weeks after the suspension of the treatment and that this tolerance affects the antinociceptive effects of repeated administration of a CB2 receptor agonist. These findings suggest that potential future analgesic drugs based on selective actions on CB2 receptor may not be a good alternative for long-term treatment in patients previously exposed to chronic cannabinoids. These results build on previous published data demonstrating that central CB1 receptor-mediated tolerance enhances tolerance to opioids (Trang et al., 2007; Garzon et al., 2009) and non-steroidal anti-inflammatory agents (Anikwue et al., 2002). Further research is needed to determine the mechanisms for this broad cross-tolerance among distinct drug classes. Additional studies are also warranted to determine whether patients with histories of cannabis or cannabinoid-based drug use for recreational or medical purposes demonstrate tolerance to common analgesic therapies.

6. Acknowledgements

Supported in part by grants DA025211 (AR-S) and DA11276 (JAD) from the National Institutes of Health (Bethesda, MD), and the American Pain Society Future Leaders in Pain Research grant. The authors declare that there are no conflicts of interest.

7. References

Alkaitis, MS., Solorzano, C., Landry, RP., Piomelli, D., DeLeo, JA., & Romero-Sandoval, EA. (2010). Evidence for a role of endocannabinoids, astrocytes and p38 phosphorylation in the resolution of postoperative pain. *PLoS One*, Vol. 5:e10891

Anikwue, R., Huffman, JW., Martin, ZL., & Welch, SP. (2002). Decrease in efficacy and potency of nonsteroidal anti-inflammatory drugs by chronic delta(9)-tetrahydrocannabinol administration. *J Pharmacol Exp Ther*, Vol. 303, No. 1, pp. 340-46

Bedi, G., Foltin, RW., Gunderson, EW., Rabkin, J., Hart, CL., Comer, SD., Vosburg, SK., & Haney, M. (2010). Efficacy and tolerability of high-dose dronabinol maintenance in HIV-positive marijuana smokers: a controlled laboratory study. *Psychopharmacology (Berl)*, Vol. 212, No. 4, pp. 675-86

Chaplan, SR., Bach, FW., Pogrel, JW., Chung, JM., & Yaksh, TL. (1994). Quantitative assessment of tactile allodynia in the rat paw. *J Neurosci Methods*, Vol. 43, No. 1, pp. 55-63

Clark, WC., Janal, MN., Zeidenberg, P., & Nahas, GG. (1981). Effects of moderate and high doses of marihuana on thermal pain: a sensory decision theory analysis. *J Clin Pharmacol*, Vol 21, pp. 299S-310S

D'Souza, DC., Ranganathan, M., Braley, G., Gueorguieva, R., Zimolo, Z., Cooper, T., Perry, E., & Krystal, J. (2008). Blunted Psychotomimetic and Amnestic Effects of Delta-9-Tetrahydrocannabinol in Frequent Users of Cannabis. *Neuropsychopharmacology*, Vol 33, No. 10, pp. 2505-16

Falenski, KW., Thorpe, AJ., Schlosburg, JE., Cravatt, BF., Abdullah, RA., Smith, TH., Selley, DE., Lichtman, AH., & Sim-Selley, LJ. (2010). FAAH-/- mice display differential tolerance, dependence, and cannabinoid receptor adaptation after delta 9-tetrahydrocannabinol and anandamide administration. *Neuropsychopharmacology*, Vol 35, No. 8, pp. 1775-1787

Jarduii, LR., Burgess, LL., Dogrul, A., Ossipov, MH., Malan, TP., Lai, J., & Porreca, F. (2002). Pronociceptive effects of spinal dynorphin promote cannabinoid-induced pain and antinociceptive tolerance. *Pain*, Vol. 98, pp. 79-88

Garzon, J., de la Torre-Madrid, E., Rodriguez-Munoz, M., Vicente-Sanchez, A., & Sanchez-Blazquez, P. (2009). Gz mediates the long-lasting desensitization of brain CB1 receptors and is essential for cross-tolerance with morphine. *Mol Pain*, Vol. 5, No. 11

Hama, A., & Sagen, J. (2009). Sustained antinociceptive effect of cannabinoid receptor agonist WIN 55,212-2 over time in rat model of neuropathic spinal cord injury pain. *J Rehabil Res Dev*, Vol. 46, No. 1, pp. 135-143

Jin, W., Brown, S., Roche, JP., Hsieh, C., Celver, JP., Kovoor, A., Chavkin, C., & Mackie, K. (1999). Distinct domains of the CB1 cannabinoid receptor mediate desensitization and internalization. *J Neurosci*, Vol. 19, No. 10, pp. 3773-3780

Lim, G., Sung, B., Ji, RR., & Mao, J. (2003). Upregulation of spinal cannabinoid-1-receptors following nerve injury enhances the effects of Win 55,212-2 on neuropathic pain behaviors in rats. *Pain*, Vol. 105, pp. 275-283

Martini, L., Thompson, D., Kharazia, V., & Whistler, JL. (2010). Differential regulation of behavioral tolerance to WIN55,212-2 by GASP1. *Neuropsychopharmacology*, Vol. 35, No. 6, pp. 1363-1373

Romero-Sandoval, A., & Eisenach, JC. (2007). Spinal cannabinoid receptor type 2 activation reduces hypersensitivity and spinal cord glial activation after paw incision. *Anesthesiology*, Vol. 106, No. 4, pp. 787-794

Romero-Sandoval, A., Nutile-McMenemy, N., & DeLeo, JA. (2008a). Spinal microglial and perivascular cell cannabinoid receptor type 2 activation reduces behavioral hypersensitivity without tolerance after peripheral nerve injury. *Anesthesiology*, Vol. 108, No. 4, pp. 722-734

Romero-Sandoval, A., Chai, N., Nutile-McMenemy, N., & DeLeo, JA. (2008b). A comparison of spinal Iba1 and GFAP expression in rodent models of acute and chronic pain. *Brain Research*, Vol. 1219, pp. 116-26

Schlosburg, JE., Blankman, JL., Long, JZ., Nomura, DK., Pan, B., Kinsey, SG., Nguyen, PT., Ramesh, D., Booker, L., Burston, JJ., Thomas, EA., Selley, DE., Sim-Selley, LJ., Liu, QS., Lichtman, AH., & Cravatt, BF. (2010). Chronic monoacylglycerol lipase blockade causes functional antagonism of the endocannabinoid system. *Nat Neurosci*, Vol. 13, No. 9, pp. 1113-1119

Selley, DE., Cassidy, MP., Martin, BR., & Sim-Selley, LJ. (2004). Long-term administration of Delta9-tetrahydrocannabinol desensitizes CB1-, adenosine A1-, and GABAB-mediated inhibition of adenylyl cyclase in mouse cerebellum. *Mol Pharmacol*, Vol. 66, No. 5, pp. 1275-1284

Sim-Selley, LJ., Schechter, NS., Rorrer, WK., Dalton, GD., Hernandez, J., Martin, BR., & Selley, DE. (2006). Prolonged recovery rate of CB1 receptor adaptation after cessation of long-term cannabinoid administration. *Mol Pharmacol*, Vol. 70, No. 3, pp. 986-996

Tanga, FY., Nutile-McMenemy, N., & DeLeo, JA. (2005). The CNS role of Toll-like receptor 4 in innate neuroimmunity and painful neuropathy. *Proc Natl Acad Sci U S A*, Vol. 102, No. 16, pp. 5856-5861

Tappe-Theodor, A., Agarwal, N., Katona, I., Rubino, T., Martini, L., Swiercz, J., Mackie, K., Monyer, H., Parolaro, D., Whistler, J., Kuner, T., & Kuner, R. (2007). A molecular basis of analgesic tolerance to cannabinoids. *J Neurosci*, Vol. 27, No. 15, pp. 4165-4177

Trang, T., Sutak, M., & Jhamandas, K. (2007). Involvement of cannabinoid (CB1)-receptors in the development and maintenance of opioid tolerance. *Neuroscience*, Vol. 146, No. 3, pp. 1275-1288

Wade, DT., Makela, P., Robson, P., House, H., & Bateman, C. (2004). Do cannabis-based medicinal extracts have general or specific effects on symptoms in multiple sclerosis? A double-blind, randomized, placebo-controlled study on 160 patients. *Mult Scler*, Vol. 10, No. 4, pp. 434-441

Yao, BB., Hsieh, G., Daza, AV., Fan, Y., Grayson, GK., Garrison, TR., El Kouhen, O., Hooker, BA., Pai, M., Wensink, EJ., Salyers, AK., Chandran, P., Zhu, CZ., Zhong, C., Ryther, K., Gallagher, ME., Chin, CL., Tovcimak, AE., Hradil, VP., Fox, GB., Dart, MJ., Honore, P., & Meyer MD. (2009). Characterization of a cannabinoid CB2 receptor-selective agonist, A-836339 [2,2,3,3-tetramethyl-cyclopropanecarboxylic acid [3-(2-methoxy-ethyl)-4,5-dimethyl-3H-thiazol-(2Z)-ylidene]-amide], using in vitro pharmacological assays, in vivo pain models, and pharmacological magnetic resonance imaging. *J Pharmacol Exp Ther*, Vol. 328, No. 1, pp. 141-151

7

Applied Radiologic Science in the Treatment of Pain: Interventional Pain Medicine

Kevin L. Wininger[1,2]
¹Orthopaedic & Spine Center, Columbus, Ohio
²Otterbein University, Westerville, Ohio
USA

1. Introduction

Accompanied by the work from innovative physician researchers and biomedical engineers who introduced new techniques and devices to expand armamentariums in interventional pain medicine in the 1990s and 2000s, the first decade of the 21st century resulted in a significant rise in the number of interventional procedures performed for pain management. For example, data from the Centers for Medicare and Medicaid Services shows a 518% increase from 1997 through 2006 in the Medicare population receiving spinal cord stimulation therapy (Manchikanti et al., 2009). Other examples include the efforts to design radiofrequency probes to target the sacroiliac joint and subsequently denervate this relatively complex but biomechanically unique structure with as little local tissue trauma as possible (Wininger, 2010); or the application of novel neuromodulation techniques to treat challenging cases of headache (Deshpande & Wininger, 2011).

The use of ionizing radiation for image construction (x-ray imaging) continues to be the standard in image guidance at many interventional pain medicine centers. Hence, the competent use of x-radiation not only benefits patients as well as physicians and ancillary staff in close proximity to the patient at the time of treatment—but from a health physics point of view also yields benefits for the general population given that recent evidence points to an overall increase in the use of radiation in medicine (Fazel et al., 2009; U.S. National Academy of Sciences, 2006). As of 2007, for example, medical sources of radiation represented the primary source of radiation exposure in the United States. Comparatively speaking, natural sources accounted for 3.0 mSv of the total dose, whereas medical sources accounted for 3.2 mSv (which was 5.9 times higher when compared to benchmark figures from 1980). The increase was primarily due to increased use of computed tomography (CT) and nuclear medicine studies. Note that medical sources were delineated as follows: 1.5 mSv from CT, 0.7 mSv from nuclear medicine, 0.6 mSv from radiography, and 0.4 mSv from interventional radiology (Johnston et al., 2011).

This chapter is intended to serve as a reference to help guide interventional pain physicians in their decision-making process concerning radiation risk management. In this context, the subject matter goes beyond the traditional emphasis placed solely on the cardinal rules of radiation safety (i.e., time, distance, and shielding) to render a systematic review of the different interventional imaging modalities used in the treatment of pain, namely fluoroscopy, CT, and ultrasound. Notably, we will center our discussion on the so-called "imaging (or 'viewing') chain" of each modality, and thus the issues surrounding image quality and signal processing relative to radiation exposure (or the lack thereof in the case of ultrasound imaging). Moreover, to develop a fundamental understanding of signal processing, key physical and mathematical concepts will be explored.

While this chapter is well-motivated allowing each section to stand alone, the subject matter is presented in such a way to promote continuity from one section to the next. We begin by focusing on fluoroscopic guidance; here analysis has been included to help establish benchmark radiation exposure for spinal cord stimulation procedures as first reported by Wininger et al. (2010). We then look closely at interventional approaches in pain medicine that utilize CT. Throughout these sections, ways to mitigate radiation dose will be considered, including recent steps to improve the shielding afforded by radiation protection apparel. Next, we provide an overview on ultrasound-guided pain medicine; here the tradeoff between spatial resolution and achievable depth of imaging is highlighted. Finally, future directions in image guidance for pain management will be surveyed, including non-ionizing radiation emitting modalities such as ultrasound imaging beyond regional anesthesia and interventional magnetic resonance imaging.

2. Fluoroscopy and interventional pain medicine

2.1 The fluoroscopic imaging chain

Overall radiographic quality is based on two principal properties, photographic quality (i.e., visibility of detail) and geometric quality (i.e., sharpness of detail) (Carlton & Adler, 2006; Bushong, 2004). Photographic quality is determined by density and contrast, whereas geometric quality is governed by recorded detail (i.e., resolution) and image distortion. In fluoroscopic image acquisition, the term "density" (a term derived from static film-based radiography) is replaced by the term "brightness" to be congruent with the language used to describe the visibility of images on a display monitor. The notion of an imaging chain makes reference to highly integrated instrumentation (together with the patient), regardless of the modality of interest. The fluoroscopic imaging chain denotes the x-ray generator, x-ray tube, collimator and filtration, table and patient, grid, image intensifier, optical coupler, and the image viewing system (Schueler, 2000). To this end, while each link in the chain is of equal importance, an understanding of fluoroscopic image quality relative to the image intensifier will be emphasized. The image intensifier functions as a "pass-through" device by converting x-rays to light (fluorescence) and then to electrons by way of its input phosphor-screen with adjoined photocathode backing (see Figure 1). This design effectively and efficiently reduces overall radiation exposure (Wang & Blackburn, 2000), and at the same time, allows physicians to dynamically view anatomy with a relatively high degree of resolution due to the total brightness gain. It is the ability to view dynamically with excellent image resolution – that underpins the role of fluoroscopy in many of the modern disciplines of medicine.

The potential for x-rays to penetrate an object (i.e., soft tissue or bone) and create an image is related to the quality of the x-ray beam as a result of the operating kilovoltage (kV) at the x-ray tube, and may simply be referred to as the "x-ray tube intensity," "tube intensity," or "tube potential." The amount of x-rays produced is related to tube current (in milliamperage (mA)) and time (in seconds (s)). Whereas the operator presets these factors in static film-based radiography, producing kilovoltage peak (kVp) and milliamperage seconds (mAs) upon exposure, this is not commonplace in fluoroscopic imaging due to automatic brightness control and real-time intended-use. Automatic brightness control is a type of automated "negative feedback" commonly set by most operators to ensure a proper amount of x-rays in order to image patients with thin to average body types. Because of its real-time imaging capability, extended exposure times are possible when operating fluoroscopy systems, and thus, the amount of tube current is substantially less compared to that used in static film-based radiography, 1 to 5 mA versus 100 to 500 mA, respectively (Carlton & Adler, 2006; Bushong, 2004). However, the physician has likely encountered degradation of recorded detail while using fluoroscopy due to a blotchy or grainy appearance that is directly related to an insufficient amount of radiation to create a uniform image (a phenomenon common to all electromagnetic imaging modalities) (Carlton & Adler, 2006). This is referred to as quantum noise or quantum mottle, as "quantum" means counted or measured. According to Carlton and Adler (2006):

> With fluoroscopy, the time factor is controlled by the length of time the eye can integrate, or accumulate, light photons from the fluoro imaging chain. Because this period is 0.2 seconds, fluoroscopy must provide sufficient photons, through mA, to avoid mottle. Quantum mottle is also a large part of video noise and is a special problem during fluoroscopy because the units operate with the minimum number of photons possible to activate the fluoro screen. The factors that influence mottle are those that affect the total number of photons arriving at the retina of the eye. This includes radiation output, beam attenuation by the subject, the conversion efficiency of the input screen, minification gain, flux gain, total brightness gain, viewing system, and the distance of the eye from the viewing system. Increasing the efficiency of any of these factors can assist in reducing quantum mottle, but the most common solution is to increase the fluoro tube mA.

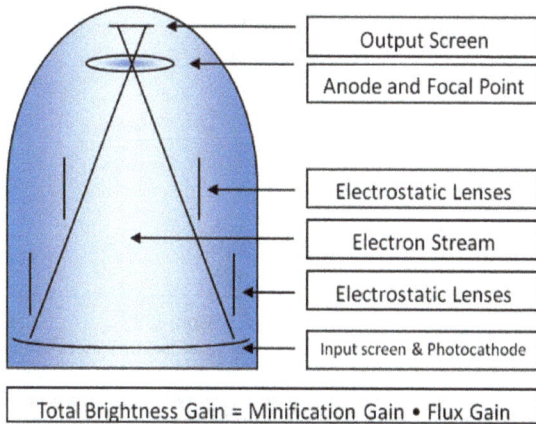

Output Screen

Anode and Focal Point

Electrostatic Lenses

Electron Stream

Electrostatic Lenses

Input screen & Photocathode

Total Brightness Gain = Minification Gain • Flux Gain

Fig. 1. Inside the image intensifier tube, x-rays photons are converted to light photons at the input screen and then to electrons at the photocathode. Flowing through the image intensifier tube the electron stream is repelled by the negatively charged electrostatic lenses and is attracted to the positively charged anode. Electrons are converted back to light at the output screen in order to proceed to the image viewing system. The output quantity of light photons is significantly greater than the input quantity of x-ray photons due to total brightness gain.

Image degradation from quantum mottle not only presents patient safety concerns due to challenges surrounding needle placement, particularly in patients with hypersthenic body habitus, but can also be a concern to the interventional pain physician and staff members inside the fluoroscopy suite, especially when team members are standing near the patient. We turn to x-ray attenuation physics to help us better understand this (McKetty, 1998). We see that in most fluoroscopically-guided pain procedures, the primary beam is directed at bony structures (i.e., material with a large content of calcium atoms, atomic number-20, which efficiently attenuates the beam) as opposed to soft tissues (i.e., material containing more atoms of carbon, oxygen, and hydrogen, producing an effective atomic number-7.4 and thus allowing more of the beam to transmit to the image intensifier). Moreover, Table 1 lists differences in the atomic numbers and densities of matter found in the makeup of the human body. It follows that in order to compensate for the attenuated beam within the field-of-view for bony imaging compared to soft tissue imaging, radiation output ramps up either as a result of adjustments to technique factors via automatic brightness control or by means of manual technique adjustments or activation of high-fluoro/boost mode by the operator. It is also important to note that most manufacturers incorporate an increase in mA during pulsed fluoroscopy to maintain equivalent image perception (Mahesh, 2001). With this in mind, a study on perceptual comparison between pulsed and continuous fluoroscopy concluded that the average absolute differences in the equivalent-perception dose is approximately 3% (Aufrichtig et al., 1994), where the equivalent-perception dose is defined as the dose of radiation in pulsed mode needed to give the visual equivalence in continuous mode. Thus, we find, importantly, an average radiation dose savings of 22%, 38%, and 49% for pulsed-15 frames per second, pulsed-10 frames per second, and pulsed-7.5 frames per second, respectively (Aufrichtig et al., 1994).

Matter	Effective Atomic Number	Density (kg/m^3)
Air	7.78	1.29
Fat	6.46	916.
Soft Tissue	7.40	n/a
*Water	7.51	1000.
Muscle	7.64	1040.
Spongy Bone	12.31	1650.
Compact Bone	13.80	1850.
Calcium	20.00	n/a

Adapted from Johns & Cunningham, 1983, and Dowd & Tilson, 1999.
*Note: x-ray output relative to the density of water serves as a baseline measure of x-ray output in the original design and calibration of x-ray producing systems as well as many radiation dose models, and may still be used to check system standards during annual physics acceptance testing. To this point, CT systems assign the number zero to water when calculating voxel/pixel brightness values (see Figure 6, CT Numbers and Hounsfield Units).

Table 1. Differences between matter in the makeup of the human body.

2.2 The physics of fluoroscopy
2.2.1 Primary radiation
When the x-ray tube is activated, electrons are "boiled off" from the wire element (i.e., a thin filament of tungsten) to form an electron cloud (see Figure 2). The wire element is strategically located opposite from the spinning target anode as part of a built-in concavity (of which the rim is slightly more negatively charged to concentrate the electrons in the

cloud) on the cathode. The number of electrons boiled off is directly related to the tube current. Occurring nearly simultaneously with tube activation, the electrons in the electron cloud are forcefully attracted to the target anode due to the potential difference between the cathode and anode. The rate of speed and the efficiency of attraction are dependent on the potential difference across the tube. When high-speed (incident) electrons strike the target, the change in kinetic energy produces only less than 1% of x-rays, with most of the change occurring in the form of heat production (99% or greater) (Dowd & Tilson, 1999). More specifically, x-rays are generated by two processes. The first process involves the interaction of electrons with the nucleus of an atom of tungsten in which the incident electron slows down to change direction (called bremsstrahlung, or "braking radiation"). Bremsstrahlung radiation is emitted from zero to the maximum energy (operating kV). The second process is a collision of the incident electron and an outer shell electron of the tungsten atom. The collision knocks the outer shell electron out of orbit (producing characteristic radiation). Characteristic radiation is the term used to reference the fact that the x-ray energy produced is related to the binding energy between the outer shell electron and the nucleus of the target atom, and is always the same for a specific target atom (again, tungsten in the case of x-ray production in fluoroscopy) (Dowd & Tilson, 1999).

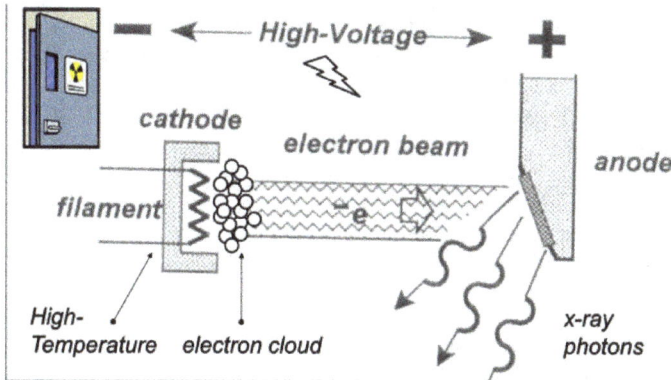

Fig. 2. A closer look inside the x-ray tube. When **tube current** is applied the filament heats up to boil off electrons into a cloud. X-rays are produced as the **tube potential** forces the incident (free) electrons to strike the target on the anode at a high-speed.

2.2.2 Secondary radiation—the patient as the point source

When x-ray photons in the primary beam pass through matter, they either pass unaltered (transmission) or undergo attenuation. Moreover, attenuated x-ray photons are either absorbed (all energy lost and the photon "dies") or scattered (some energy lost and the photon changes direction). The x-ray photons which are absorbed are primarily responsible for patient radiation exposure (via the photoelectric effect) and those photons which scatter are responsible for occupational radiation exposure (via Compton scattering). Note: when tube potential increases the photoelectric effect decreases *greatly* and the percentage of Compton interactions decreases *slightly*. (Dowd & Tilson, 1999). We will further elucidate the significance of the patient as the point source when discussing radiation risk management in fluoroscopy (or otherwise briefly stated, the occupational exposure due to secondary radiation emanating from the patient due to the interactions between the primary beam and the patient).

2.3 Fluoroscopically-guided pain medicine procedures

Nearly all interventional pain treatments and techniques evolved using fluoroscopic guidance. This was, in part, due to the capability of fluoroscopy systems to render high resolution images of bony anatomy (and adjacent tissues) to target pain generators. Today, with the versatility afforded by mobile C-arms (Tuohy et al., 1997), together with continued fidelity of the images rendered, the fluoroscope remains the principal modality for pain medicine image guidance. As a resulting consequence of this history, the literature not only contains several articles on the pros and cons of imaging techniques (for example, see Kapural and Goyle, 2007), but also contains multiple and diverse reports on radiation exposure associated with interventional pain procedures.

Notably, data collected on fluoroscopy time (the traditional metric used for clinical radiation management) serves to benchmark performance (Balter, 2006). While this parameter (fluoroscopy time) plays an essential role in the development of suitable registries to catalog radiation exposure levels according to the different pain procedures being performed, it may also be said that it is simply an awareness of this parameter by the physician that is inherent to optimization strategies in health physics (Shahabi, 1999). Table 2 presents the fluoroscopy times reported for the more common interventional pain medicine procedures using mobile multi-directional fluoroscopy systems (i.e., the conventional mobile C-arm). Other data noteworthy to collect includes: dose settings employed (operator chosen) and patient body mass. It is this additional information along with fluoroscopy time which may be used to calculate patient radiation dose received (i.e., entrance skin exposure). Table 3 shows fluoroscopy time as well as radiation dose using mobile multi-directional systems or biplanar systems for vertebral augmentation procedures.

Botwin 2001 2002 2003	*Wininger 2010	Zhou 2003	Manchikanti 2002	Manchikanti 2003a	Manchikanti 2003b	
–	–	–	13.2	8.9	12.5	Per Procedure
–	–	–	7.7	4.9	7.5	Per Patient
–	–	81.5	–	4.5	5.8	Facet Nerve Blocks
–	–	–	5.9	–	–	Cervical
–	–	–	5.5	–	–	Thoracic
–	–	–	5.7	–	–	Lumbar
–	–	50.6	–	–	7.5	Sacroiliac Joint Blocks
–	–	46.6	3.75	2.7	3.7	Epidurals
–	–	–	–	–	–	Interlaminar
12.6	–	–	–	–	–	Caudal
–	–	–	8.8	–	–	TFESI – Cervical
15.2	–	–	10.9	–	–	TFESI – Lumbar
–	–	–	12.7	–	–	Medial Branch Block
57.2	–	146.8	–	–	–	Discography
–	133.4	–	–	–	–	Spinal Cord Stimulation

*Wininger et al. also reported calculations on entrance skin exposure.

Table 2. Fluoroscopy time (in seconds) using mobile multi-directional systems.

Cullines 2003	Buszczyk 2006	**Perisinakis 2004	***Villavicencio 2005	***Izadpanah 2009	Thoracic Spine
522	216	609	81.3	175	Total Fluoroscopy Time
–	100	203	–	–	Total Patient *ESE*
–	32	–	–	–	*ESE* – AP Imaging
–	68	–	–	–	*ESE* – Lateral Imaging
–	–	3598	–	1245	Total DAP
–	–	2294	–	–	DAP – AP Imaging
–	–	1304	–	–	DAP – Lateral Imaging
–	–	–	–	–	Effective Dose/Minute
236	–	–	–	–	Physician Hand

**without or ***with 3D navigation in vertebroplasty or kyphoplasty procedures.
Fluoroscopy time (in seconds); patient entrance skin exposure (*ESE*) and dose area product (DAP, a calculation of stochastic risk for the patient [Vano et al., 2001]) (in centiGray); physician total and hand exposure (in microSieverts/minute).

Table 3. Radiation exposure associated with biplanar systems or multi-directional systems.

Inter-procedural variance compared to fluoroscopy times observed in Tables 2 and 3 may be attributed to differences in procedural techniques, level of experience, and/or physician preferences in imaging assistance, as well as attenuation physics relative to image quality. To illustrate this last point, we consider spinal imaging. During spinal imaging, two common challenges associated with image quality exist: 1) highly radiolucent vertebral bodies, particularly against the imaged lung field, creating excess image brightness in the region of interest, and 2) large body habitus with resultant poor image quality. In the former, tight collimation with the paired leaves shutters drawn close to the spine and continuous-mode imaging may help compensate for poor contrast resolution due to the vertebral bodies lacking enough cortical bone density to effectively attenuate the beam (i.e., low beam attenuation) (Johns & Cunningham, 1983). Subsequently, overriding automatic brightness control by manually ramping down tube current (mA) during tightly collimated bony imaging can help improve image resolution, especially for extremely radiolucent vertebral bodies. Alternatively, a manual adjustment to monitor/display window contrast may effectively improve image quality. To compensate for poor image quality secondary to large body habitus (i.e., a highly attenuated beam with resultant image granularity), it too may be necessary to operate the fluoroscope in continuous mode to increase the overall radiation at the image intensifier rather than disengaging the low dose feature. This strategy may improve image contrast while limiting patient exposure if a "manual beam on/off" operator technique is used, e.g., while panning or moving the C-arm between anteroposterior/oblique positioning to keep region of interest in the field of view.

2.4 Radiation risk management/safety

In recent years the assessment of radiation dose has received increased scrutiny; notably, the evaluation of deterministic effects, for which the severity of effects will vary according to the dose received and for which dose thresholds usually exist (e.g., radiation induced skin injuries) (Balter, 2006 & 2008). Moreover, dose assessment has seemingly evolved from an academic enterprise to a clinical endeavour. Direct influence on clinical practice is appreciated by The Joint Commission's recent decision to add unexpectedly prolonged fluoroscopic exposure to its list of reviewable sentinel events, as well as their suggestion to follow-up qualifying events with a period of over six-months to one-year to monitor cumulative skin dose (The Joint Commission, n.d.). While fluoroscopy time alone provides inadequate skin dose estimates (Balter, 2006; Balter, 2008), the evaluation of incident air kerma (x-ray exposure to the skin, previously referred to as entrance skin exposure) is possible by simplistic modeling (Balter, 2008; American Association of Physicists in Medicine (AAPM), 2001; Bushong, 2004).

In part with its approach to minimally invasive treatments and therapeutic procedures, interventional medicine is the one branch of medicine which, in its practice, is riddled with concepts that stem from physics. It may be further stated that physicians, even interventionally-trained physicians, may feel as though they are not able to translate applicable literature into everyday practice without possessing a doctorate in the physical sciences. For example, radiation dose models can be complicated as there exists many nuances when talking about dose, and the units of measure are not intuitive. However, both radiation safety and radiation protection are fundamental considerations for the interventional pain physician, and are equally paramount responsibilities in the interventional pain practice. In the view of the author, physicians who utilize fluoroscopic guidance will find that keeping radiation exposure, and therefore radiation dose, as low as reasonably achievable (given the acronym ALARA) is a challenge that is not insurmountable. This goal is achieved by exploitation of the principles unique to image acquisition in fluoroscopy, together with radiologic physics and applied radiobiology (Dowd & Tilson, 1999), and a suitable quality assurance program. Thus, by first laying out the conversion between the basic units of measure in radiation physics,

$$1\ R \approx 1\ rad = 10\ mGy = 10\ mSv$$

this section will strive to provide the interventional pain physician with information on radiation risk management which may be readily acted on and implemented.

Entrance skin exposure is the radiation exposure to the skin measured in Roentgen (R) or milliRoentgen (mR) at the point of skin entrance for the nominal patient (i.e., 30 cm from the image intensifier). The measurement is made without the contributions from scatter radiation. In compliance with physics acceptance testing, the fluoroscopic tube potentials (kVp) under automatic brightness control should operate at/or between 70 and 90 kVp with 3.8 cm of aluminum (~15 cm of water or acrylic plastic) attenuation material. This produces measured fluoroscopic exposure rates in the range of 1.0 to 4.0 R/minute for all magnification modes (fields of view) for continuous mode in the normal dose setting (AAPM, 2001; Bushong, 2004). The lower portion of the exposure range accounts for the largest field of view (least magnification), and the upper portion of the exposure range accounts for the smallest field of view (most magnification). The name of the quantity which corresponds to entrance skin exposure and which is recognized by the International Commission on Radiation Units and Measurements is incident air kerma (Balter, 2008), and the unit of measurement is milligray (mGy). (Note: 1 R = 1 Roentgen = 2.58×10^{-4} coulombs/kg-m of air at standard temperature and pressure, and 1 R = 8.76 mGy [milligray].)

The dedicated use of the low dose setting (which provides 40% or more dose reduction compared to the normal dose setting, Smiddy et al., 1996; Davies et al., 2006), when paired with pulsed fluoroscopy (which provides 50% dose reduction at 7.5 frames per second, Aufrichtig et al., 1994) promotes optimal radiation risk management. This impact is best observed by a closer inspection of the work by Wininger et al. (2010) on radiation exposure in spinal cord stimulation [trialing] procedures. The authors point out that although pulsed fluoroscopy was utilized differently during cases #3 and #43, the fluoroscopy time for each case was recorded as 198.9 seconds. Analysis between actual settings used and hypothetical use variances for the low dose setting and the pulsed mode feature, based on simplistic modeling, illustrated how fluoroscopy time alone may lead to inadequate skin dose assessments. In other words, analysis of incident air kerma derived from the actual settings revealed that case #43 incurred 39.4% more skin exposure than case #3. Hypothetically, if neither the low dose feature nor pulsed fluoroscopy had been utilized, the resultant incident air kerma (i.e., 38.7 mGy) would have approximated the actual estimates derived for fluoroscopy times greater than 300 seconds (i.e., approximately double) for this procedure (i.e., 25.7–43.7 mGy). However, because the earliest deterministic threshold is 2.0 Gy, the level associated with transient erythema (Geleijns & Wondergem, 2005), research indicates that induction of deterministic insults (such as skin injuries) is highly unlikely during interventional pain medicine procedures. *Rather, in interventional pain medicine, the prime objective is to safeguard to the degree possible (i.e., ALARA) against low doses of x-radiation (U.S. National Academy of Sciences, 2006; Little et al., 2009).*

With respect to quality assurance programs for fluoroscopy systems, it is important to address mechanical and electrical safety in addition to radiation safety and image quality. Moreover, such programs are particularly important for mobile systems due to the various uses and locations in which these units are intended to perform. Given that mobile units are often the more commonly utilized systems in pain management applications, a quality assurance protocol is essential. However, due to differences between mobile systems from the various manufacturers, as well the different regulations overseeing radiologic licensure in the various jurisdictions the reader finds him- or herself in, an outline of such program is beyond the scope of this chapter. The reader is, therefore, referred to Tuohy et al. (1997) who tackled these issues and made several key recommendations.

Reports on occupational incurred dose from scatter radiation are typically based on radiation exposure to standardized phantoms, thus representing the symmetrical ideal "small lumbar" spine. This methodology, however, may potentially underestimate the amount of occupational radiation exposure since body habitus does not always lend itself to symmetry and body size varies from patient to patient. Hence, Whitworth (n.d.) performed scatter radiation vector analysis on the lumbar spines of five cadavers to better parallel the general experience of the interventional pain physician and those team members inside the fluoroscopy suite. The study employed an OEC 9800 mobile C-arm with automatic brightness control engaged. Radiation exposure was recorded using Geiger Mueller techniques (measurements are shown in Table 4).

OEC 9800	mrem/hour	kV	mA
High Level/Boost Fluoro	204	71	3.9
Normal Dose	111	70	2.2
Low Dose	56	72	0.76
Low Dose + Collimation	15	74	0.82
Pulsed-8 frames per second	7	76	0.86

Meter set at 17 inches above the floor and 12 inches lateral to the image intensifier.

Table 4. Scatter radiation measurements: imaging the lumbar spine of a cadaver with 21.5 body mass index.

Four important concepts were drawn from the resulting data set, as follows:

- Scatter radiation is exponential with increasing kilovoltage (kV) and linear with increasing mA;
- Collimation reduces scatter radiation by 50% or more;
- Use of low dose reduces scatter radiation by 50-75%; use of pulsed mode reduces scatter radiation by 65-90%; and
- Scatter radiation drops 50% every 6 inches away from the image intensifier.

It is interesting to pair the data set obtained by Whitworth with a law in radiophysics which aptly describes the phenomenon of scatter radiation in a meaningful way: as kilovoltage increases the photoelectric effect decreases *greatly* and the percentage of Compton interactions decreases *slightly*. Thus, Whitworth actually observed the following. As tube potential (kVp) increases, fewer x-rays interact with tissue, and therefore less scatter is created. However, the scatter that is created has higher energy and is more likely to reach the image intensifier [or nearby dosimeter(s)] than to interact with the patient's body. This makes increased kVp a radiation protection tool that must be counterbalanced with image concerns (Dowd & Tilson, 1999). See Table 5.

Tube Potential Kilovoltage (kVp)	Secondary Radiation (The Patient as the Point Source)		Total Number of Interactions in 1mm Tissue
	Total Number of Photoelectric Effects	Total Number of Compton Scatter/ Coherent Interactions	
50	500 (50%)	500 (50%)	1000
90	165 (33%)	335 (67%)	500

Adapted from Dowd & Tilson, 1999.

Table 5. Effects of x-ray tube potential (kilovoltage) on secondary radiation generated.

In many interventional pain suites, "lead aprons" are the principal shield for radiation protection of personnel. In addition, it should be noted that a table skirt substantially decreases occupational radiation levels—since the majority of scatter radiation is produced under the fluoroscopy table (for fluoroscopes/C-arms with under-table x-ray tubes) in the form of backscatter. Thus, significant reduction to scatter radiation is gained from the combined pair, as each scattering incidence results in x-radiation energy levels of only 1/1000 of that prior to the episode (Dowd & Tilson, 1999). Moreover, largely as a consequence of complaints of back pain over time from the wearers of lead aprons (Christodoulou et al., 2003), lead equivalent aprons became the apron-of-choice among interventionalists, and recently, "lead free" aprons have emerged in the marketplace. Such alternative materials include tin, iodine, barium, and antimony, or any combination thereof. Such "lead free" alternatives offer significant weight reduction, compared to primarily-leaded aprons, and equivalent radiation protection (Finnerty, 2005) (see Table 6). As part of an occupation radiation safety program, it is suggested that the reader ensure annual inspections of aprons are performed and rejection criteria established. Practical rejection criteria have been offered by Stam and Pillay (2008).

It is known that the dominant hand of the interventionalist receives the highest dose of radiation. It is interesting to note that a new type of sterilizable, radiation protection glove (primarily composed of tungsten) was recently tested among surgeons during a variety of cases, including micro-discectomy (Back et al., 2004). In terms of radiation protection, results revealed that the glove was superior to all other gloves in the marketplace, attenuating 90% of x-rays (see Table 6), and radiation dose to the dominant hand was reduced to less than the dose received by the non-dominant hand.

Aprons (0.25 mm)		Aprons (0.50 mm)			
Pure lead	Lead equivalent	Pure lead	Lead equivalent	"Lead-free"	
Attenuation at 70 kVp					
95%	92% 89-95%	99%	98-99%	n/a 98.1-98.3%	Mean Range
Transmission at 70 kVp					
	8% 5-11%		1% 1-2%		Mean Range
Attenuation at 100 kVp					
85%	83% 79-87%	95%	95% 93-96%	n/a 93.2-93.9%	Mean Range
Transmission at 100 kVp					
	17% 13-31%		5% 4-7%		Mean Range
Gloves – supplier or *type, and quoted decrease at 80 kVp					
*Tungsten		Henleys Medical (3 STAR)	Henleys Medical (2 STAR)	Henleys Medical (1 STAR)	F&L Medical Products Co.
90%		65%	57%	32%	25%

Adapted from Back et al., 2005; Christodoulou et al., 2003; and Clasper & Pinks, 1995.

Table 6. Radiation protection apparel.

Risks of cataract development due to radiation exposure to the eyes have been investigated in interventionalists, with no conclusive evidence to date. However, the use of lead-based glasses is advocated, especially when the risk of "rescatter" (radiation which emanates from within the interventionalist's head, or so-called tertiary exposure) is considered (Cousin et al. 1987). As pointed out in a review on exposure risks of interventional pain physicians, studies demonstrate a decrease in transmission rates of 70-90% with appropriate eyewear ("lead" glasses) (Fish et al., 2011). Moreover, because it is the patient that is the point source of occupational radiation risk coupled with the proximity of the interventional pain physician to the patient, positioning the monitor to require the interventionalist to look 90° (from the patient) with eyewear with side shields could further help reduce eye exposure. As stated by Fish et al. (2011), "…It is extremely vital for the interventionalist to be cognizant of his/her surroundings. This reiterates the importance of increasing the distance between the physician and the source of the radiation, it also emphasizes decreasing the amount of exposure time, which can both drastically reduce unnecessary radiation via scatter."

2.5 Special report: Radiation exposure during spinal cord stimulation mapping: A new data set

Summary of Background Data: The increase in exposure to low-dose radiation from the growing use of medical imaging has raised concerns about cumulative dose among the general population (Fazel et al., 2009; U.S. National Academy of Sciences, 2006; Little et al., 2009), and accordingly, dose assessment has received increased scrutiny (Balter, 2008). Conversely, unique among implantable devices, some spinal cord stimulation systems utilize integrated technology to perform "electronic fluoroscopy" to assess device orientation (i.e., the leads) without irradiation (Kosek et al., 2006). Recently, however, a first look at radiation exposure from spinal cord stimulation [trialing] procedures was published to help benchmark radiation exposure reference levels for this procedure (Wininger et al., 2010). Although estimated exposure was negligible, data on patient size was unavailable and the source-to-skin distance (SSD) was not taken into account due to simplistic modeling.

Objective: To address the aforementioned limitations, radiation exposure was reexamined by the author for a new patient population.

Methods: 106 dual parallel lead spinal cord stimulation trialing procedures [using either multiple-independent current-controlled systems or constant-voltage systems] in the non-university, outpatient setting, from October 2008 to October 2009, were studied prospectively. Body mass index (BMI) measurements were retrieved. The *fluoroscopy system automatically tabulated total fluoro-time (in seconds) per case, and partitioned the absolute time- and the percentage of time allocated to- pulsed and continuous-mode imaging. High dose fluoroscopy, or "boost" mode, was not used. A study specific ‡personal dosimeter was worn by the physician. For the dose model, radiation output was measured with a §dosimeter/ion chamber located 30 cm from the image intensifier, along the central axis of an anteroposterior projected beam, and calculated based on the following equation.

$$ESE_{pat} = ESE_{pha} \cdot \left[\frac{O_{pha}}{O_{pat}} \cdot \left(\frac{SSD_{pat}}{SSD_{pha}} \right)^2 \right] \cdot t_{flu}$$

Where ESE_{pat} and ESE_{pha} are skin exposure to the patient and †phantom; O_{pha} and O_{pat} are radiation output for phantom and patient exposure (in Röentgens); SSD_{pat} and SSD_{pha} are the distances from the x-ray source to the skin for the patient and phantom; and t_{flu} is fluoro-time (converted to minutes). Note: incident air kerma is measured in milligray (mGy) and is converted from ESE_{pat} by applying a factor of 8.76 mGy to 1 Röentgen. Incident air kerma estimates were stratified according to SSD and low dose mode engaged/disengaged.

Results:

Total fluoroscopy time:
  Mean: 71.7 seconds
  (standard deviation: 34.9 seconds)
  Range: 19.5 seconds to 166.6 seconds

Percentage pulsed imaging:
    Mean: 33.4%
    Range: 1.80% to 75.2%
    Mode: 55.4% (compiled % most frequent)
Source-to-skin distance:
    Mean: not reported
    Range: 43 cm to 50 cm
Body mass index:
    n = 54 females
    Mean: 31.54 kg/m^2
    Range: 18.46-53.32 kg/m^2
    n = 52 males
    Mean: 29.65 kg/m^2
    Range: 17.03-42.45 kg/m^2
Incident air kerma:
    Mean: 8.33 mGy
    Range: 1.53 mGy to 32.0 mGy
Physician dosimeter:
Whole body cumulative dose: 73 mrem

Discussion:

1. Figure 3 shows the descriptive statistical summary for fluoroscopy time. Seven outliers were identified in each data set. Notably, less variance around the median value occurred with the new data (i.e., the interquartile range was reduced by 47.4%).
2. Accounting for outliers, total fluoroscopy time was normally distributed.
    * Figure 4 compares the grouped subsets—based on one minute intervals.
3. Mean total fluoroscopy time was 46.3% less (71.7 seconds compared to 133.4 seconds). However, it is noted that outliers from the previous data set had not been removed in the reporting of that data, and thus mean total fluoroscopy time for the previous data set was artificially inflated.
4. Percentage pulsed imaging was equivalent.
5. Patient radiation exposure was reduced: 1.53 − 32.0 mGy compared to 1.8 − 43.7 mGy.
6. Patient size ranged from mildly underweight to morbidly obese according to BMI (as defined by the World Health Organization, n.d.). The mean BMI, by gender, bordered pre-obese and obese.
    * Note: trending increase in body weight among the U.S. population paired with concern about cumulative dose trends (Yanch et al., 2009; Fazel et al., 2009) underscore the need to obtain accurate reference levels on radiation exposure, as such exposure will, in general, be higher for patients with greater body mass.
7. Estimates for incident air kerma were stratified according to various SSDs, see Figure 5.

Conclusions:

Radiation exposure from spinal cord stimulation trialing procedures remains negligible despite the likelihood, as suggested here, for this therapy to be used in a patient population with a greater risk for increased irradiation based on BMI valuations.

Acknowledgements:

The author thanks Siva Gopal, PhD, Otterbein University, for his constructive instruction in descriptive statistical methods.

Footnotes:

*OEC 9800 Super-C, GE Healthcare, Salt Lake City, UT, USA.

†Phantom: 3.8 cm of aluminum.

‡Badge report, study specific: Luxel, optically stimulated luminescence dosimetry, LANDAUER, Glenwood, IL, USA.

§Radiation meter – Model 1515 with converter model 1050U and ion chamber model 10X6-6M, Radcal Co., Monrovia, CA, USA.

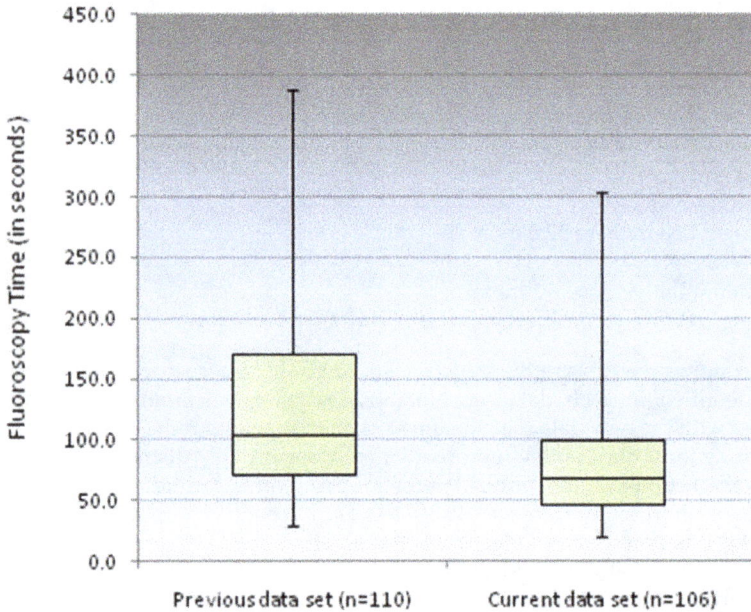

	Previous data set (n=110)	Current data set (n=106)
Interquartile Range	98.9	52.0
Lower Fence	-76.6	-30.8
Upper Fence	319.1	177.2
Outliers	321.1	208.9
	329.3	217.7
	336.2	236.3
	343.8	239.4
	373.1	294.0
	387.2	299.7
	387.4	304.0

Fig. 3. Box plots comparing previous and current fluoroscopy time data sets for spinal cord stimulation mapping procedures. Note: Because all data (both sets) were obtained from the same interventional spine team, inter- and intra- procedural variability was minimized.

Number of SCS trialing procedures / time intervals (fluoro-time in seconds)

⊔ Previous data set (n=110)   ■ Current data set (n=106)

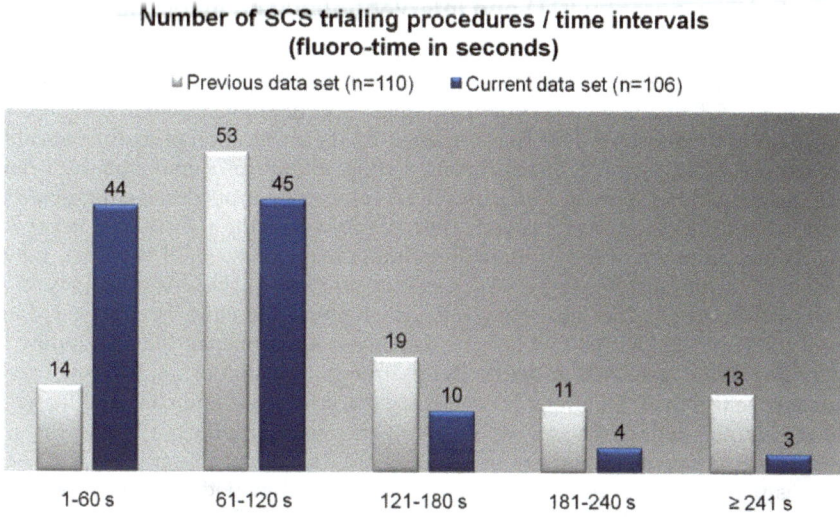

Fig. 4. Bar chart comparing the prior and new data sets with respect to fluoroscopy time during percutaneous spinal cord stimulation mapping procedures.

Skin Dose Model (adapted from physics acceptance testing)

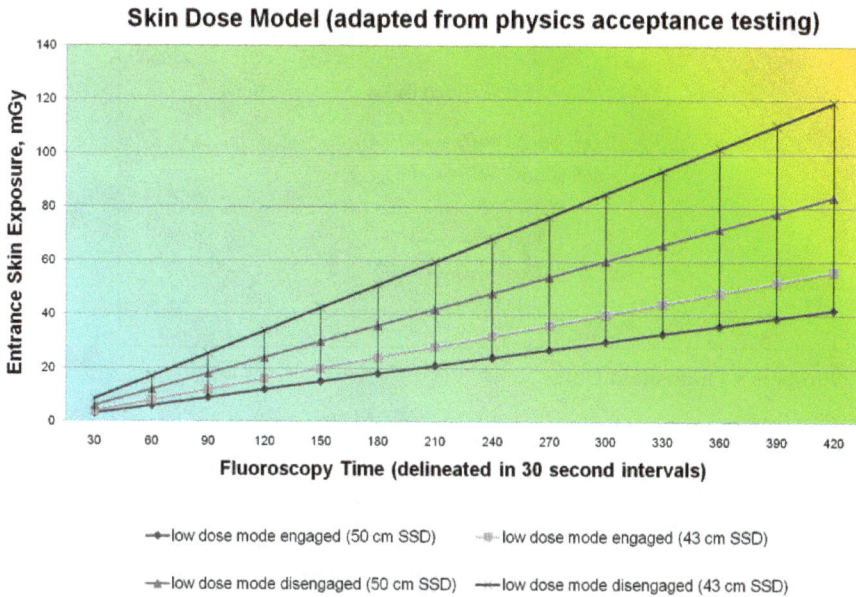

Fluoroscopy Time (delineated in 30 second intervals)

→ low dose mode engaged (50 cm SSD)   ─■─ low dose mode engaged (43 cm SSD)

→ low dose mode disengaged (50 cm SSD)   ── low dose mode disengaged (43 cm SSD)

Fig. 5. ESE_{pat} to anterior chest: 50 kg. adult patient accounting for one dose reduction feature, i.e., the low dose mode, either "on" or "off" for stratified SSDs (either 43 cm or 50 cm) in percutaneous spinal cord stimulation mapping. (Note: valuations represent continuous-mode imaging, no beam collimation.)

3. Computed Tomography (CT) and interventional pain medicine

3.1 The CT imaging chain

Although the underlying physical concepts are, for the most part, the same (such as x-ray production), the CT imaging chain offers a higher level of sophistication compared to the imaging chain of fluoroscopy. This is exemplified by the application of mathematical filters selected for a desired level of image reconstruction to control signal/quantum noise to optimize image quality (Sprawls, 1992), and most commonly applied using high-pass filters to control edge artifacts. According to Barnes (1992), while the CT scanner is capable of dividing its measurement of tissue attenuation into a range of 4,096 CT numbers, the eye is not capable of distinguishing this much detail in an image. The image display of a CT scanner represents only 256 levels of gray, which must therefore be mapped onto the portion of the Hounsfield scale that is to be displayed. Adjustments called "window level" and "window width" are used to define this mapping. Selection of the window level (i.e., brightness) specifies the CT number for centering the gray scale, and choice of the window width (i.e., contrast) defines the range of CT numbers over which the gray scale is to extend. These adjustments can be thought of as defining the "slope" of the gray scale. When the gray scale is placed at a window level of 100 and the window width is set at 500, the gray scale permits display of CT numbers from -150 to +350. All CT numbers below the lower limit of the window width are displayed as black, and all those above the upper limit are displayed as white on the image (see Figure 6).

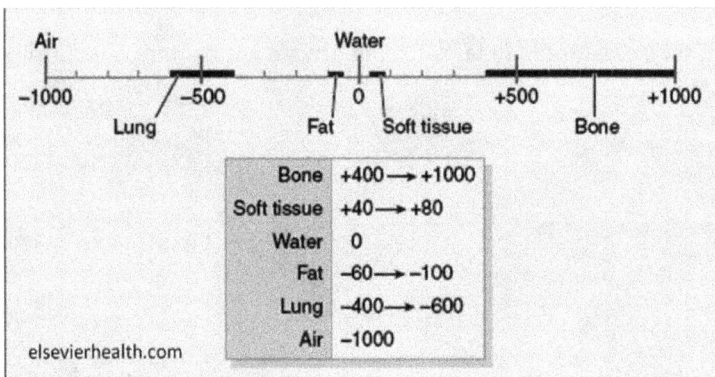

Fig. 6. CT Numbers = Hounsfield Units.

3.2 The mathematics of CT physics

The language of mathematics not only permeates all scientific study, but the very application of mathematics itself allows exploration to occur at the limits-of-discovery to find answers to questions that vex human nature. To this end, it is through a mathematical framework that physicists talk about dosimetry—with various selected examples on dosimetric methods in CT given in Table 7. Moreover, computational models for CT scanning enable testing of quality control algorithms to ultimately help reduce overexposure errors (Ferreira et al., 2010). This section will serve as a mathematical primer to highlight the physics behind image acquisition/signal processing of CT scanning to allow interventional pain physicians to gain deeper insight into this modality, and through this appreciation, demystify the process of CT imaging.

First Author	Title of Article	Citation: Journal Year;Volume:Page
Balter	Why (Continue to) Study Physics?	Radiographics 1992;12:609
Rothenberg	Radiation Dose in CT	Radiographics 1992;12:1225
McNitt-Gray	Topics in CT: Radiation Dose in CT?	Radiographics 2002;22:1541
Bauhs	CT Dosimetry: Comparison of Measurement Techniques and Devices	Radiographics 2008;28:245
Huda	Converting Dose-Length Products to Effective Dose at CT	Radiology 2008;248:995

Table 7. Select references on the physics of CT appearing in the journals of the Radiological Society of North America.

Although the subject matter on this topic is diverse, no truly rigorous mathematical justification of a tomographic algorithm exists (Shepp & Kruskal, 1978). For this reason a generalized derivation (that of inverting the Radon transform, as this is the widely accepted technique to describe how we recapture the information lost to attenuated x-ray photons) will be described in plain mathematical language. In addition, where noted, Wolfram *Mathematica* — the online computational engine, Wolfram|Alpha™ — was used to plot the traditional representative line equations of the x-ray photons. It is also important to note that in order to simplify the derivation the following three constraints will be made. First, we will ignore the playoff between Cartesian and polar coordinate representations, i.e., the 2-dimensional xy-plane versus spherical or circular symmetry. Second, we will not account for adjustments in the derivation for cone beam and/or fan-beam CT constructs due to their mathematical complexities (Note: the fan-beam third generation CT scanner, see Figure 7, is the most commonly utilized type of scanner.) Finally, discrete numerical analysis will not be

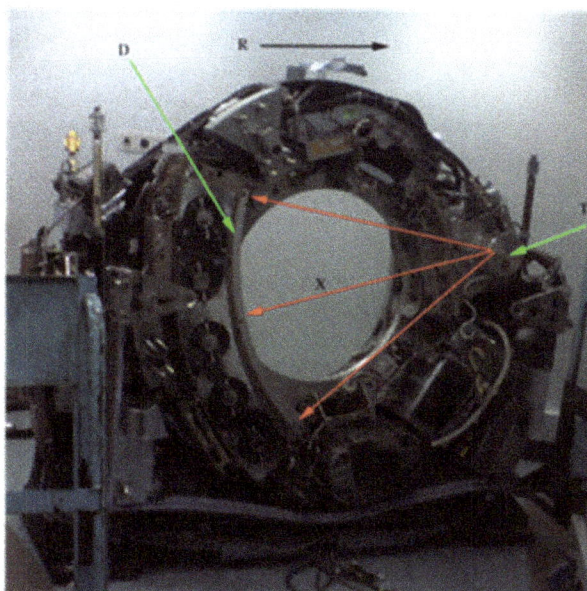

Fig. 7. Third generation "fan-beam" CT scanner.

addressed. To this end, the steps necessary to invert the Radon transform with respect to the parallel beam model (and thus most enthusiastically applicable to first and second generation CT scanners will constitute the balance of this section. It is the hope that such insight will complement the physician's knowledge-base when carrying out CT-guided pain procedures.

The set up

The underlying theme in this mathematical application is a signal processing challenge, and the set up for the analysis is straightforward. We have a 2-dimensional slice of a region of variable density (the patient), and the goal as applied to CT scanning is to reconstruct the resulting x-ray signal (the image) after repeatedly passing x-rays through the region at different angles of initial projection (the CT gantry). More concisely stated, we are measuring the resultant signal at different trajectory lines by accumulating (integrating) the signal after projecting x-ray photons through the region. Hence, the approach reconstructs the densities of the materials interacting with the x-ray photons (Johns & Cunningham, 1983), to ultimately assign density values according to the Hounsfield unit scale of CT numbers for data acquisition/image processing (Jackson & Thomas, 2004). Such modeling serves as an engineering template for trouble-shooting in the event of errors, such as equipment failure or computer algorithm failures, which may lead to radiation overdose of the patient.

Given that the approach resolves signal processing by means of calculating line integrals to recover the intensity of the x-ray signal (i.e., capture the data lost to attenuated or scattered x-rays), a comparison may be made to the inverse square law which estimates beam intensity from known initial conditions, the intensity of- and distance from- the beam (Carlton & Adler, 2006). However, the comparison is rudimentary at best because the central and interesting feature of the model applicable here, i.e., the Radon transform and its inverse, lies in the fact that we are *strictly* calculating the intensity of the exit/secondary beam based *solely* on a known intensity of the primary beam.

It is important to understand that the Radon transform refers to a special case of the Fourier transform; and the Fourier transform is a limiting case of the Fourier series (Boyce & DiPrima, 2005; Bracewell, 1986). This means whereas a Fourier series is the mathematical instrument used when evaluating periodic phenomena (Boyce & DiPrima, 2005), a Fourier transform is reserved for the study of phenomena that is nonperiodic (Bracewell, 1986). Thus, the choice of the application of a "transform" is an intuitively simple decision, given that x-ray photons in the exit beam strike the image receptor in burst-like impulses that are mostly nonperiodic rather than periodic in fashion. In mathematical terms, burst-like physical phenomena that are almost periodic are known as line impulses. *The concept of the line impulse will be a key point expanded upon below.*

The derivation of the mathematical model can be relatively easy to follow since the steps involved are pragmatic to imaging tasks carried out in the CT suite. We begin by a detailed inspection of representative x-ray trajectories relative to the CT gantry (i.e., the family of parallel lines), and then compare the suitability of two different proposed coordinate systems for the model.

Lines/family of lines

Refer to Figure 8 for a depiction of the CT gantry with the x-ray beam drawn as a family of parallel lines though the region. Each representative x-ray trajectory (i.e., the parallel lines) can be written in the slope-intercept form of a line.

$$y = mx + b \qquad -\infty < b < \infty , \qquad 0 \leq m < \infty$$

In this form, the coordinates of the lines in the xy-plane are the points (m,b), "m" the slope of the line and "b" the y-intercept. However, this coordinate system breaks down as "m" and "b" vary because the formula is not valid for vertical lines, such that a vertical slope is not defined (Larson et al., 2007). Therefore, a more suitable coordinate system is required to parameterize a line (and all families of parallel lines), and therefore, it is interesting to look at what a family of parallel lines may have in common (see Figure 9).

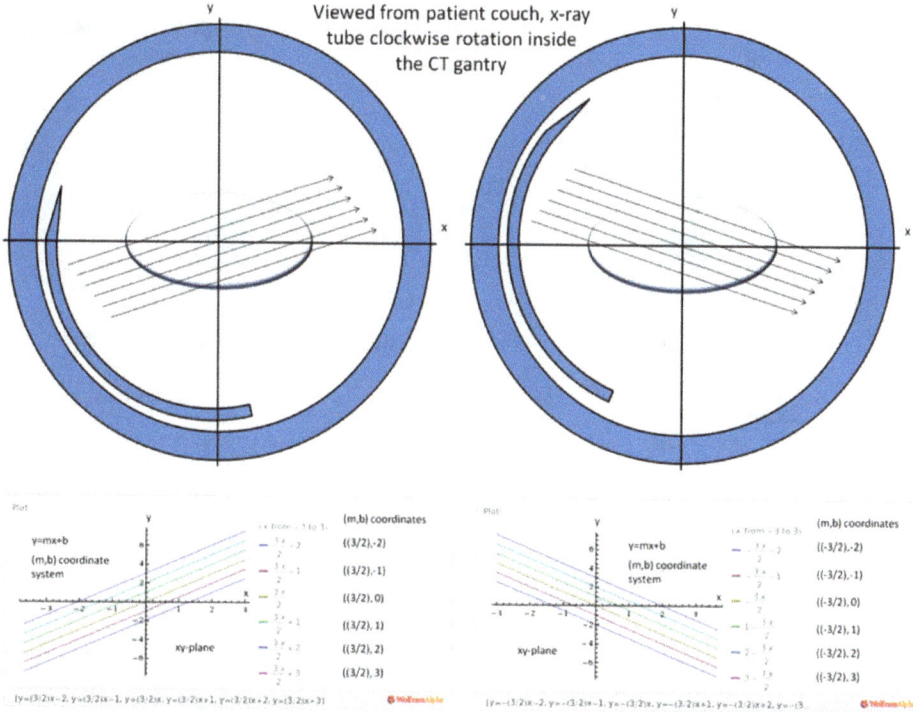

Fig. 8. (Top left) Gantry of CT scanner showing trajectories of x-rays [long arrows] emitted as lines/family of parallel lines. (Top right) Illustrated clockwise rotation of the x-ray tube inside the gantry. (Bottom left/right) Representative, corresponding line equations written in the slope-intercept form y=mx+b in the xy-plane. The (m,b) coordinates are given by the line equations.

Referring to Figure 9, one such identified commonality is that each line has the same angle to the horizontal axis, the x_1-axis. Thus, we will call this angle, the angle φ (phi). Specifically, it is the normal vectors of these lines that have the same angle to the x_1-axis. However, to better identify locations of lines, we need more than just the angle to the x_1-axis. To single-out a line we look at its distance ρ (rho) from the line passing through the origin (see Figure 9). Thus, with these parameters, the distance ρ (rho) and the angle φ (phi), we have successfully established an unambiguous coordinate system that is not flawed by the non-existence issue of a vertical slope. The *Cartesian equation of the line for the model*, is now specified by a given coordinate pair (ρ,φ) in the form:

$$x \cdot n = x_1 \cos \varphi + x_2 \sin \varphi = \rho$$

where both **x** and **n** are vectors, each defined in the following way, $x=\langle x_1,x_2 \rangle$ and $n=\langle \cos(\varphi),\sin(\varphi) \rangle$, and the line equation is derived by vector multiplication, in this case by using the dot product method, where it is said that **x** is dotted with **n**.

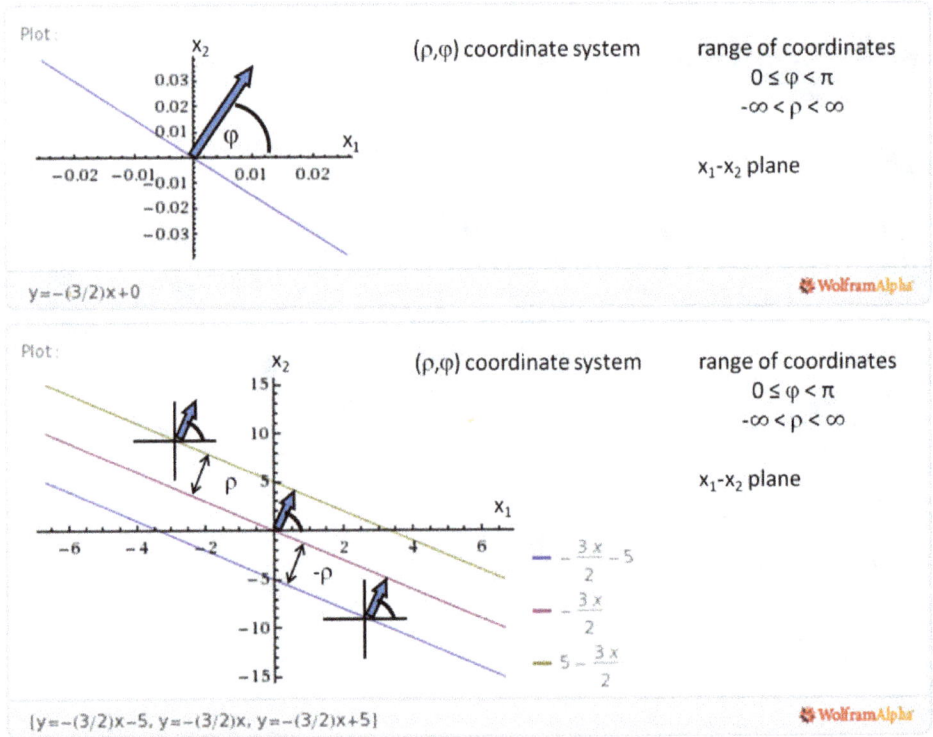

Fig. 9. A better-suited coordinate system (ρ,φ) for the model. (Top panel) Arrow demonstrating the unit normal vector associated with the line passing through the origin, and oriented with an angle phi (φ) to the x_1-axis in the x_1-x_2 plane. (Bottom panel) A family of 3-parallel lines and their unit normal vectors [arbitrarily placed on the lines] showing signed distances rho (ρ) from the origin [double ended arrows]. By convention, distances are positive [i.e., positive rho (ρ)] when measured *in the direction of the normal vector from the line passing through the origin to associated parallel lines*. In a similar fashion, distances are negative [i.e., negative rho (-ρ)] when measured *from the line passing through the origin to parallel lines spatially existing opposite to the direction established for the normal vector*. Rho (ρ) is zero at the line passing through the origin. (Note: the unit normal vectors are not drawn to scale, and when compared to Figure 8, the xy-plane has been renamed the x_1-x_2 plane.)

Line impulse

Accordingly, it is necessary to account for the nonperiodic nature of the signal concentrated along each trajectory taken by the x-ray photons, and this is accomplished by considering the line impulse (Bracewell, 1986). The line impulse describes the physical phenomena of x-ray photons striking the image receptor in the CT gantry. To define the line impulse mathematically, we first need to set the *Cartesian equation of the line for the model* to zero as shown.

$$\rho = x_1 \cos \varphi + x_2 \sin \varphi \xrightarrow[\text{set to zero}]{} \rho - x_1 \cos \varphi - x_2 \sin \varphi = 0$$

The resultant equation, specifically the left hand side of the new equation above, then becomes a function of delta, denoted by δ, on the right hand side (Bracewell, 1986).

$$\rho - x_1 \cos \varphi - x_2 \sin \varphi \xrightarrow{\text{becomes}} \delta(\rho - x_1 \cos \varphi - x_2 \sin \varphi)$$

The delta function δ, is the classical way to approach the line impulse, and has advantageous implications for dimensionality and integration of a line (Figure 10) (Bracewell, 1986). Such line integrals have a domain of infinity on the line and zero off the line (Bracewell, 1986).

$$\int_L \mu = \iint_{\mathcal{R}^2} \mu(x_1, x_2)\, \delta(\rho - x_1 \cos \varphi - x_2 \sin \varphi)\, dx_1\, dx_2$$

line impulse

The line integral, denoted by L, of the function μ (mu). The single integral is the 1-dimensional case for the line.

Integrating the function μ (mu) against the delta function δ concentrated on the line. The double integral is representative of a plane, denoted by R^2, the 2-dimensional case for the region.

Fig. 10. Expansion of the line integral to an integral of a plane (2-dimensional space) containing the line impulse. The above notations of the integrals, L and R^2, are understood to have domains or "boundaries" from negative infinity ($-\infty$) to infinity (∞).

The Radon transform

Equipped with a suitable coordinate system and having addressed the line integral with respect to the line impulse, we are ready to introduce the computational steps central to the mathematical model, inverting the Radon transform. As we do this, it is important to first point out what is varying as we work through the computations, i.e., to identify the variables associated with the integrand (those terms being integrated).

As shown below in Figure 11, superimposition of the useful/suitable coordinate system (as described earlier) onto a representative cross-sectional image (the region of interest) will help identify the variable.

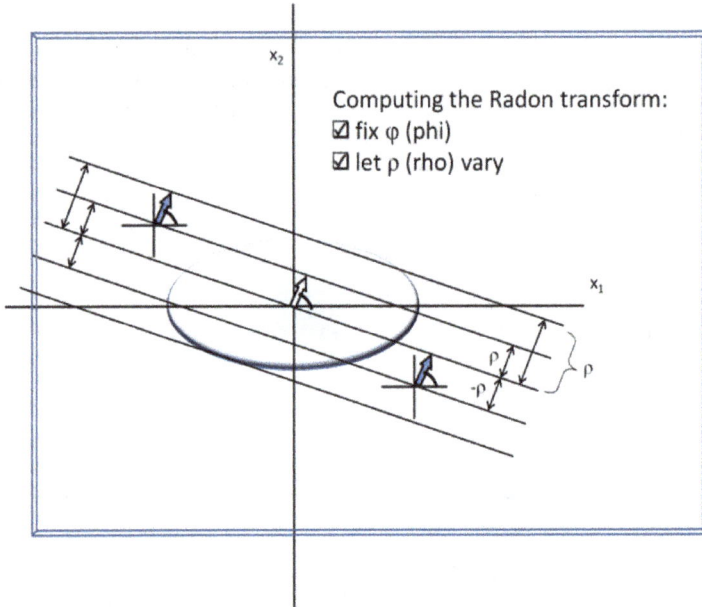

Fig. 11. Notice what this family of parallel lines has in common, each line has the same angle φ (phi) to the x_1-axis. Thus, the variable to use with respect to integrating the constituent integrals of the Radon transform (and those integrals contributing to the Fourier transform) is the distance ρ (rho) of a line from the line passing through the origin.

Looking at Figure 11, think in terms of what it means to fix φ (phi) and let ρ (rho) vary. This means the family of parallel lines will be defined by the angle made with the x_1-axis, and only the distance of a line from the line going through the origin will be of concern. In other words, the angle is fixed, it does not change, allowing ρ (rho) to be the variable as we accumulate (integrate) data. Thus, the Radon transform R can now be introduced by rewriting the equation from Figure 10 in greater detail (Bracewell, 1986), in relation to the signal/function μ (mu), where μ (mu) is a function of ρ (rho) and φ (phi), as shown below. *Note: in this and the remaining sections, the x-ray signal will be written as the function μ (mu).*

$$\mathcal{R}\mu(\rho,\varphi) = \int_{L(\rho,\varphi)} \mu = \int_{-\infty}^{\infty}\int_{-\infty}^{\infty} \mu(x_1,x_2)\, \delta\, (\rho - x_1 \cos\varphi - x_2 \sin\varphi)\, dx_1\, dx_2$$

Accordingly, both the line integral L and the double integral above are more concisely expressed here than that seen in Figure 10. With respect to the line integral, it is now written as a function of ρ (rho) and φ (phi), and the limits of integration (-∞ to ∞) are explicitly stated for the double integral.

As discussed earlier the Radon transform is a special case of the Fourier transform, thus it is accurate to write the Fourier transform F with respect to ρ (rho) (denoted by the subscript ρ) as a function of the Radon transform R, as seen in the following notation (Bracewell, 1986).

$$\mathcal{F}_\rho\big(\mathcal{R}\mu(\rho,\varphi)\big) = \int_{-\infty}^{\infty} e^{-2\pi i r \rho}\,\big(\mathcal{R}\mu(\rho,\varphi)\big)\,d\rho$$

The significance of this step is that we are now accounting for the spatial domain, denoted by the letter "r" in the complex exponential, $e^{-2\pi i r \rho}$ (Boyce & DiPrima, 2005). In reality, the derivation for this mathematical application (as we strive to understand it in the context of CT) is concerned with two domains, the spatial domain and the frequency domain, and moreover, both are present/available in the complex exponential, $e^{-2\pi i r \rho}$.

$$\mathcal{F}_\rho\big(\mathcal{R}\mu(\rho,\varphi)\big) = \int_{-\infty}^{\infty} e^{-2\pi i r \rho}\,\big(\mathcal{R}\mu(\rho,\varphi)\big)\,d\rho$$

$$= \int_{-\infty}^{\infty} e^{-2\pi i r \rho}\left(\int_{-\infty}^{\infty}\int_{-\infty}^{\infty} \mu(x_1,x_2)\,\delta\,(\rho - x_1\cos\varphi - x_2\sin\varphi)\boxed{dx_1\,dx_2}\;\boxed{d\rho}\right)$$

The right hand side of the Fourier transform $\mathcal{F}$ equality (top equation) contains the Radon transform $\mathcal{R}$ (underscored). It is subsequently rewritten (underscored) as the function μ (mu), as seen in Figure 3, to evaluate the line impulse delta function δ (i.e., bursts of x-ray phenomena). Then, the selected (boxed) terms are switched to rearrange the order of integration and evaluate the single integral first (illustrated below).

$$= \int_{-\infty}^{\infty}\int_{-\infty}^{\infty} \mu(x_1,x_2)\left(\int_{-\infty}^{\infty} e^{-2\pi i r \rho}\,\delta\,(\rho - x_1\cos\varphi - x_2\sin\varphi)d\rho\right)dx_1\,dx_2$$

With the terms now rearranged and grouped together, the equation is set up to integrate the 1-dimensional Fourier transform (the single integral in parentheses), in order that we may later deal with the 2-dimensional Fourier transform (the double integral) to recover the densities contained in the function μ (mu), along the line/family of lines (i.e., the information concentrated in the trajectories of the x-rays in the exit beam). **Note: the delta function δ remains in place, ready to be integrated.**

Fig. 12. Illustrative drawing to explain the way in which the dimensionality of the model is handled as the mathematical derivation unfolds.

Refer to Figure 12 which shows the critical steps on how dimensionality is dealt with in the model. The 1-dimensional component is evaluated first, as described in Figure 12, and is rewritten below in bold type face for emphasis, note the left hand side of the equation below.

$$\int_{-\infty}^{\infty} e^{-2\pi i r \rho}\,\delta\,(\rho - (x_1\cos\varphi + x_2\sin\varphi))d\rho = e^{-2\pi i r (x_1\cos\varphi + x_2\sin\varphi)}$$

We see that the integral equates to the complex exponential, $e^{-2\pi i r (x_1\cos\varphi + x_2\sin\varphi)}$, which is rewritten after distributing the "r".

$$e^{-2\pi i r(x_1 \cos\varphi + x_2 \sin\varphi)} = e^{-2\pi i(x_1 r \cos\varphi + x_2 r \sin\varphi)}$$

To finish simplifying the complex exponential, we introduce the concept of dual variables, in that (x_1 is paired with ξ_1) and (x_2 is paired with ξ_2), where ξ_1 and ξ_2 are each constants defined in the following way:

$$\xi_1 = r \cos\varphi \quad \text{and} \quad \xi_2 = r \sin\varphi$$

Although it is noted that each of these equalities above suggest implementation of polar coordinates (the coordinate system employed for spherical/circular symmetry), they are not intended to do so in this derivation. The equalities merely serve as a means to express the complex exponential more simply with dual variables, as follows:

$$= e^{-2\pi i(x_1\xi_1 + x_2\xi_2)}$$

It is now important to emphasize what has been derived thus far, and what computational steps remain. The above result is the answer to the evaluation of the 1-dimensional integral described in Figure 12 (that integral involving the line impulse, which has now been computed). The remaining computational steps involve the actual processes to recover the values of the densities μ (mu), i.e., to reconstruct the densities from the region, by inverting the Radon transform as a function of the Fourier transform over 2-dimensional region.

Inverting the Radon transform

To invert the Radon transform, we first plug the result of the 1-dimensional integral (as derived above and in bold type face below) back into the original Fourier transform which we set up earlier. This is shown below. We now have the 2-dimensional Fourier transform of μ (mu), i.e., the double integral, set up to integrate first with respect to dx_1 and then with respect to dx_2.

$$\mathcal{F}_\rho\big(\mathcal{R}\mu(\rho,\varphi)\big) = \int_{-\infty}^{\infty} \int_{-\infty}^{\infty} \mu(x_1, x_2)\, e^{-2\pi i(x_1\xi_1 + x_2\xi_2)}\, dx_1\, dx_2$$

Hence, to best convey the details of the final computation step, it is of certain benefit to pause in order to recapitulate the entire mathematical derivation up to this point.

1.   A suitable coordinate system (ρ,φ) was found.
2.   φ (phi) was fixed to let ρ (rho) vary, where φ (phi) is the angle that each line in the family of parallel lines makes with the x_1-axis, and ρ (rho) represents the values of distances of these lines from the line passing through the origin.
3.   The 1-dimensional Fourier transform of the corresponding Radon transform was found with respect to ρ (rho), resulting in the 2-dimensional Fourier transform of μ (mu).
     a.   In principle the problem is solved. We have measured the Radon transform, i.e., the line integral of μ (mu) along the family of parallel lines.
     b.   Because we know the 1-dimensional transform expression and the values which emerge, those associated with $\left[\,e^{-2\pi i(x_1\xi_1 + x_2\xi_2)}\right]$, we can now compute the Fourier transform with respect to ρ (rho) (Bracewell, 1986).

By computing the Fourier transform with respect to ρ (rho), we get the 2-dimensional Fourier transform with respect to μ (mu). This means that we can find μ (mu) by taking the inverse of the 2-dimensional Fourier transform of what was found:

$$\mathcal{F}\mu(\xi_1,\xi_2) = \mathbb{G}(\xi_1,\xi_2) \xrightarrow{recovers\ \mu} \mu = \mathcal{F}^{-1}\mathbb{G}(\xi_1,\xi_2)$$

where $\mathbb{G}(\xi_1,\xi_2)$ equals ($e^{-2\pi i(x_1\xi_1+x_2\xi_2)}$), the known values of the 1-dimensional Fourier transform. By taking the inverse of the signal/function μ (mu) (we recover the lost data contained in the trajectory lines of the x-ray photons passing through the region of interest), and we are able to reconstruct the densities of the region (Bracewell, 1986). That is to say, we now have μ (mu). *In turn, this enables the CT scanner to assign density values according to the Hounsfield unit scale of CT numbers for data acquisition/image processing* (Jackson & Thomas, 2004).

In summary, the goal of this section was to familiarize interventional pain physicians with the equations that ultimately underscore quality control algorithms for CT scanners and provide a footprint to build quality assurance protocols for CT scanning to help reduce risks of radiation overexposure. Accordingly, the derivation presented here represents the mathematical framework employing the parallel beam model. Ideally, to make the model practical, and to implement it numerically, discrete versions need to be rooted in the steps above, and certain computation issues, such as the playoff between Cartesian and polar coordinate representations, need to be dealt with.

Acknowledgements: The author thanks Stanford University Engineering for open access to EE261 The Fourier Transform and Its Applications as taught by Brad Osgood, PhD, as well as acknowledges John Labowsky for his technical critique of this section.

3.3 Triplanar imaging in pain medicine procedures: Conventional-CT guidance and CT-fluoroscopy

In the 1990s conventional-CT guidance began to be used by interventionally-trained pain physicians for chronic benign spinal pain (Aguirre et al., 2005; Gangi et al., 1998). During this period, algorithms were also developed to establish CT-fluoroscopy, which introduced a real-time feature to this modality (Daly & Templeton, 1999). Accordingly, CT-fluoroscopy has become a powerful imaging tool (Meleka, 2005). To this point, interventional pain techniques have been proposed and studied under this imaging technique, such as treatment of coccydynia by targeting the ganglion impar (Datir et al., 2010) or the efficacy of lumbar sympathetic blocks (Schmid, 2006). Interestingly, the literature remains sparse for pain procedure-specific dosimetry reports relative to CT, although Table 8 highlights the work in this area by Wagner (2004a, 2004b). In this light, the interested reader performing CT-guided pain procedures (or interested in being trained for such procedures) may wish to initiate dosimetry studies, since all radiologic based procedures should be evaluated specifically and the knowledge gained disseminated to help follow ALARA principles for patients and personnel radiation exposure (and hence, optimize health physics strategies).

3.4 Radiation risk management/safety

While CT-fluoroscopy may decrease patient absorbed dose by 94% compared to conventional CT (Meleka et al., 2005), others argue that the radiation exposure may not be justified, especially when other modalities can be used which eliminate the need for such exposure altogether, such as CT-guided (Thoumas et al., 1999) versus ultrasound-guided (Gruber & Bodner, 2004) pudendal nerve blocks. In cases were CT guidance has shown to be clearly beneficial, the lower doses associated with CT-fluoroscopy have been attributed to

148 Pain Management

intermittent exposure techniques and/or exposure parameters, such as lower tube current (Meleka et al., 2005). Moreover, strategies have also emerged to help reduce occupational radiation dose. For example, the use of lead shields, or as previously discussed, the use of lead aprons. In addition, the use of needle holders, when feasible during the procedure, avoids physician hand placement directly into the x-ray beam (Kato, 1996).

Kato 1996	Wagner 2004a	Wagner 2004b	CT-Fluoroscopy
			• Lumbar Selective Nerve Root Block
–	2	–	CT-Fluoroscopy Time
–	7.3	–	o Patient Effective Dose
–	390	–	o Effective Dose (Total) Physician
			• Lumbar Epidural
		Not specified	CT-Fluoroscopy Time
–	–	> 1	o Effective Dose (Physician/Procedure)
–	–	75	o Effective Dose (Total) Physician
			• Effective Dose (given in microSieverts per second)
1140	–	–	o Physician Hand

Key: CT-Fluoroscopy time (in seconds); effective dose (in microSieverts).

Table 8. CT-Fluoroscopy exposure metrics.

4. Ultrasound and interventional pain medicine

4.1 The ultrasound imaging chain

Continued research in the area of medical imaging has led to the development of compact and durable ultrasound scanners with improved imaging capabilities. Nevertheless, the basic instrumentation and underlying principles of this modality remain the same. The ultrasound imaging chain is considered a "closed" loop made up of the following links: a transmitter, a transducer, a receiver, and the image viewing system (Aldrich, 2007). Note that the physical phenomenon behind image creation is the piezoelectric effect, or stated more explicitly it is the effect on and induced by deformations of piezoelectric crystals embedded within materials housed inside the transducer which enables mechanical energy to be transformed into ultrasonic impulses—and vice versa for signal processing.

Upon interaction with tissue, ultrasonic waveforms may be 1) transmitted through the tissue, 2) undergo reflection (echo) or refraction (bending) at tissue boundaries, or 3) the acoustic energy may be attenuated. Surfaces that **reflect** these sound waves are classified as either *specular reflectors* or *scattering reflectors*. An example of the former is the needle, whereas an example of the latter is the interface between neural and adjacent tissues. Thus, it is the reflected sound waves (i.e., the available energy contained in the echoes collected at the transducer) which contribute to a meaningful image. **Refracted** sound waves are those which change direction due to slight differences at the boundary (i.e., edge) between two tissue types. We note that such waves may not contribute to successful imaging if a significant amount of the propagated waveform is lost. Finally, with similarities which evoke comparisons to the attenuated x-ray beam, the attenuation of sound beams conveys a loss of energy as the ultrasonic waveforms are absorbed by the tissue. According to Sites et al. (2007):

> While attenuation can have a profound negative impact on image quality, there are two important adjustments that can be made on the ultrasound machine that help to overcome

some of the effects of attenuation. First, most machines allow the operator to artificially increase (or decrease) the signal intensity of the return echoes from all points in the displayed field. This is accomplished by adjusting the gain control higher to increase the overall brightness. Second, most machines offer the operator the ability to control gain independently at specified depth intervals. This is known as time gain compensation. The time gain compensation should be progressively increased as the depth of penetration increases in order to compensate for the corresponding loss of signal intensity.

It is also interesting to note that *attenuation is inversely related to waveform frequency*, and that this relationship is nontrivial with respect to image resolution (i.e., recorded detail or the ability to distinguish between objects) and ultrasound physics. In the following subsection, which highlights the physics behind ultrasound imaging, we will further explore this relation to better understand the clinical impact of sound wave attenuation.

4.2 Waveform propagation in tissue: The physics of ultrasound

Based on waveform physics, that is, frequency, amplitude, and wavelength, the principles of ultrasound are unified by the foregoing description. A pulse of sound is emitted from a source (i.e., the transducer) and travels outward through a medium. If an object reflects the wave, then acoustic energy travels back to the source and is detected as an echo at the source. Thus, at a known speed (the speed of sound of the surrounding medium), the waveform travels a distance equal to twice the distance from the source to the reflected object (Kane, 2009). The basic equation follows:

$$L = (V_S \cdot T)/2$$

where L is twice the distance from the source to the object, V_S is the speed of sound of the surrounding medium, and T is time. Note: the average value of V_S in soft tissue is 1540 m/s. The ultrasound scanner records the time required for each pulse to return, and then uses the speed of sound to calculate the distance of the object. See Figure 13. Echo intensity is indicated by plotting a variety of intensities on the monitor subsequent to a gray-scale (white to gray to black). Thus, brightness is a consequence of a mapping of echo intensity versus position; hence this viewing algorithm/mode is named B-scan, where "B" means brightness.

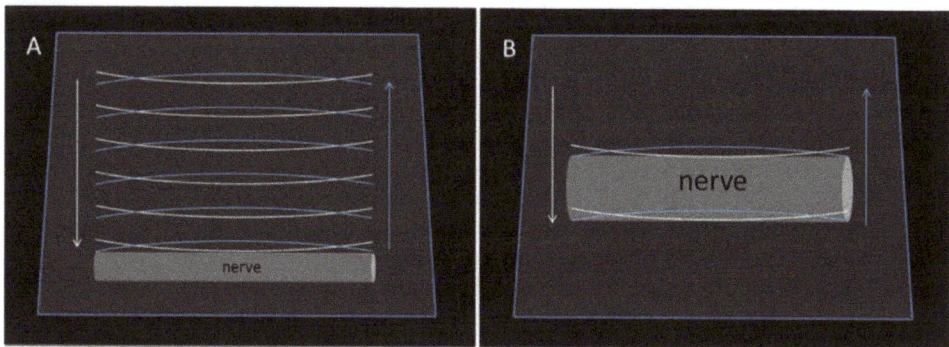

Fig. 13. Panel-A shows a target nerve (or scattering reflector) and direction of travel of incident sound waves (white) and echoes (blue). Panel-B shows a zoomed-in view of the same nerve to more closely exhibit the reflection of sound waves from near and far tissue borders (with respect to the transducer).

As emphasized in the above subsection, a nontrivial inverse relationship exists between attenuation and waveform frequency. We will now look more closely at this relation.

The most important aspects of ultrasound image resolution are those which govern axial, lateral, and temporal resolution—*in which all three together comprise spatial resolution*. **Axial resolution** is the ability to distinguish two structures at different depths, parallel to the direction of the ultrasound beam. Furthermore, it is approximately equal to one half of the ultrasound pulse length. In other words, if the distance between two objects is greater than one half of the pulse length, then the objects will appear as two distinct structures. It follows that higher waveform frequencies (short pulse lengths) produce the best axial resolution. However, because of the existing inverse relationship, higher frequency waveforms are more readily attenuated, and thus, tissue penetration is sacrificed. **Lateral resolution** is the ability to distinguish two structures at the same depth, perpendicular to the direction of the ultrasound beam. High frequency and focused ultrasound beams produce the narrowest beams, thus maximizing lateral resolution, but once again tissue penetration is sacrificed. Finally, **temporal resolution** relates to frame rate, and therefore, the ability to distinguish between real-time imaging and motion artifacts. During nerve blocks in regional anesthesia for example, motion artifacts occur with movement of the probe/transducer, or during needle insertion, or with injection of the anesthetic agent. Ultimately, temporal resolution is limited by the sweep speed (activation of the piezoelectric crystals) of the ultrasound beam, which in turn is limited by the speed of sound in tissue. Attempts to control temporal resolution consist of 1) increasing the sweep speed or 2) decreasing the scanning angle (applicable to phased array probes only). The first option decreases the lateral resolution, and the second option decreases the field of view. Thus, not only do we see an interconnected relationship with respect to image resolution, but at present, adjustments available to try to improve resolution are restrained by the laws of waveform physics. That is to say, despite the progress made in ultrasound equipment and technology (which we will highlight in the accompanying discussion on regional anesthesia), ultrasound imaging is, in reality, a tradeoff between spatial resolution and achievable depth of imaging (Sites et al., 2007).

4.3 Ultrasound guidance in pain medicine: Regional anesthesia

The use of ultrasound for image guidance in regional anesthesia has several practical benefits (Sites et al., 2009), the foremost being that ionizing radiation is not necessary for image production enabling ultrasound machines to be highly portable. Case series and small-scaled outcomes studies with respect to nerve blocks have purported shortened procedure times and faster block onset; increased patient satisfaction; and fewer block-related complications (Marhofer & Chan, 2007). As far as limitations, there are two primary considerations: 1) resolution and image quality vary inversely with depth of penetration, as previously discussed; and 2) needle tracking for in-plane needle entry is a challenge in part because the needle is not visible on the monitor (Marhofer & Chan, 2007). However, with respect to in-plane needle tracking, one company (SonoSite, Inc.) has developed an ultrasound system to remedy this problem. By sending out a "secondary beam" at a 45° angle from the transducer for perpendicular beam-to-needle alignment established outside the region of interest, needle visualization is optimized. This enables the physician to see the needle's approach to the target nerve within the field of view. In addition, to help improve therapeutic accuracy of ultrasound-guided pain medicine, the ultrasound characteristics of needles have been described (Maecken et al., 2007), "echo-friendly" needle designs have been developed (Deam, 2007), and the benefits of three-dimensional (3D) ultrasound imaging has been investigated (Teleglass et al., 2007, Foxall, et al., 2007). Moreover, cutting edge ultrasonic technological advances have introduced image-enhanced tissue staining to remotely palpate the target nerve of interest using acoustic radiation force imaging to both improve accuracy and limit variability in regional anesthesia (Palmeri et al., 2008; Nightingale et al., 2001).

4.4 Risk management: Ultrasound safety
While there are no known absolute contraindications in ultrasound imaging, the position of The U.S. Food and Drug Administration (FDA) (n.d.) concerning ultrasound safety follows.

Ultrasound imaging has been used for over 20 years and has an excellent safety record. It is non-ionizing radiation, so it does not have the same risks as x-rays or other types of ionizing radiation. Even though there are no known risks of ultrasound imaging, it can produce effects on the body. When ultrasound enters the body, it heats the tissues slightly. In some cases, it can also produce small pockets of gas in body fluids or tissues (cavitation). The long-term effects of tissue heating and cavitation are not known.

For a more in-depth discussion on tissue sensitivity relative to interpreting risk from exposure to ultrasound imaging, the reader is encouraged to study the report on this topic issued by members of the World Federation for Ultrasound in Medicine and Biology Safety Committee (Barnett et al., 1997).

5. Future directions in interventional pain medicine

5.1 *The promise of real-time three-dimensional (3D) fluoroscopy
While CT-fluoroscopy offers unique viewing perspectives with overall imaging capabilities (as discussed in the earlier section, "Triplanar Imaging in Pain Medicine Procedures: Conventional-CT Guidance and CT-Fluoroscopy"), interestingly, real-time 3D imaging has not been reported. Conversely, although real-time 3D ultrasound has been show to be beneficial in regional anesthesia (as cited in the above section, "Ultrasound guidance in Pain Medicine: Regional Anesthesia"), ultrasound imaging does not offer the allure that fluoroscopy enjoys with respect to image resolution, particularly of bony anatomy.

Technology is currently available to fit mobile C-arm fluoroscopy systems with 3D imaging capabilities (Stübig et al., 2009; Izadpanah et al., 2009; Villavicencio et al., 2005). (Note: current fluoroscopy systems creating 3D imagery are limited to $150° - 360°$ with mechanical orientation or manipulation or post-processing.) Notably, the limiting factor in the utility of these systems under most interventional pain protocols is image construction time. However, one company, Imaging3 Inc., claims to have developed signal processing algorithms to produce 3D high-resolution fluoroscopic images in *real-time* via its "Dominion" platform. (Note: at the time of this publication, this device has *not* received FDA clearance.) The design is built around a dedicated O-arm — a gantry similar to that used in CT — to allow continuous 360° rotation of the x-ray tube and scintillation detector with on-demand imaging of the patient under continuous or pulsed fluoroscopy. (See the earlier discussion on radiation risk management in fluoroscopy to review the advantages of pulsed fluoroscopy.) This approach is expected to allow imaging of the patient from any frame of reference or angulation. Intended use is anticipated by the company to be procedures in which multiple frames of reference are required. From a pain medicine perspective, real-time 3D fluoroscopic guidance may be possible for discography, vertebral augmentation, percutaneous lumbar decompression, facet rhizotomy, or intradiscal electrothermal therapy.

In addition, it is projected that the Dominion will offer a multi-modal feature to give physicians the ability to view cross-sectional anatomy by emulating CT, using a cone-beam CT model.

*Note: neither the author nor anyone known to the author has any relationship with any of the companies mentioned in this subsection. This includes but is not limited to financial, consulting, and business relationships. All information was obtained through company filings and/or press releases and/or marketing literature.

5.2 *Interventional magnetic resonance imaging (MRI)

This section presents a brief discussion on the concept of MRI-guided procedures. Whereas the use of MRI for this purpose is in its infancy, the intent of MRI-guided/interventional scanning is to assist physicians during intra-operative, and diagnostic and therapeutic procedures using magnetic-compatible instrumentation. The Fonar 360™ MRI unit represents the cutting edge in technology for this vision. The Fonar 360™ is a specialized MRI design with the field and gradient magnets encapsulated in the ceiling and floor of a dedicated, monolithic room. In this capacity, the enlarged room-sized magnet and the 360° access to the patient permits full-fledged medical teams to walk into the room (i.e., "inside the magnet") to interact with the patient. The first unit was installed at the Nuffield Orthopaedic Centre in Oxford, United Kingdom.

Another developer, MRI Interventions Inc., a medical device maker focusing on interventional MRI applications, has obtained FDA clearance on their ClearPoint® system which is designed to enable minimally invasive procedures in the brain—namely to facilitate image guidance for the introduction of deep brain stimulation leads—utilizing a hospital's existing MRI suite. On this note, although to date the use of deep brain stimulation for pain is limited due to lackluster outcomes (Levy et al., 1987; Coffey, 2001; Hamani et al., 2006), research is ongoing to find appropriate surgical candidates and areas in the brain conducive to long-term efficacy for conditions with a central pain aspect. Such targeted brain centers currently under investigation are the ventral capsule/ventral striatum in thalamic pain syndrome (U.S. National Institutes of Health [NIH], NCT 01072656). On another note, the introduction of deep brain stimulation systems with "steerable" field currents (the VANTAGE trial) (NIH, NCT 01221948) may ultimately prove clinically advantageous in such approaches to pain management.

Finally, our discussion on interventional MRI would be incomplete without reference made to patient care and concerns about biologic effects relative to exposure to MRI. Hence, we refer the reader to the collection of work by Frank Shellock. On this point, we encourage the reader to begin with Shellock and Cruse (2004) to gain an overview on tissue sensitivity associated with gradient magnetic fields, acoustic noise, and radiofrequency fields/radiation in MRI.

*Note: neither the author nor anyone known to the author has any relationship with any of the companies mentioned in this subsection. This includes but is not limited to financial, consulting, and business relationships. All information was obtained through company filings and/or press releases and/or marketing literature.

5.3 Ultrasound imaging: Beyond regional anesthesia

With ultrasound guidance for nerve blocks in regional anesthesia established, intriguing applications of this modality in pain medicine are beginning to surface. For example, ultrasound guidance for trigger point injection therapy has been shown to be comparable to electromyographic guidance (Boiwin et al., 2008). One advantage of this technique is that in the cervicothoracic area, the physician can see the lungs in order to guard against inadvertent procedure-induced pneumothorax. In other applications, the use of ultrasound was also recently documented as the modality of choice to facilitate placement of percutaneous leads in two peripheral nerve stimulation trialing procedures to treat ilioinguinal neuralgia (Carayannopoulos et al., 2009). This marked a new era in ultrasound-guided pain medicine, as well as technical improvement and refinement of a surgical technique. Likewise, image guidance with ultrasound in pain procedures traditionally reserved for x-ray producing modalities (fluoroscopy) have been reported. The evidence for this is gleaned from reports on real-time ultrasound-guided epidural injections (Karmakar, 2009), and even the introduction of current procedural terminology codes for transforaminal epidural injections and paravertebral/facet injections.

However, more compelling evidence for the versatility of ultrasound in pain medicine is found in its utility in pain-related physical rehabilitation (a role for this modality which is in its infancy) (Peolsson & Brodin, 2009; Primack, 2010; Wininger, 2010). It is well recognized that when musculoskeletal injuries/syndromes induce pain, use of the involved body part (such as the shoulder for example) becomes limited, which may in turn cause more pain and more limited use and a vicious cycle is started, possibly leading to physical limitation that negatively influences the quality of life of the patient. Alternatively, qualitative and quantitative description of musculoskeletal tissue dynamics and coordination during real-time procedures is possible through ultrasound imaging via tissue velocity imaging. This technique may be used to scrutinize both intra-muscular and inter-muscular coordination patterns (Peolsson & Brodin, 2009). Dynamic imaging using ultrasound to assess shoulder impingement syndromes is another example of pain-related physical rehabilitation ultrasound use (Bureau et al., 2006). To this point, it is noteworthy to mention that researchers have looked into how the overall utility of musculoskeletal ultrasound imaging impacts MRI. It was discovered that selective substitution of musculoskeletal ultrasound for MRI can result in significant cost savings to the health care system, but issues related to accuracy, variability, education and competence need to be further addressed (Jacobson, 2009).

6. References

AAPM. Cardiac catheterization equipment performance. (2001). American Association of Physicists in Medicine. Report Series No. 70.

Aguirre DA, Bermudez S, & Diaz OM. (2005). Spinal CT-guided interventional procedures for management of chronic back pain. *J Vasc Interv Radiol*, vol. 16, no. 5, pp. 689-697.

Aldrich JE. (2007). Basic physics of ultrasound imaging. *Crit Care Med*, vol. 35, no. 5, pp. S131-S137.

Aufrichtig R, Xue P, Thomas CW, Gilmore GC, & Wilson DL. (1994). Perceptual comparison of pulsed and continuous fluoroscopy. *Med Phys*, vol. 21, no. 2, pp. 245-256.

Back DL, Hilton AI, Briggs TW, Scott J, Burns M, & Warren P. (2005). Radiation protection for your hands. *Injury*, vol. 36, no. 12, pp. 1416-1420.

Barnes JE. (1992). Characteristics and control of contrast in CT. *Radiographics*, vol. 12, no. 4, pp. 825-837.

Barnett SB, Rott HD, ter Haar GR. Ziskin MC, Maeda K. (1997). The sensitivity of biological tissue to ultrasound. *Ultrasound Med Biol*, vol. 23, no. 6, pp. 805-812.

Balter S. (2006). Methods for measuring fluoroscopic skin dose. *Pediatr Radiol*, vol. 36, suppl. 2, pp. 136-140.

Balter S. (2008). Capturing patient doses from fluoroscopically based diagnostic and interventional systems. *Health Phys*, vol. 95, no. 5, pp. 535-540.

Boszczyk BM, Bierschneider M, Panzer S, et al. (2006). Fluoroscopic radiation exposure of the kyphoplasty patient. *Eur Spine J*, vol. 15, no. 3, pp. 347-355.

Botwin KP, Freeman ED, Gruber RD, et al. (2001). Radiation exposure to a physician performing fluoroscopically guided caudal epidural steroid injections. *Pain Physician*, vol. 4, no. 4, pp. 343-348.

Botwin KP, Thomas S, Gruber RD, et al. (2002). Radiation exposure of the spinal interventionalist performing fluoroscopically guided transforaminal epidural steroid injections. *Arch Phys Med Rehabil*, vol. 83, no. 5, pp. 697-701.

Botwin KP, Fuoco GS, Torres FM, et al. (2003). Radiation exposure to the spinal interventionalist performing lumbar discography. *Pain Physician*, vol. 6, no. 3, pp. 295-300.

Botwin KP, Sharma K, Saliba R, & Patel BC. (2008). Ultrasound-guided trigger point injections in the cervicothoracic musculature: a new and unreported technique. *Pain Physician*, vol. 11, no. 6, pp. 885-889.

Boyce WE, DiPrima RC. (2005). *Elementary Differential Equations*. 8th ed. John Wiley & Sons, Inc; Hoboken, NJ.

Bracewell RN. (1986). *The Fourier Transform and Its Applications*. 3rd ed. McGraw Hill. Singapore.

Bureau NJ, Beauchamp M, Cardinal E, & Brassard P. (2006). Dynamic sonography evaluation of shoulder impingement syndrome. *AJR Am J Roentgenol*, vo. 187, no. 1, pp. 216-220.

Bushong SC. (2004). Radiation protection procedures. In: Bushong SC, ed. *Radiologic Science for Technologists: Physics, Biology, and Protection*. 8th ed. pp. 583-601, Mosby Inc., St. Louis, Mo.

Carayannopoulos A, Beasley R, & Sites B. (2009). Facilitation of percutaneous trial lead placement with ultrasound guidance for peripheral nerve stimulation trial of ilioinguinal neuralgia: a technical note. *Neuromodulation*, vol. 12, no. 4, pp. 296-301.

Carlton RR, Adler AM. (2006). *Principles of Radiographic Imaging: An Art and a Science*. 4th ed. Clifton Park, NY: Thomson Delmar.

Clasper JC, Pinks T. (1995). Technical note: an assessment of x-ray protective gloves. *Br J Radiol*, vol. 68, no. 812, pp. 917-919.

Christodoulou EG, Goodsitt MM, Larson SC, Darner KL, Satti J, & Chan HP. (2003). Evaluation of the transmitted exposure through lead equivalent aprons in a radiology department, including the contribution from backscatter. *Med Phys*, vol. 30, no. 6, pp. 1033-1038.

Coffey RJ. (2001). Deep brain stimulation for chronic pain: results of two multicenter trials and a structured review. *Pain Med*, vol. 2, no. 3, pp. 183-192.

Cousin AJ, Lawdahl RB, Chakraborty DP, & Koehler RE. (1987). The case for radioprotective eyewear/facewear. Practical implications and suggestions. *Invest Radiol*, vol. 22, no. 8, pp. 688-692.

Daly B, Templeton PA. (1999). Real-time CT fluoroscopy: evolution of an interventional tool. *Radiology*, vol. 211, no. 2, pp. 309-315.

Datir A, Connell D. (2010). CT-guided injection for ganglion impar blockade: a radiological approach to the management of coccydynia. *Clin Radiol*, vol. 65, no. 1, pp. 21-25.

Davies AG, Cowen AR. Kengyelics SM, et al. (2006). X-ray dose reduction in fluoroscopically guided electrophysiology procedures. *PACE*, vol. 29, no. 3, pp. 262-271.

Deam RK, Kluger R, Barrington MJ, & McCutcheon CA. (2007). Investigation of a new echogenic needle for use with ultrasound peripheral nerve blocks. *Anaesth Intensive Care*, vol. 35, no. 4, pp. 582-586.

Deshpande KK, Wininger KL. (2011). Feasibility of combined epicranial temporal and occipital neurostimulation: treatment of a challenging case of headache. *Pain Physician*, vol. 14, no. 1, pp. 37-44.

Dowd SB, Tilson ER. (1999). *Practical Radiation Protection and Applied Radiobiology.* 2nd ed. Philadelphia, Pa: Saunders.

Fazel R, Krumholz HM, Wang Y, et al. (2009). Exposure to low-dose ionizing radiation from medical imaging procedures. *N Eng J Med*, vol. 361, no. 9, pp. 849-857.

Feinglass NG, Clendenen SR, Torp KD, Wang RD, Castello R, & Greengrass RA. (2007). Real-time three-dimensional ultrasound for continuous popliteal blockade: a case report and image description. *Anesth Analg*, vol. 105, no. 1, pp. 272-274.

Ferreira CC, Galvão LA, Veira JW, Maia AF. (2010). Validation of an exposure computational model to computed tomography. *Brazilian Journal of Physics Médica*, vol. 4, no. 1, pp. 19-22.

Finnerty M, Brennan PC. (2005). Protective aprons in imaging departments: manufacturer stated lead equivalence values require validation. *Eur Radiol*, vol. 15, no. 7, pp. 1477-1484.

Fish DE, Kim A, Ornelas C, Song S, & Pangarkar S. The risks of radiation exposure to the eyes of the interventional pain physician. *Radiology Research and Practice*, vol. 2011. Article ID 609537, 5 pages, 2011. doi:10.1155/2011/609537.

Foxall GL, Hardman JG, Bedforth NM. (2007). Three-dimensional, multiplanar, ultrasound-guided, radial nerve block. *Reg Anesth Pain Med*, vol. 32, no. 6, pp. 516-521.

Gangi A, Dietemann JL, Mortazavi R, Pfleger D, Kauff C, & Roy C. (1998). CT-guided Interventional procedures for pain management in the lumbosacral spine. *Radiographics*, vol. 18, no. 3, pp. 621-633.

Geleijns J, Wondergem J. (2005). X-ray imaging and the skin: Radiation biology, patient dosimetry and observed effects. *Rad Prot Dos*, vol. 114, no. 1-3, pp. 121-125.

Kapural L, Goyle A. (2007). Imaging for provocative discography and minimally invasive percutaneous procedures for treatment of discogenic lower back pain. *Tech Reg Anesth Pain Manag*, vol. 11, no. 2, pp. 73-80.

Gruber H, Bodner G. (2004). Why CT guided? [comment]. *AJR Am J Roentgenol*, vol. 182, no. 3, p. 824.

Hamani C, Schwalb JM, Rezai AR, Dostrovsky JO, Davis KD, Lozano AM. (2006). Deep brain stimulation for chronic neuropathic pain: long-term outcome and the incidence of insertional effect. *Pain*, vol. 125, no. 1, pp. 188-196.

Izadpanah K, Konrad G, Südkamp NP, & Oberst M. (2009). Computer navigation in balloon kyphoplasty reduces the intraoperative radiation exposure. *Spine*, vol. 34, no. 12, pp. 1325-1329.

Jackson S, Thomas R. (2004). Introduction to CT physics. *Cross-Sectional Imaging Made Easy.* p. 7, Churchill Livingston; Edinburgh, Scotland. 2004.

Jacobson JA. (2009). Musculoskeletal ultrasound: focused impact on MRI. *AJR Am J Roentgenol*, vol. 193, no. 3, pp. 619-627.

Johns HE, Cunningham JR. (1983). The interaction of ionizing radiation with matter. In: *The Physics of Radiology.* 4th ed. pp. 133-164, Thomas, Springfield, IL.

Johnston J, Killion JB, Vealé B, & Comello R. (2011). U.S. technologists' radiation exposure perceptions and practices. *Radiol Technol*, vol. 82, no. 4, pp. 311-320.

Kallmes DF, O E, Roy SS, et al. (2003). Radiation dose to the operator during vertebroplasty: prospective comparison of the use of 1-cc syringes versus an injection device. *AJNR Am J Neuroradiol*, vol. 24, no. 6, pp. 1257-1260.

Kane SA. (2009). *Introduction to Physics in Modern Medicine*. 2nd ed. Boca Raton, Fl: CRC Press.

Karmaka MK, Li X, Ho AM, Kwok WH, & Chui PT. (2009). Real-time ultrasound-guided paramedian epidural access: evaluation of a novel in-plane technique. *Br J Anaesth*, vol. 102, no. 6, pp. 845-854.

Kato R, Katada K, Anno H, Suzuki S, Ida Y, Koga S. (1996). Radiation dosimetry at CT fluoroscopy: physician's hand dose and development of needle holders. *Radiology*, vol. 201, no. 2, pp. 576-578.

Kosek P, Morgan D, Dunn J, et al. Electronically generated lead (EGL) scan: report of first clinical use. [abstract]. *North American Neuromodulation Society*. Dec. 7-9, 2006.

Levy RM, Lamb S, & Adams JE. (1987). Treatment of chronic pain by deep brain stimulation: long term follow-up and review of the literature. *Neurosurgery*, vol. 21, no. 6, pp. 885-893.

Larson R, Hostetler B, & Edwards BH. (2007). Calculus: Early Transcendental Functions. 4th ed. Houghton Mifflin Company; Boston, MA.

Little MP, Wakeford R, Tawn EJ, Bouffler SD, & Berrington de Gonzalez A. (2009). Risks associated with low doses and low dose rates of ionizing radiation: why linearity may be (almost) the best we can do. *Radiology*, vol. 251, no. 1, pp. 6-12.

Maecken T, Zenz M, & Grau T. (2007). Ultrasound characteristics of needles for regional anesthesia. *Reg Anesth Pain Med*, vol. 32, no. 5, pp. 440-447.

Mahesh M. (2001). Fluoroscopy: patient radiation exposure issues. *Radiographics*, vol. 21, no. 4, pp. 1033-1045.

Manchikanti L, Cash KA, Moss TL, & Pampati V. (2002). Radiation exposure to the physician in interventional pain management. *Pain Physician*, vol. 5, no. 4, pp. 385-393.

Manchikanti L, Cash KA, Moss TL, & Pampati V. (2003a). Effectiveness of protective measures in reducing risk of radiation exposure in interventional pain management: a prospective study. *Pain Physician*, vol. 6, no. 3, pp. 301-305.

Manchikanti L, Cash KA, Moss TL, Rivera J, & Pampati V. (2003b). Risk of whole body radiation exposure and protection measures in fluoroscopically guided interventional techniques: a prospective evaluation. *BMC Anesthesiol*, vol. 3, no. 1, p. 2.

Manchikanti L, Singh V, Pampati V, Smith HS, & Hirsch J. (2009). Analysis of growth of interventional techniques in managing chronic pain in the Medicare population: A 10-year evaluation from 1997 to 2006. *Pain Physician*, vol. 12, no. 1, pp. 9-34.

Marhofer P, Chan VWS. (2007). Ultrasound-guided regional anesthesia: current concepts and future trends. *Anesth Analg*, vol. 104, no. 5, pp. 1265-1269.

McKetty MH. (1998). The AAPM/RSNA physics tutorial for residents. X-ray attenuation. *Radiographics*, vol. 18, no. 1, pp. 151-163.

Meleka S, Patra A, Minkoff E, & Murphy K. (2005). Value of CT fluoroscopy for lumbar facet blocks. *AJNR Am J Neuroradiol*, vol. 26, no. 5, pp. 1001-1003.

Nightingale KR, Palmeri ML, Nightingale RW, & Trahey GE. (2001). On the feasibility of remote palpation using acoustic radiation force. *J Acoust Soc Am*, vol. 110, no. 1, pp. 625-634.

Ortiz AO, Natarajan V, Gregorius DR, & Pollack S. (2006). Significantly reduced radiation exposure to operators during kyphoplasty and vertebroplasty procedures: methods and techniques. *AJNR Am J Neuroradiol*, vol. 27, no. 5, pp. 989-994.

Palmeri ML, Dahl JJ, MacLeod D, Grant S, & Nightingale KR. Regional anesthesia guidance using acoustic radiation force imaging. [abstract]. Proceedings of the Seventh International Conference on the Ultrasonic Measurement and Imaging of Tissue Elasticity. Oct. 27-30, 2008.

Peolsson M, Brodin LA. (2009). Functional musculoskeletal ultrasound. *European Musculoskeletal Review*, vol. 4, no. 2, pp. 102-107.

Perisinakis K, Damilakis J, Theocharopoulos N, Papadokostakis G, Hadjipavlou A, & Gourtsoylannis N. (2004). Patient exposure and associated radiation risks from fluoroscopically-guided vertebroplasty or kyphoplasty. *Radiology*, vol. 232, no. 3, pp. 701-701.

Primack SJ. (2010). A physiatrist's perspective on musculoskeletal ultrasound. *Phys Med Rehabil Clin N Am*, vol. 21, no. 3, pp. 645-650.

Schmid MR, Kissling RO, Curt A, Jaschko G, & Hodler J. (2006). Sympathetic skin response: monitoring of CT-guided lumbar sympathetic blocks. *Radiology*, vol. 241, no. 2, pp. 595-602.

Schueler BA. (2000). The AAPM/RSNA physics tutorial for residents: general overview of fluoroscopic imaging. *Radiographics*, vol. 20, no. 4, pp. 1115-1126.

Sentinel Event Policy and Procedures. The Joint Commission website. http://www.jointcommission.org/assets/1/18/Radiation_Overdose.pdf. Accessed June 21, 2008.

Shahabi S. Radiation safety/protection and health physics. (1999). In: Dowd SB, Tilson ER, eds. *Practical Radiation Protection and Applied Radiobiology*. 2nd ed. pp. 167-196, Saunders, Philadelphia, Pa.

Shellock FA, Crues JV. (2004). MR procedures: biologic effects, safety, and patient care. *Radiology*, vol. 232, no. 3, pp. 635-652.

Shepp LA, Kruskal JB. (1978). Computerized tomography: the new medical x-ray technology. *Am Math Mon*, vol. 85, no. 6, pp. 420-439.

Sites BD, Brull R, Chan VWS, et al. (2007). Artifacts and pitfall errors associated with ultrasound-guided regional anesthesia. Part I: Understanding the basic principles of ultrasound physics and machine operations. *Reg Anesth Pain Med*, vol. 32, no. 5, pp. 412-418.

Sites BD, Chan VW, Neal JM, et al. (2009). The American Society of Regional Anesthesia and Pain Medicine and the European Society of Regional Anaesthesia and Pain Therapy joint committee recommendations for education and training in ultrasound-guided regional anesthesia. *Reg Anesth Pain Med*, vol. 34, no. 1, pp. 40-46.

Smiddy PF, Quinn AD, Freyne PJ, Marsh D, & Murphy JM. (1996). Dose reduction in double contrast barium enema by use of low fluoroscopic current. *Br J Radiol*, vol. 69, no. 825, pp. 852-854.

Sprawls P. AAPM tutorial. (1992). CT image detail and noise. *Radiographics*, vol. 12, no. 5, pp. 1041-1046.

Stam W, Pillay M. (2008). Inspection of lead aprons: a practical rejection model. *Health Phys*, vol. 95, suppl. 2, pp. S133-S136.

Stübig T, Kendoff D, Citak M, et al. (2009). Comparative study of different intraoperative 3-D image intensifiers in orthopedic trauma care. *J Trauma*, vol. 66, no. 3, pp. 821-830.

Thoumas D, Leroi AM, Mauillon J, et al. (1999). Pudendal neuralgia: CT-guided pudendal nerve block technique. *Abdom Imaging*, vol. 24, no. 3, pp. 309-312.

Tuohy B, Marsh DM, O'Reilly G, Dowling A, Cooney P, & Malone JF. (1997). Quality assurance programme applied to mobile C-arm fluoroscopy systems. *Eur Radiol*, vol. 7, no. 4, pp. 534-541.

U.S. Food and Drug Administration Radiation Emitting Products: Radiation Emitting Products and Procedures: Medical Imaging: Ultrasound Imaging: http://www.fda.gov/Radiation-EmittingProducts/RadiationEmittingProductsandProcedures/MedicalImaging/ucm115357.htm. n.d.

U.S. National Academy of Sciences, National Research Council, Committee to Assess Health Risks from Exposure to Low Levels of Ionizing Radiation. Health Risks from Exposure to Low Levels of Ionizing Radiation. BEIR VII Phase 2. Washington, DC: National Academies Press, 2006.

U.S. National Institutes of Health. Safety study of deep brain stimulation to manage thalamic pain syndrome. Identifier: NCT01072656. Clinical Trials website. http://clinicaltrials.gov. Accessed May 16, 2011

U.S. National Institutes of Health. Vercise implantable stimulator for treating Parkinson's disease (VANTAGE). Identifier: NCT01221948. Clinical Trials website. http://clinicaltrials.gov. Accessed May 16, 2011.

Vano E, Gonzalez L, Ten JI, et al. (2001). Skin dose and dose-area product values for interventional cardiology procedures. *Br J Radiol*, vol. 74, no. 877, pp. 48-55.

Villavicencio AT, Burneikiene S, Bulsara KR, & Thramann JJ. (2005). Intraoperative three-dimensional fluoroscopy-based computerized tomography guidance for percutaneous kyphoplasty. *Neurosurg Focus*, vol. 18, no. 3, p. E3.

Wagner AL. (2004a). Selective lumbar nerve root blocks with CT fluoroscopic guidance: technique, results, procedure time, and radiation dose. *AJNR Am J Neuroradiol*, vol. 25, no. 9, pp. 1592-1594.

Wagner AL. (2004b). CT fluoroscopy-guided epidural injections: techniques and results. *AJNR Am J Neuroradiol*, vol. 25, no. 10, pp. 1821-1823.

Wang J, Blackburn TJ. (2000). The AAPM/RSNA physics tutorial for residents: x-ray image intensifiers for fluoroscopy. *Radiographics*, vol. 20, no. 5, pp. 1471-1477.

Whitworth ML. Fluoroscopy scatter radiation studies of the lumbar spine. In: Interventional Spine. Volume 5, Issue 5. Kentfield, Ca: International Spine Intervention Society, n.d.

Wininger KL. (2010). The lumbosacral spine: kinesiology, physical rehabilitation, and interventional pain medicine. *Clinical Kinesiology*, vol. 64, no. 3, pp. 22-50.

Wininger KL, Deshpande KK, & Deshpande KK. (2010). Radiation exposure in percutaneous spinal cord stimulation mapping: a preliminary report. Pain Physician, vol. 13, no. 1, pp. 7-18.

World Health Organization. The WHO Global Database on Body Mass Index. BMI Classification website. http://apps.who.int/bmi/index.jsp?introPage=intro_3.html. n.d.

Yanch JC, Behrman RH, Hendricks MJ, & McCall JH. (2009). Increased radiation dose to overweight and obese patients from radiographic examinations. *Radiology*, 2009, vol. 252, no. 1, pp. 128-139.

Zhou Y, Singh N, Abdi S, Wu J, Crawford J, Furgang FA. (2005). Fluoroscopy radiation safety for spine interventional pain procedures in university teaching hospitals. *Pain Physician*, vol. 8, no. 1, pp. 49-53.

Part 2

Acute Pain

8

Local Anesthetic Agents in Arthroscopy

Joseph Baker
Cappagh National Orthopaedic Hospital
Ireland

1. Introduction

Arthroscopy is performed with increasing frequency on a number of joints. In the lower limb the role of knee arthroscopy is well established with procedures enabling more accurate diagnosis and treatment of a myriad of conditions including but not being limited to meniscal injury and articular surface defects. Hip and ankle arthroscopy are less widely performed. However, despite this their use can be expected to increase as indications are better developed and techniques honed.

While surgical technique often determines outcome in the long-term, analgesic control can significantly affect the patient's satisfaction following a procedure as well as the overall acceptability of a procedure. Arthroscopic procedures in particular have enabled many procedures to be performed on a day case basis where as more traditional surgical interventions may have required at least an overnight hospital stay. This trend toward day case surgery also emphasizes the importance of optimum analgesic control.

Traditionally intra-articular analgesic agents have been used following arthroscopic procedures as an augment to post-operative pain control. Classically these include the typical local anesthetic agents but also alternatives such as morphine. Recently however, the potential for deleterious effects of the intra-articular analgesics on the articular cartilage has been reported in a number of experimental studies, which has caused concern among practicing arthroscopic surgeons. The purpose of this chapter is to review the potential intra-articular analgesic agents used for pain control following lower limb arthroscopy and to also provide an up-to-date review of the evidence for the potential chondrotoxic effect of these agents.

2. Analgesic agents

Classical local anesthetic agents can be classified into the esters and amides. Amides including lignocaine and bupivacaine among others have commonly been used in arthroscopy. Local anesthetics block action potential initiation and propagation along sensory pathways by blocking the sodium channel transmembrane pores. Their activity is increased in alkaline conditions and this enables them to penetrate the nerve sheath and axonal membrane.

Other agents to have been trialed as intra-articular agents include opiates or opiate related substances (e.g. morphine, tramadol), non-steroidal anti-inflammatory medications, benzodiazepines and NMDA-receptor antagonists (e.g. magnesium sulfate) among others.

2.1 Hip and ankle arthroscopy

Numerous studies have assessed the ability of local anesthetic agents to provide pain control following arthroscopic procedures in the lower limb. A vast majority of these have focused on the knee and only a few have reported the use of local anaesthetic following hip and ankle arthroscopy(Middleton et al., 2006, Baker et al., 2011c).

Of these two studies both found that intra-articular local anaesthetic was superior to either placebo or local anesthetic infiltrated around the arthroscopic portals (Table 1). The paucity of data here reflects the relative infancy of hip and ankle arthroscopy compared to knee arthroscopy and highlights the need for further work – hip arthroscopy in particular requires significant force to overcome the intra-articular negative pressures and can result in significant post-operative pain(Baker et al., 2011a).

Author	Setting	Number	Key findings
(Baker et al., 2011c)	RCT	73	Intra-articular bupivacaine superior to peri-portal bupivacaine at controlling pain following HIP arthroscopy
(Middleton et al., 2006)	RCT	35	Intra-articular bupivacaine was superior to saline placebo in reducing post-operative VAS pain scores and need for supplemental analgesia following ANKLE arthroscopy

Table 1. Studies assessing the benefit of intra-articular analgesic agents following hip and ankle arthroscopy

2.2 Knee arthroscopy

Numerous studies have attempted to establish the ideal intra-articular analgesic for pain control following knee arthroscopy (for a summary of these studies see Table2). The studies selected for inclusion here predominantly include those that use an intra-articular analgesic following surgery in a bolus dose fashion. Some studies that use it prior to surgery are also included for comparison sake particularly where comparison is later made with a bolus given following surgery. This section focuses on intra-articular analgesia given as an augment following surgery performed under general anesthesia or spinal anesthesia.

Although many studies have found that classical local anesthetic agents are of benefit following knee arthroscopy a randomized controlled trial reported by Townsend et al noted that intra-articular bupivacaine was no more effective that bupivacaine infiltrated around the portal sites(Townshend et al., 2009). This equivalence takes on even more importance with the reported potential for the toxic effect on articular cartilage of bupivacaine and other similar agents.

In general local anesthetics have been shown to be effective compared to placebo although this is not necessarily the case if the surgery is performed under spinal anesthetic when it appears the additional use of an intra-articular agent is negated by the spinal block(Santanen et al., 2001).

Non-steroidal anti-inflammatory medications have been trialed as intra-articular agents but are not in wide spread use. A single study has found that tenoxicam was superior to bupivacaine following surgery but this was only with regards analgesic consumption – the reported pain scores were still similar(Cook et al., 1997). It was similarly found that lornoxicam resulted in lower pain scores than did bupivacaine in a randomized controlled trial of 40 patients(Fagan et al., 2003). The use of an anti-inflammatory into the joint cavity may play a role in pain control particularly when a significant inflammatory component to the intra-articular pathology is found(Izdes et al., 2003).

When compared to opiate type analgesia (intravenous) was shown in one study to provide quicker onset of analgesia but was not significantly better at 24 hours after surgery(Franceschi et al., 2001). The benefit of morphine as an intra-articular analgesic is questionable however as noted later and this perhaps reflects poorly on ropivacaine.

Combinations of amide local anesthetics with other agents have been tried and this may represent the optimum way to control pain although at this point in time it is unknown. A combination of magnesium sulfate and bupivacaine was shown to be superior to either agent in isolation, which were again superior to placebo with regard pain scores following knee arthroscopy(Elsharnouby et al., 2008). These findings are supported by another study that also included morphine in the intra-articular cocktail but again found that a combination of agents was superior to any of the agents given in isolation(Farouk and Aly, 2009). A combination of bupivacaine with fentanyl was shown to be superior to bupivacaine in isolation following knee arthroscopy in a randomized trial including 33 patients(Jawish et al., 1996). Despite these promising reports in combinations of an amide local anesthetic and an opiate type agent others have failed to find this multimodal approach any better than placebo alone(Aasbo et al., 1996). While pain intensity or pain scale score is a frequent measure in these studies, the actual need for additional analgesia is a limiting factor with regard the ability to perform a procedure as a day case or not and may reflect a more practical end-point for further research.

Despite a small number of studies suggesting that morphine provides adequate analgesic control following knee a recent review of these studies has suggested that of the higher quality studies, most had a negative finding not in favor of its use as an intra-articular analgesic agent(Rosseland, 2005, Drosos et al., 2002). The key point of this review was that post-operative pain intensity was no less in the morphine treated groups than the placebo treated groups in the well-designed studies. This review is supported by a study by the same author group that found only those with intense pain after arthroscopy had any benefit from intra-articular morphine(Rosseland et al., 1999).

Other agents have been studied in with some success including midazolam (increased the time to first analgesia after surgery compared to placebo), clonidine (additive effect with bupivacaine compared to bupivacaine alone) and neostigmine (more effective when compared to morphine)(Batra et al., 2008, Tamosiunas et al., 2005, Yang et al., 1998). Unfortunately these agents have been studies in a very limited capacity and a clear conclusion in unable to be drawn as their effectiveness.

Author	Setting	Number	Key findings
(Aasbo et al., 1996)	RCT	107	Patients randomised to receive either: bupivacaine (20ml of 2.5mg/ml) + morphine (3mg); bupivacaine (20ml of 2.5mg/ml) alone; morphine (3mg) alone; or isotonic saline – no differences between the groups with regard analgesic requirement post-surgery
(Al-Metwalli et al., 2008)	RCT	60	Intra-articular dexmedetomidine (α-2-adrenergic agonist) given via the intra-articular route resulted in less post-operative pain and analgesic requirement than either dexmedetomidine given intravenously or intra-articulat and intravenous placebo (saline)
(Alagol et al., 2004)	RCT	210	Intra-articular tramadol at doses 50-100mg provided good post-operative analgesia with the higher doe more effectuve. The intra-articular route was more effective than the intravenous route.
(Batra et al., 2008)	RCT	60	Intra-articular midazolam (50 or 75µg/kg) provided superior, albeit briefly, analgesic control compared to saline placebo. Time to first analgesic requirement was 4.7 and 4.6 hours compared to 0.7.

Author	Setting	Number	Key findings
(Buerkle et al., 2000)	RCT	60	Patients given **morphine** (1mg) and **clonidine** (150µg) intra-articularly in combination had lower VAS pain scores at 2 hours post-surgery and lower need for rescue analgesia compared to groups given either agent in isolation or saline placebo
(Calmet et al., 2004)	RCT	80	Following arthroscopic meniscectomy, patients receiving intra-articular **ketorolac** (60mg) had better post-operative pain control and less need for rescue analgesia compared to those receiving 10ml of 0.25% **bupivacaine**, 1mg of **morphine** or normal saline placebo.
(Cepeda et al., 1997)	RCT	112	Intra-articular and subcuticular **morphine** (10mg) and intraarticuular **bupivacaine** (20ml 0.5%) were compared with noraml saline placebo. Single dose morphine by either route provided superior pain conrol with lower pain scores at 6- and 3-hours post-surgery.
(Colbert et al., 1999)	RCT	88	Patients receiving intra-articular **tenoxicam** had lower pain scores at 30-180 minutes post-surgery and required less analgesia later than thos receiving the same drug intravenously.
(Convery et al., 1998)	RCT	60	Patients given 5mg **ketorolac** with 20ml of 0.25% **bupivacaine** into the joint after surgery provided similar analgesic control to 10mg ketorolac given intravenously with 20ml of 0.25% **bupivacaine** given into the joint.
(Cook et al., 1997)	RCT	63	Patients received either 40ml solution containing only normal saline, 0.25% **bupivacaine** or 20mg **tenoxicam** at the end of knee arthroscopy. Less analgesia was needed by the tenoxicam group but subjective pain reporting was similar in all groups.
(Dalsgaard et al., 1993)	RCT	52	Patients receiving 1mg of **morphine** intrarticularly at the end of surgery had lower pain scores at 8- and 24-hours after surgery and used less paracetamol compared to those receiving saline placebo.
(Drosos et al., 2002)	RCT	30	No significant difference seen in VAS pain scores between patients receiving intra-articular saline, 5mg **morphine** or 15mg **morphine** following diagnostic arthroscopy or arthroscopic meniscectomy.
(Elhakim et al., 1999)	RCT	60	Patients randomised to receive either saline placebo; 2% **lidocaine** and 10mg **pethidine**, or; 2% **lidocaine**, 10mg **pethidine** and 20mg **tenoxicam**. Combination of all three agents resulted in lower VAS pain scores for longer and less need for analgesic use.
(Elsharnouby et al., 2008)	RCT	108	Patients receiving 1g **magnesium sulfate** and 0.25% **bupivacaine** (20ml total) had significantly lower VAS pain scores and longer time to first analgesic use than thos receiving either agent in isolation or placebo.
(Eren et al., 2008)	RCT	90	Patients receving either 8mg **lornoxicam** or 50mg **bupivacaine** had less analgesic consumption after surgery than those receiving plcebo. Pain rating were lower for those receinving the lornoxicam than thos receiving the bupivacaine.
(Fagan et al., 2003)	RCT	40	Patients receiving pre-emptive injection of **bupivacaine with adrenaline** showed a trend toward needing less analgesia in the recovery room than those receiving the injection at completion of surgery.
(Farouk and Aly, 2009)	RCT	80	A combination of **magnesium** (150mg) and **morphine** (2mg) with 20 ml of 0.25% **bupivacaine** provided superior analgesic control (lower VAS scores and longer time to first analgesic) than either agent alone with bupivacaine or bupivacaine alone.

Author	Outline	Number	Key findings
(Franceschi et al., 2001)	RCT	90	**Ropivacaine** (75mg in 20ml saline) had quicker onset of effective analgesia post-opeatively than **morphine** (2mg in 20ml saline) with lower VAS pain scores in the first 4 hours and equivalent control in the first 24 hours.
(Goodwin et al., 2005, Goodwin and Parker, 2005)	RCT	50	**Bupivacaine with epinephrine** and **morphine** or **bupivacaine with epinephrine** alone given either pre- or post-operatively resulted in lower pain scores and narcotic onsumption than with epinephrine alone. There was a trend toward superior control in those receiving the injection pre-operatively.
(Goodwin and Parker, 2005)	RCT		Combinations of **bupivacaine, morphine** and **epinephrine** given pre- or post-surgery resulted in similar pain control.
(Grabowska-Gawel et al., 2003)		56	Patients received either 10ml 0.5% **bupivacaine** or 5mg **morphine** in normal saline. Mean time to rescue analgesia was shorter in the bupivacaine group but there was no difference in reported VAS pain scores.
(Graham et al., 2000)	RCT	36	Intra-articular analgesia given at completion of arthroscopy was equivalent to pre-operative intravenous regional analgesia with respect to post-opertive pain control
(Gupta et al., 1999)	RCT	100	Knee arthroscopy performed under LA (prilocaine (5mg/ml). **Morphine** (3mg), **ketorolac** (30mg) or a combination of the two was given at completion of surgery. A combination of morphine and ketorolac provided significantly superior analgesia than morphine alone or placebo.
(Hege-Scheuing et al., 1995)	RCT	59	**Morphine** (1mg) given either intra-articularly or intravenously at the end of arthroscopy had equivalent analgesic benefit.
(Izdes et al., 2003)	RCT	90	Patients receiving intra-articular **piroxicam** (20mg) and 25ml of 0.25% **bupivacaine** had longer analgesic duration in cases where synovial inflammation was confirmed present than when not present.
(Jacobson et al., 2006)	RCT	120	**Levobupivacaine** (5mg/ml) significantly reduced the need for analgesia in the first 24 hours post-surgery compared to **levobupivacaine** (2.5mg/ml) and **lidocaine** (10mg/ml) with **adrenaline**.
(Jaureguito et al., 1995)	RCT		Knee arthroscopy [performed under LA. Patients receiving intra-articular **morphine** (4mg) had lower VAS pain scores than those receiving 0.25% **bupivacaine** or saline placebo. Less supplemental pain medication was needed by the morphine group.
(Jawish et al., 1996)	RCT	33	Patients receiving a combination of 0.25% **bupivacaine** with 50µg of **fentanyl** had reduced post-operative pain for at least 9 hours post-surgery when compared to patients receiving 0.25% **bupivacaine** alone or saline placebo.
(Joshi et al., 1992)	RCT	20	Patients receiving intra-articular **morphine** (5mg) following knee arthroscopy had lower VAS pain scores and needed less rescue analgesia than those recevinig saline placebo. Low serum morphine metabolites suggested that the morphine was acting locally.
(Joshi et al., 1993)	RCT	40	Intra-articular **morphine** (5mg) either in isolation or incombination with 25ml of 0.25% **bupivacaine** resulted in significantly lower pain scores and need for supplementary analgesia than **bupivacaine** in isolation or saline placebo.

Author	Setting	Number	Key findings
(Juelsgaard et al., 1993)	RCT	47	There was no difference in reposrted VAS pain scores or acetaminophen use in the 48 hours after knee arthroscopy in patients receiving either 2 or 4mg of intra-articular **morphine** after surgery
(Kanbak et al., 1997)	RCT		Patients receiving 5mg **morphine** intra-articularly after arthroscopy had superior pain control in the 24 hours after surgery compared to those receiving 1mg **morphine** or saline placebo.
(Karaman et al., 2009)	RCT	40	No significant difference was found in control of post-operative pain and analgesic requirement between patients receiving 20ml of 0.5% **levobupivacaine** and 20ml of 0.5% **bupivacaine.**
(Kligman et al., 2002)	RCT	60	Infiltration of **morphine** (1mg) into the synovial tissue or outer third of meniscal tissue resulted in better pain control (lower VAS pain scores and less analgesic use) post-arthroscopy than if morphine (1mg) was given by the intra-articular route.
(Lundin et al., 1998)	RCT	50	Intra-articular **bupivacaine** 0.25% (40ml) with the addition of **morphine** 1mg compared to **bupivacaine** alone. Lower VAS pain scores noted with the addition of morphine in the 24 hours after surgery but no difference in supplementary analgesic use.
(Niemi et al., 1994)	RCT	80	Patients underwent knee arthroscopy under either spinal or LA (1% lidocaine with adrenaline) blockade. Intra-articular **morphine** (1mg) given at the end of the procedure resulted in reduced rescue analgesia requirement in the group that had LA block.
(Pooni et al., 1999)	RCT	107	Patients randomized to receive either intra-articular **bupivacaine** or **fantanyl** after knee arthroscopy reported similar pain scores except at 2-hours post-surgery when bupivacaine was superior
(Raj et al., 2004)	RCT	40	Patients receinving 10mg **morphine** intra-articularly repoted lower pain scores between 4- and 24-hours post-surgery and consumed less analgesia than patients receiving 10mg morphine via the intramuscular route.
(Rasmussen et al., 2002)	RCT	60	Patients randomized to receive either saline placebo; 150mg **bupivacaine** and 4mg **morphine**, or; 150mg **bupivacaine**, 4mg **morphine** and 40mg **methylprednisolone** intra-articulalry at the end of surgery.Bupivacaine with mprhine was effective at reducing pain and duration of immobilization, the addition of methylprednisolone futher reduce dpain and use of analgesics.
(Rautoma et al., 2000)	RCT	200	Pre-operative per oral diclofenac reduced post-operative pain scores compared to the intra-articular **ropivacaine** given at the time of surgery. Arthoscopy performed under spinal anaesthesia.
(Richardson et al., 1997)	RCT		Intra-articular morphine (1mg) was superior to bupivacaine (100mg) at reducing pain scores and need for supplementary anlgesia at 6- and 24-hours post-surgery. An intra-articular dose of 5mg morphine was more effective thatn 1mg intra-articular or 5mg intravenous at reducing VAS pain scores.
(Rosseland et al., 2004)	RCT	60	Intra-articular **saline** (1 or 10ml) was given following surgery via an intra-articular catheter in patients with at least moderate pain. Within 1 hour VAS pain scores reduced from 50 to 27 on a 100mm scale with both volumes.
(Rosseland et al., 2003)	RCT	40	Intra-articular **saline** (10ml) or **morphine** (2mg in 10ml saline) was given following surgery via an intra-articular catheter in patients with at least moderate pain. Equivalent improvements in pain intesnity were found in both groups.

Author	Design	Number	Key findings
(Rosseland et al., 1999)	RCT	90	Only patients with more intense pain after arthroscopy had beneift from intra-articular **morphine** (2mg) with regard reduced pain intensity and analgesia requirement. In most patients **morphine** (1 or 2mg) was equivalent to saline placebo.
(Samoladas et al., 2006)	RCT	60	Patientes received either 10 or 20ml of 7.5mg/ml **ropivacaine**. Both provided excellent pain control for two hours, however after that the lower dose group reported increased pain and need for supplementary analgesia.
(Santanen et al., 2001)	RCT	100	Knee arthroscopy performed under spinal anaesthesia. 20ml of 0.5% **ropivacaine** failed to reduce VAS pain scores or need for rescue analgesia when compared to saline control.
(Solheim et al., 2006)	RCT	40	Patients received intra-articular **morphine** (5mg) or saline placebo via intra-articular catheter 1 hour post-surgery if they developed at least moderate pain. Morphine was of no greater benefit than saline. Timing of catheter removal did not influence the outcome.
(Souza et al., 2002)	RCT	60	Patients receiving either saline placebo, 10ml 0.25% **bupivacaine**, 2mg **morphine** or 100μg **fentanyl** intra-articularly at the end of arthroscopy did not differ significantly in reported pain intensity.
(Tamosiunas et al., 2005)	RCT	48	Patients receiving 20ml of 0.5% **bupivacaine** with the addition of 1μg/kg of **clonidine** controlled post-operative pain more effectivley than **bupivacaine** in isolation or placebo.
(Townshend et al., 2009)	RCT	137	Patients receiving 20ml of 0.5% bupivacaine either intra-articulalry or infiltrated around the portals reported equivalent pain scores at 1-hour post-surgery.
(VanNess and Gittins, 1994)	RCT	81	Patients receiving intra-artticular **morphine** (2mg) reported significantly less pain and lower analgesic requirements in the 24-hours after surgery than those receiving 30ml of 0.25% **bupivacaine with epinephrine.**.
(Varrassi et al., 1999)	RCT	48	Intra-articular **buprenorphine** (100μg) and intra-articular **bupivacaine** (50mg) resulted in lower VAS pain scores in the 6-hours after surgery than intra-articular saline or intra-muscular buprenorphine. Analgesic use was less in thoe treated with intra-articular **buprenorphine** or **bupivacaine.**
(Vranken et al., 2001)	RCT	60	**Sufentanil** (5 or 10μg) given intra-articulalry resulted in lower VAS pain scores than in control (intravenous sufentanil). Post-operative analgesic use was also lower in the treatment group.
(White et al., 1990)	RCT		Patients treated with **prilocaine with adenaline** reported prolonged time to first dose of oral analgesia but overall there was no difference in pain scores.
(Yang et al., 1998)	RCT	60	Patients receiving intra-articular **neostigmine** (500μg) had lower VAS pain scores 1-hour after surgery and had longer lasting duration of analgesia compared to those receiving intra-articular **morphine** (2mg) or saline placebo. No significant effects were seen with neostigmine 125 or 250μg.
(Zeidan et al., 2008)	RCT	90	Intra-articular administration of **tramadol** (100mg) and 0.25% **bupivacaine** to 20ml vloume had lower VAS scores, longer time to rescue analgesia and less analgesic use in the first 24-hours compared to when either agent was given in isolation.

Table 2. Studies assessing the benefit of intra-articular analgesic agents following knee arthroscopy. Treatments are in bold.

In summary a myriad of agents have been studied for their potential use in attenuating post-operative pain following knee arthroscopy. While the amide local anesthetic agents are the most widely studied their continuing benefit and use is questionable as portal infiltration has been shown to be as effective at providing pain control for a procedure that is generally very well tolerated. Knee arthroscopy performed under local anesthetic is a different entity although far less frequent.

Hip and ankle arthroscopy are far less studied and the ideal intra-articular agent is uncertain in these joints. A multi-model intra-articular analgesic bolus may be the best approach in these joints that require significant traction and subsequent injury to the capsule that can cause greater discomfort after surgery.

2.3 The potential for articular chondrocyte toxicity

The potential for deleterious effects of local anesthetic agents on articular chondrocytes was increasingly noted with the use of arthroscopic pain pumps following glenohumeral arthroscopy(Busfield and Romero, 2009, Hansen et al., 2007, Solomon et al., 2009). Increasingly however studies are alerting the practicing clinician to the potential for toxic effects secondary to amide local anesthetics given as a single bolus injection. Most of these are laboratory-based studies. Although some have questioned the relevance given the long use of intra-articular local anesthetic without seemingly any complication the serve as a caution.

The aim of this section is to provide an over view of the basic science evidence on the potential for local anesthetic agents to cause articular chondrocyte toxicity.

2.3.1 In vitro reports

A number of different laboratory modesl utilizing cell lines from a variety of animal species have been used in the study of local anaesthetic toxicity. A toxic effect in canine chondrocytes exposed to bupivacaine 0.5% using a proven in vitro model by Anz et al. They reported an almost 100% reduction in cell viability after two days exposure to bupivacaine. Bupivacaine conferred an anti-inflammatory effect in their study, evidenced by reduced nitric oxide and PGE rise in the presence of interleukin-1, but their conclusion maintained that continuous exposure to bupivacine resulted in a clear toxic effect toward the canine chondrocytes(Anz et al., 2009). Again using a canine osteochondral model the toxic effect of bupivacaine was again confirmed, with or without the addition of methylparaben(Hennig et al., 2010). Exposure to the local anaesthetic alone for 5 or 30 minutes caused significant cell death, although this was only significant statistically at the 30 minute exposure.

Miyazaki et al demonstrated a concentration dependent reduction in bovine chondrocyte viability after treatment with lidocaine (0.125, 0.25, 0.5 or 1%) (Miyazaki et al., 2011). Glycosaminoglycan (GAG)content of the cells was also noted to be reduced as the concentration of the local anaesthetic was increased. GAG and lactate production were higher in the cells treated with 0.5 and 1% lidocaine. The authors felt that this finding conferred a reparative response by the cells.

Using bovine articular chondrocytes in alginate bead cultures Karpie et al exposed these to 1 or 2% lidocaine for 15 to 60 minutes(Karpie and Chu, 2007). A dose and time dependent increase in cell toxicity was reported. An intact surface on the osteochondral core or variation in the pH of the treatments (pH 7.4, 7.0, 5.0) failed to confer any protective effect (this is in contrast to other studies – see below). Others have also reported time and concentration dependent reductions in cell viability using a bovine disc model(Lo et al., 2009). In this case osteochondral cores were harvested from the radiocarpal joint of cows and these were treated with either lidocaine (1%), bupivacaine (0.25%) or ropivacaine (0.5%).

The toxic effects of bupivacaine (0.125%, 0.5% and 0.5%) on the the articular chondrocyte from a bovine cell line were well demonstrated (Chu et al., 2008). Cells were cultured in a 3-dimensional alginate-bead culture. Specimens were exposed for 15, 30 or 60 minutes and analysis was performed at 1 and 24 hours and at 1 week. A clear time and concentration dependent respose to the local anaetshetic treatments was observed. Treatment with 0.125% bupivacaine for 15 minutes was not significantly different to the saline control. Almost complete loss of cell viability was noted with 0.5% bupivacaine. Analysis of osteochondral cores with an intact superficial cell layer suggested that an the superficial layer of the articular cartilage provided some protective benefit when intact. This may be significant in deciding during surgery whether or not intra-articular analgesic agents are safe to administer.

To test the respective toxic effects on chondrocytes of lidocaine, mepivacaine and bupivacaine Park et al used an equine model (Park et al., 2011). Bupivacaine (0.5%) was the most toxic of the agents used with cell viability reduced to 29 +/- 8% after 30 minutes. Cell viability after treatment with saline was 96%. Lidocaine and mepivacaine were both less toxic with mepivacine exerting the least toxic effect of the three.

A number of studies have used human cell lines which is arguably more useful for the extrapolation of results into clinical pratice. Dragoo et al used a custom made bioreactor to mimic the metabolism of synovial fluid to simulate the use of a pain pump following arthroscopic surgery(Dragoo et al., 2008). They found that both lignocaine (1%) and bupivacaine (0.25 or 0.5%) resulted in reduced cell viability but that the rates of necrosis were noted with the presence of epinephrine. Cell viability was similar at 24 and 48 hours in the bupivaine group, but there was a greater toxic effect seen at 72 hours. Further work using the same bioreactor model demonstrated that epineprhine, at levels of 1:100000-200000, conferred no significant increase in cell death compared to acidic media with a pH of 4.5-5.0 and local anaesthetics in combination with epinephrine (Dragoo et al., 2010). The authors suggest that local anaesthetic agents containing epinephrine should be used with caution as these are often titrated to a low pH.

Syed et al reported significant toxic effects of bupivacaine either alone or in combination with triamcinolone in a monlayer culture model using human articular chondrocytes (Syed et al., 2011). When the treatments were administered to the osteochondral plug with an intact surface however, the toxic effect of bupivacaine in isolation was no more than that of the control – again suggesting there is a benefit to an intact articular surface with regard exposure to potentially toxic agents.

Using chondrocytes harvested from osteoarthritic human knees it was demonstrated that exposure to lidocaine, bupivacaine or ropivacaine for 24 or 120 hours resulted in significant levels of cell death(Grishko et al., 2010). In the lignocaine 2% group massive necrosis was seen at 24 hours. After 120 hours exposure there were significant dereases in cell viability in all treatments groups with the exception of those cells treated with 0.2% ropivacaine. As viability decreased a concomitant rise in cell apoptosis was noted.

Jacobs et al harvested human articular chondrocytes from the knees of human tissue donors or patients undergoing total knee arthroplasty(Jacobs et al., 2011). They treated the articular chondrcytes with either 1% or 2% lidocaine with or without epinephrine and used saline as a control. Cell death between 91-99% was seen for each of the three treatments. A prolonged exposure time was also associated with higher rates of cell death.

Ropivacaine 0.5% was found to be significantly less toxic to human chondrocytes than bupivacaine 0.5% (Piper and Kim, 2008). Normal human articular cartilage was harvested from the femoral head or tibial plateau in in patients underoing surgical procedures. Full thickness explants and cultured chondrocytes were treated with either ropivacaine or bupivacaine for 30 minutes. Cell viability in the explant cultures fell to 95% and 78% after treatment with ropivacaine and bupivacaine respectively. Viability in the cell cultures fell to 64% and 37%. The viability of the cells in the explant cultures treated with ropivacaine did not differ significantly to that in the controls treated with saline. Ropivacaine may therefore confer a much more acceptable risk than bupivacaine – an important consideration if using it as an intra-articular agent following arthroscopy.

However, others failed to find a difference between these two agents using a simple monolayer culture model. Both ropivacaine and bupivacaine conferred simlar toxic effects to the articular chondrocytes either in isolation or if they were used in combination with magnesium sulfate(Baker et al., 2011b, Baker et al., 2011d). Lignocaine combined with magnesium sulfate was less toxic than either ropivacaine, bupivacaine or levobupivacaine combined with magnesium suflate after an exposure time of only 15 minutes(Baker et al., 2011b).

A useful finding for the practicing surgeon in the studies that have assessed human cells in in vitro settings is the recurrent finding that ropivacaine is less toxic than bupivacaine(Baker et al., 2011b, Baker et al., 2011d, Piper and Kim, 2008). If ropivacaine confers a less toxic effect, then as long as it provides equally efficacious analgesic control, then these studies support its use. Notably, Piper et al also found ropivacaine to be less toxic in the explant culture with cells embedded in an intact matrix, potentially a better representation of the in vivo state.

2.3.2 In vivo studies

In vivo models shoulde in theory provide the best simulation of what may happen in pratcice. However, consideration needs to be given to the culture model used and also the species studied. Arguably the ideal model is unknown to date and no human in vivo studies at the time of writing have been able to demonstrate a lasting deleterious effect of local anaesthetic on articular chondrocytes.

The effect of a single intra-articular injection of 0.5% bupivacaine into a stifle joint compared to 0.9% saline control was studied(Chu et al., 2010). Six months following injection gross and histological appearances showed that the chondral surfaces remained intact. They diod note howeevr, that there was a reduction in chondrocyte density of up to 50% in the joint treated with local anaesthetic compared to the saline control.

In an in vivo rabbit study three groups recieved continuous infusions of either saline, bupivacaine or bupivacaine with epinephrine over 48 hours(Gomoll et al., 2006). One week after treatment the animals were sacrificed and osteochondral and synovial samples analysed. Bupivacaine with or without epinephrine resulted in cell viability reduction by 20 to 32%. Histological analysis was worse in both treatment gourps compared to saline control.

A similar treatment regime did not result in long term changes in articular cartilage(Gomoll et al., 2009). When the rabbits were sacrificed three months after the infusion of the saline of local anaesthetic there was no significant difference found between treatment and control groups. An increase in cartilage metabolism in the treatment groups was noted suggesting that the cartilage was undergoing a reparative process. This study provides conflicting information to the earlier one noted by Chu et al creating more difficulty in ascertaining the true chronic effect of intra-articular local anaesthetic use.

In another, histological changes in rabbit knee joint articular cartilage have been reported (Dogan et al., 2004). Knees were injected with either 0.9% saline, bupivacaine or neostigmine. Histological analysis performed at 1, 2 and 10 days confirmed more toxic changes in both treatment groups compared to saline control.

2.3.3 The mechaisn of local anaesthetic mediated chondroctoxicity

Despite a number of studies reporting the potential toxic effects the mechanism by which these agents exert their effect is uncertain. Mitochondrial dysfunction is thought to be a key factor in articular chondrocyte death(Grishko et al., 2010). Grishko et al demonstrated mitochondrial DNA damage and a reduction in ATP and mitochondrial protein levels in response to treatment with a variety of local anaesthetics at varying concentrations.

In another study cells exposed to lidocaine or bupivacine in isolation had rates of cell death just over 10%(Bogatch et al., 2010). When the local anaesthetics were mixed with the cell culture medium this rate rose to over 96% in each instance. Crystal formation was seen when the bupivacine was mixed with culture medium. Acididc phosphate buffered saline resulted in increased cell death only when the acidity was increased to a pH less than 3.4. Based on these results the authors propose an incompatibility between the synovial fluid and the local anaesthetic is responsible for the majority of chondrocyte death rather than the local anaesthetic agent itself.

3. Summary

A number of different agents have been trialed as intra-articular analgesic agents following arthroscopy in the lower limb. Many of the reported trials have focussed on the use of amide local anaesthetic sgents as these are the most widely used in clinical practice. Depsite multiple studies there is no agent that appears clearly superior to the rest. Bupivacaine or ropivacaine appear the most likely to offer the greatest analgesic control by this route and a small number of studies are supportive of a multi-modal infiltration. Magnesium sulfate for one may be an ideal synergist.

Although Townsend et al have offered evidence that intra-articular local anaesthetc can be avoided in knee arthroscopy without compromising analgesic control, the ideal mode of analgesic control in hip and ankle arthroscopy is still uncertain. Recent reports of chondrolysis in shoulder arthroscopy prompted a number of investigations in the potential toxic effect that amide local anaesthetcis may have on articular chondrocytes.

Ropivacaine appears to less toxic than bupivacaine and a combination of ropivacaine and magnesium has also been suggested as a more acceptable alternative approach to intra-articular local anaesthesia(Baker et al., 2011b, Webb and Ghosh, 2009). The potential diffculties in applying laboratory findings to the clinical setting has been noted(Webb and Ghosh, 2009). In the arthroscopic setting, a number of variables including the articular surface disease state, the dilutional effect of the arthroscopic fluid and absorbance of injected agents into surrounding synovium and adjacent soft tissues could all modify the effect the local anaesthetic has on the articular chondrocyte. The potential for toxic effects on articular chondrocytes by local anaesthetic needs to be further investigated.

4. References

Aasbo, V., Raeder, J. C., Grogaard, B. & Roise, O. 1996. No additional analgesic effect of intra-articular morphine or bupivacaine compared with placebo after elective knee arthroscopy. *Acta Anaesthesiol Scand,* 40, 585-8.

Al-Metwalli, R. R., Mowafi, H. A., Ismail, S. A., Siddiqui, A. K., Al-Ghamdi, A. M., Shafi, M. A. & El-Saleh, A. R. 2008. Effect of intra-articular dexmedetomidine on postoperative analgesia after arthroscopic knee surgery. *Br J Anaesth,* 101, 395-9.

Alagol, A., Calpur, O. U., Kaya, G., Pamukcu, Z. & Turan, F. N. 2004. The use of intraarticular tramadol for postoperative analgesia after arthroscopic knee surgery: a comparison of different intraarticular and intravenous doses. *Knee Surg Sports Traumatol Arthrosc,* 12, 184-8.

Anz, A., Smith, M. J., Stoker, A., Linville, C., Markway, H., Branson, K. & Cook, J. L. 2009. The effect of bupivacaine and morphine in a coculture model of diarthrodial joints. *Arthroscopy,* 25, 225-31.

Baker, J. F., Byrne, D. P., Hunter, K. & Mulhall, K. J. 2011a. Post-operative opiate requirements after hip arthroscopy. *Knee Surg Sports Traumatol Arthrosc,* 19, 1399-402.

Baker, J. F., Byrne, D. P., Walsh, P. M. & Mulhall, K. J. 2011b. Human chondrocyte viability after treatment with local anesthetic and/or magnesium: results from an in vitro study. *Arthroscopy,* 27, 213-7.

Baker, J. F., McGuire, C. M., Byrne, D. P., Hunter, K., Eustace, N. & Mulhall, K. J. 2011c. Analgesic control after hip arthroscopy: a randomised, double-blinded trial comparing portal with intra-articular infiltration of bupivacaine. *Hip Int,* 21, 373-377.

Baker, J. F., Walsh, P. M., Byrne, D. P. & Mulhall, K. J. 2011d. In vitro assessment of human chondrocyte viability after treatment with local anaesthetic, magnesium sulphate or normal saline. *Knee Surg Sports Traumatol Arthrosc.*

Batra, Y. K., Mahajan, R., Kumar, S., Rajeev, S. & Singh Dhillon, M. 2008. A dose-ranging study of intraarticular midazolam for pain relief after knee arthroscopy. *Anesth Analg,* 107, 669-72.

Bogatch, M. T., Ferachi, D. G., Kyle, B., Popinchalk, S., Howell, M. H., Ge, D., You, Z. & Savoie, F. H. 2010. Is chemical incompatibility responsible for chondrocyte death induced by local anaesthetics? *Am J Sports Med,* 38, 520-6.

Buerkle, H., Huge, V., Wolfgart, M., Steinbeck, J., Mertes, N., Van Aken, H. & Prien, T. 2000. Intra-articular clonidine analgesia after knee arthroscopy. *Eur J Anaesthesiol,* 17, 295-9.

Busfield, B. T. & Romero, D. M. 2009. Pain pump use after shoulder arthroscopy as a cause of glenohumeral chondrolysis. *Arthroscopy,* 25, 647-52.

Calmet, J., Esteve, C., Boada, S. & Gine, J. 2004. Analgesic effect of intra-articular ketorolac in knee arthroscopy: comparison of morphine and bupivacaine. *Knee Surg Sports Traumatol Arthrosc,* 12, 552-5.

Cepeda, M. S., Uribe, C., Betancourt, J., Rugeles, J. & Carr, D. B. 1997. Pain relief after knee arthroscopy: intra-articular morphine, intra-articular bupivacaine, or subcutaneous morphine? *Reg Anesth,* 22, 233-8.

Chu, C. R., Coyle, C. H., Chu, C. T., Szczodry, M., Seshadri, V., Karpie, J. C., Cieslak, K. M. & Pringle, E. K. 2010. In vivo effects of single intra-articular injection of 0.5% bupivacaine on articular cartilage. *J Bone Joint Surg Am,* 92, 599-608.

Chu, C. R., Izzo, N. J., Coyle, C. H., Papas, N. E. & Logar, A. 2008. The in vitro effects of bupivacaine on articular chondrocytes. *J Bone Joint Surg Br,* 90, 814-20.

Colbert, S. T., Curran, E., O'Hanlon, D. M., Moran, R. & McCarroll, M. 1999. Intra-articular tenoxicam improves postoperative analgesia in knee arthroscopy. *Can J Anaesth,* 46, 653-7.

Convery, P. N., Milligan, K. R., Quinn, P., Scott, K. & Clarke, R. C. 1998. Low-dose intra-articular ketorolac for pain relief following arthroscopy of the knee joint. *Anaesthesia,* 53, 1125-9.

Cook, T. M., Tucker, J. P. & Nolan, J. P. 1997. Analgesia after day-case knee arthroscopy: double-blind study of intra-articular tenoxicam, intra-articular bupivacaine and placebo. *Br J Anaesth,* 78, 163-8.

Dalsgaard, J., Felsby, S., Juelsgaard, P. & Frokjaer, J. 1993. [Analgesic effect of low-dose intra-articular morphine after ambulatory knee arthroscopy]. *Ugeskr Laeger,* 155, 4166-9.

Dogan, N., Erdem, A. F., Erman, Z. & Kizilkaya, M. 2004. The effects of bupivacaine and neostigmine on articular cartilage and synovium in the rabbit knee joint. *J Int Med Res,* 32, 513-9.

Dragoo, J. L., Korotkova, T., Kanwar, R. & Wood, B. 2008. The effect of local anesthetics administered via pain pump on chondrocyte viability. *Am J Sports Med,* 36, 1484-8.

Dragoo, J. L., Korotkova, T., Kim, H. J. & Jagadish, A. 2010. Chondrotoxicity of low pH, epinephrine, and preservatives found in local anesthetics containing epinephrine. *Am J Sports Med,* 38, 1154-9.

Drosos, G. I., Vlachonikolis, I. G., Papoutsidakis, A. N., Gavalas, N. S. & Anthopoulos, G. 2002. Intra-articular morphine and postoperative analgesia after knee arthroscopy. *Knee,* 9, 335-40.

Elhakim, M., Nafie, M., Eid, A. & Hassin, M. 1999. Combination of intra-articular tenoxicam, lidocaine, and pethidine for outpatient knee arthroscopy. *Acta Anaesthesiol Scand,* 43, 803-8.

Elsharnouby, N. M., Eid, H. E., Abou Elezz, N. F. & Moharram, A. N. 2008. Intraarticular injection of magnesium sulphate and/or bupivacaine for postoperative analgesia after arthroscopic knee surgery. *Anesth Analg,* 106, 1548-52, table of contents.

Eren, M., Koltka, K., Koknel Talu, G., Asik, M. & Ozyalcin, S. 2008. [Comparison of analgesic activity of intraarticular lornoxicam, bupivacaine and saline after knee arthroscopy]. *Agri,* 20, 17-22.

Fagan, D. J., Martin, W. & Smith, A. 2003. A randomized, double-blind trial of pre-emptive local anesthesia in day-case knee arthroscopy. *Arthroscopy,* 19, 50-3.

Farouk, S. & Aly, A. 2009. A comparison of intra-articular magnesium and/or morphine with bupivacaine for postoperative analgesia after arthroscopic knee surgery. *J Anesth,* 23, 508-12.

Franceschi, F., Rizzello, G., Cataldo, R. & Denaro, V. 2001. Comparison of morphine and ropivacaine following knee arthroscopy. *Arthroscopy,* 17, 477-80.

Gomoll, A. H., Kang, R. W., Williams, J. M., Bach, B. R. & Cole, B. J. 2006. Chondrolysis after continuous intra-articular bupivacaine infusion: an experimental model investigating chondrotoxicity in the rabbit shoulder. *Arthroscopy,* 22, 813-9.

Gomoll, A. H., Yanke, A. B., Kang, R. W., Chubinskaya, S., Williams, J. M., Bach, B. R. & Cole, B. J. 2009. Long-term effects of bupivacaine on cartilage in a rabbit shoulder model. *Am J Sports Med,* 37, 72-7.

Goodwin, R. C., Amjadi, F. & Parker, R. D. 2005. Short-term analgesic effects of intra-articular injections after knee arthroscopy. *Arthroscopy,* 21, 307-12.

Goodwin, R. C. & Parker, R. D. 2005. Comparison of the analgesic effects of intra-articular injections administered preoperatively and postoperatively in knee arthroscopy. *J Knee Surg,* 18, 17-24.

Grabowska-Gawel, A., Gawel, K., Hagner, W. & Bilinski, P. J. 2003. Morphine or bupivacaine in controlling postoperative pain in patients subjected to knee joint arthroscopy. *Ortop Traumatol Rehabil,* 5, 758-62.

Graham, N. M., Shanahan, M. D., Barry, P., Burgert, S. & Talkhani, I. 2000. Postoperative analgesia after arthroscopic knee surgery: a randomized, prospective, double-blind study of intravenous regional analgesia versus intra-articular analgesia. *Arthroscopy*, 16, 64-6.

Grishko, V., Xu, M., Wilson, G. & Pearsall, A. W. t. 2010. Apoptosis and mitochondrial dysfunction in human chondrocytes following exposure to lidocaine, bupivacaine, and ropivacaine. *J Bone Joint Surg Am*, 92, 609-18.

Gupta, A., Axelsson, K., Allvin, R., Liszka-Hackzell, J., Rawal, N., Althoff, B. & Augustini, B. G. 1999. Postoperative pain following knee arthroscopy: the effects of intra-articular ketorolac and/or morphine. *Reg Anesth Pain Med*, 24, 225-30.

Hansen, B. P., Beck, C. L., Beck, E. P. & Townsley, R. W. 2007. Postarthroscopic glenohumeral chondrolysis. *Am J Sports Med*, 35, 1628-34.

Hege-Scheuing, G., Michaelsen, K., Buhler, A., Kustermann, J. & Seeling, W. 1995. [Analgesia with intra-articular morphine following knee joint arthroscopy? A double-blind, randomized study with patient-controlled analgesia]. *Anaesthesist*, 44, 351-8.

Hennig, G. S., Hosgood, G., Bubenik-Angapen, L. J., Lauer, S. K. & Morgan, T. W. 2010. Evaluation of chondrocyte death in canine osteochondral explants exposed to a 0.5% solution of bupivacaine. *Am J Vet Res*, 71, 875-83.

Izdes, S., Orhun, S., Turanli, S., Erkilic, E. & Kanbak, O. 2003. The effects of preoperative inflammation on the analgesic efficacy of intraarticular piroxicam for outpatient knee arthroscopy. *Anesth Analg*, 97, 1016-9, table of contents.

Jacobs, T. F., Vansintjan, P. S., Roels, N., Herregods, S. S., Verbruggen, G., Herregods, L. L. & Almqvist, K. F. 2011. The effect of Lidocaine on the viability of cultivated mature human cartilage cells: an in vitro study. *Knee Surg Sports Traumatol Arthrosc*.

Jacobson, E., Assareh, H., Cannerfelt, R., Anderson, R. E. & Jakobsson, J. G. 2006. The postoperative analgesic effects of intra-articular levobupivacaine in elective day-case arthroscopy of the knee: a prospective, randomized, double-blind clinical study. *Knee Surg Sports Traumatol Arthrosc*, 14, 120-4.

Jaureguito, J. W., Wilcox, J. F., Cohn, S. J., Thisted, R. A. & Reider, B. 1995. A comparison of intraarticular morphine and bupivacaine for pain control after outpatient knee arthroscopy. A prospective, randomized, double-blinded study. *Am J Sports Med*, 23, 350-3.

Jawish, D., Antakly, M. C., Dagher, F., Nasser, E. & Geahchan, N. 1996. [Intra-articular analgesia after arthroscopy of the knee]. *Cah Anesthesiol*, 44, 415-7.

Joshi, G. P., McCarroll, S. M., Cooney, C. M., Blunnie, W. P., O'Brien, T. M. & Lawrence, A. J. 1992. Intra-articular morphine for pain relief after knee arthroscopy. *J Bone Joint Surg Br*, 74, 749-51.

Joshi, G. P., McCarroll, S. M., O'Brien, T. M. & Lenane, P. 1993. Intraarticular analgesia following knee arthroscopy. *Anesth Analg*, 76, 333-6.

Juelsgaard, P., Dalsgaard, J., Felsby, S. & Frokjaer, J. 1993. [Analgesic effect of 2 different doses of intra-articular morphine after ambulatory knee arthroscopy. A randomized, prospective, double-blind study]. *Ugeskr Laeger*, 155, 4169-72.

Kanbak, M., Akpolat, N., Ocal, T., Doral, M. N., Ercan, M. & Erdem, K. 1997. Intraarticular morphine administration provides pain relief after knee arthroscopy. *Eur J Anaesthesiol*, 14, 153-6.

Karaman, Y., Kayali, C., Ozturk, H., Kaya, A. & Bor, C. 2009. A comparison of analgesic effect of intra-articular levobupivacaine with bupivacaine following knee arthroscopy. *Saudi Med J*, 30, 629-32.

Karpie, J. C. & Chu, C. R. 2007. Lidocaine exhibits dose- and time-dependent cytotoxic effects on bovine articular chondrocytes in vitro. *Am J Sports Med*, 35, 1621-7.

Klinman, M., Draushln, A., N Khannehr, J., Vahod, R. & Hellman, M. 2002. Intra-synovial, compared to intra-articular morphine provides better pain relief following knee arthroscopy menisectomy. *Can J Anaesth*, 49, 380-3.

Lo, I. K., Sciore, P., Chung, M., Liang, S., Boorman, R. B., Thornton, G. M., Rattner, J. B. & Muldrew, K. 2009. Local anesthetics induce chondrocyte death in bovine articular cartilage disks in a dose- and duration-dependent manner. *Arthroscopy*, 25, 707-15.

Lundin, O., Rydgren, B., Sward, L. & Karlsson, J. 1998. Analgesic effects of intra-articular morphine during and after knee arthroscopy: a comparison of two methods. *Arthroscopy*, 14, 192-6.

Middleton, F., Coakes, J., Umarji, S., Palmer, S., Venn, R. & Panayiotou, S. 2006. The efficacy of intra-articular bupivacaine for relief of pain following arthroscopy of the ankle. *J Bone Joint Surg Br*, 88, 1603-5.

Miyazaki, T., Kobayashi, S., Takeno, K., Yayama, T., Meir, A. & Baba, H. 2011. Lidocaine cytotoxicity to the bovine articular chondrocytes in vitro: changes in cell viability and proteoglycan metabolism. *Knee Surg Sports Traumatol Arthrosc*.

Niemi, L., Pitkanen, M., Tuominen, M., Bjorkenheim, J. M. & Rosenberg, P. H. 1994. Intraarticular morphine for pain relief after knee arthroscopy performed under regional anaesthesia. *Acta Anaesthesiol Scand*, 38, 402-5.

Park, J., Sutradhar, B. C., Hong, G., Choi, S. H. & Kim, G. 2011. Comparison of the cytotoxic effects of bupivacaine, lidocaine, and mepivacaine in equine articular chondrocytes. *Vet Anaesth Analg*, 38, 127-33.

Piper, S. L. & Kim, H. T. 2008. Comparison of ropivacaine and bupivacaine toxicity in human articular chondrocytes. *J Bone Joint Surg Am*, 90, 986-91.

Pooni, J. S., Hickmott, K., Mercer, D., Myles, P. & Khan, Z. 1999. Comparison of intra-articular fentanyl and intra-articular bupivacaine for post-operative pain relief after knee arthroscopy. *Eur J Anaesthesiol*, 16, 708-11.

Raj, N., Sehgal, A., Hall, J. E., Sharma, A., Murrin, K. R. & Groves, N. D. 2004. Comparison of the analgesic efficacy and plasma concentrations of high-dose intra-articular and intramuscular morphine for knee arthroscopy. *Eur J Anaesthesiol*, 21, 932-7.

Rasmussen, S., Lorentzen, J. S., Larsen, A. S., Thomsen, S. T. & Kehlet, H. 2002. Combined intra-articular glucocorticoid, bupivacaine and morphine reduces pain and convalescence after diagnostic knee arthroscopy. *Acta Orthop Scand*, 73, 175-8.

Rautoma, P., Santanen, U., Avela, R., Luurila, H., Perhoniemi, V. & Erkola, O. 2000. Diclofenac premedication but not intra-articular ropivacaine alleviates pain following day-case knee arthroscopy. *Can J Anaesth*, 47, 220-4.

Richardson, M. D., Bjorksten, A. R., Hart, J. A. & McCullough, K. 1997. The efficacy of intra-articular morphine for postoperative knee arthroscopy analgesia. *Arthroscopy*, 13, 584-9.

Rosseland, L. A. 2005. No evidence for analgesic effect of intra-articular morphine after knee arthroscopy: a qualitative systematic review. *Reg Anesth Pain Med*, 30, 83-98.

Rosseland, L. A., Helgesen, K. G., Breivik, H. & Stubhaug, A. 2004. Moderate-to-severe pain after knee arthroscopy is relieved by intraarticular saline: a randomized controlled trial. *Anesth Analg*, 98, 1546-51, table of contents.

Rosseland, L. A., Stubhaug, A., Grevbo, F., Reikeras, O. & Breivik, H. 2003. Effective pain relief from intra-articular saline with or without morphine 2 mg in patients with moderate-to-severe pain after knee arthroscopy: a randomized, double-blind controlled clinical study. *Acta Anaesthesiol Scand*, 47, 732-8.

Rosseland, L. A., Stubhaug, A., Skoglund, A. & Breivik, H. 1999. Intra-articular morphine for pain relief after knee arthroscopy. *Acta Anaesthesiol Scand*, 43, 252-7.

Samoladas, E. P., Chalidis, B., Fotiadis, H., Terzidis, I., Ntobas, T. & Koimtzis, M. 2006. The intra-articular use of ropivacaine for the control of post knee arthroscopy pain. *J Orthop Surg Res*, 1, 17.

Santanen, U., Rautoma, P., Luurila, H. & Erkola, O. 2001. Intra-articular ropivacaine injection does not alleviate pain after day-case knee arthroscopy performed under spinal anaesthesia. *Ann Chir Gynaecol*, 90, 47-50.

Solheim, N., Rosseland, L. A. & Stubhaug, A. 2006. Intra-articular morphine 5 mg after knee arthroscopy does not produce significant pain relief when administered to patients with moderate to severe pain via an intra-articular catheter. *Reg Anesth Pain Med*, 31, 506-13.

Solomon, D. J., Navaie, M., Stedje-Larsen, E. T., Smith, J. C. & Provencher, M. T. 2009. Glenohumeral chondrolysis after arthroscopy: a systematic review of potential contributors and causal pathways. *Arthroscopy*, 25, 1329-42.

Souza, R. H., Issy, A. M. & Sakata, R. K. 2002. [Intra-articular analgesia with morphine, bupivacaine or fentanyl after knee video-arthroscopy surgery.]. *Rev Bras Anestesiol*, 52, 570-80.

Syed, H. M., Green, L., Bianski, B., Jobe, C. M. & Wongworawat, M. D. 2011. Bupivacaine and Triamcinolone May Be Toxic To Human Chondrocytes: A Pilot Study. *Clin Orthop Relat Res*.

Tamosiunas, R., Brazdzionyte, E., Tarnauskaite-Augutiene, A. & Tranauskaite-Keraitiene, G. 2005. [Postoperative analgesia with intraarticular local anesthetic bupivacaine and alpha2-agonist clonidine after arthroscopic knee surgery]. *Medicina (Kaunas)*, 41, 547-52.

Townshend, D., Emmerson, K., Jones, S., Partington, P. & Muller, S. 2009. Intra-articular injection versus portal infiltration of 0.5% bupivacaine following arthroscopy of the knee: a prospective, randomised double-blinded trial. *J Bone Joint Surg Br*, 91, 601-3.

VanNess, S. A. & Gittins, M. E. 1994. Comparison of intra-articular morphine and bupivacaine following knee arthroscopy. *Orthop Rev*, 23, 743-7.

Varrassi, G., Marinangeli, F., Ciccozzi, A., Iovinelli, G., Facchetti, G. & Ciccone, A. 1999. Intra-articular buprenorphine after knee arthroscopy. A randomised, prospective, double-blind study. *Acta Anaesthesiol Scand*, 43, 51-5.

Vranken, J. H., Vissers, K. C., de Jongh, R. & Heylen, R. 2001. Intraarticular sufentanil administration facilitates recovery after day-case knee arthroscopy. *Anesth Analg*, 92, 625-8.

Webb, S. T. & Ghosh, S. 2009. Intra-articular bupivacaine: potentially chondrotoxic? *Br J Anaesth*, 102, 439-41.

White, A. P., Laurent, S. & Wilkinson, D. J. 1990. Intra-articular and subcutaneous prilocaine with adrenaline for pain relief in day case arthroscopy of the knee joint. *Ann R Coll Surg Engl*, 72, 350-2.

Yang, L. C., Chen, L. M., Wang, C. J. & Buerkle, H. 1998. Postoperative analgesia by intra-articular neostigmine in patients undergoing knee arthroscopy. *Anesthesiology*, 88, 334-9.

Zeidan, A., Kassem, R., Nahleh, N., Maaliki, H., El-Khatib, M., Struys, M. M. & Baraka, A. 2008. Intraarticular tramadol-bupivacaine combination prolongs the duration of postoperative analgesia after outpatient arthroscopic knee surgery. *Anesth Analg*, 107, 292-9.

9

Multimodal Analgesia for Postoperative Pain Management

G. Ulufer Sivrikaya
Sisli Etfal Training and Research Hospital,
Department of 2nd Anesthesiology and Reanimation, Istanbul,
Turkey

1. Introduction

The experience of pain is complex, multifaceted, and "an unpleasant sensory and emotional experience," as defined in part by the International Association for the Study of Pain. It is a personal, subjective experience that involves sensory, emotional and behavioral factors associated with actual or potential tissue injury (Rawal). The differential behavior response to surgical incision can be influenced by many variables including global (i.e., personality, gender, age, cultural background, pre-existing pain syndromes, genetic makeup, kind and type of surgical approach, cultural background) and specific (i.e., fear, anxiety, depression, anger, and coping) psychological factors (Eccleston, 2001). Only by considering all concomitant factors can physicians provide optimal treatment.

Millions of surgeries are performed on an annual basis, necessitating the frequent use of acute postoperative pain management. There are many types of surgery and, with few exceptions, all are painful. Fear of uncontrolled pain is among the primary concerns of many patients who are about to undergo surgery.

One of the most important factors in determining when a patient can be safely discharged from a surgical facility, and that also has a major influence on the patient's ability to resume his/her normal activities of daily living, is the adequacy of postoperative pain control. Pain is a predictable part of the postoperative experience. Unrelieved postoperative pain may result in clinical and psychological changes that increase morbidity and mortality as well as costs and that decrease quality of life (Carr& Goudas, 1999).

The guidelines for acute pain management in the perioperative setting published in 1992 and 1995 (Acute Pain, 1992; American Pain, 1995; Practice Guidelines, 1995) promoted aggressive treatment of acute pain and educate patients about the need to communicate unrelieved pain. Nonetheless these guidelines appear to have had little influence on practice patterns or on improved pain control for patients. In a study of Warfield and Kahn (Warfield&Kahn, 1995) they found three of four patients reported experiencing pain after surgery, and 80% of these patients rated pain after surgery as moderate to extreme. Since their study, newer drugs, techniques and protocols for postoperative pain management have been developed, and minimally invasive surgical techniques, such as endoscopic procedures, are used more frequently. These changes in practice patterns thought that they could affect the management of postoperative pain and patient attitudes about pain. But in a recent study (Apfelbaum, 2003) that assessed patients' postoperative pain experience and the status of acute pain management in a random sample, approximately 80 percent of patients said (not very different the previous study mentioned above) they experienced acute pain after surgery. The authors concluded that; despite an increased focus on pain management programs and the development of new standards for pain management, many patients continue to experience intense pain after surgery.

Effective and appropriate pain management requires a proactive approach using a variety of treatment modalities to obtain an optimal outcome with respect to facilitating rapid recovery and returning to full function, allowing early discharge from hospital, improving quality of life for the patient and reducing morbidity (Rawal).   Protocols for postoperative pain treatment should be made with considering patients' needs, surgical indications, and institutional resources. It is important to use effective state-of-the-art techniques combined with hospital protocols for early rehabilitation and recovery.

Many options are available for the treatment of postoperative pain, including systemic (i.e., opioid and nonopioid) analgesics and regional (i.e., neuraxial and peripheral) analgesic techniques. Multimodal analgesia is achieved by combining different analgesics that act by different mechanisms and at different sites in the nervous system, resulting in additive or synergistic analgesia with lowered adverse effects of sole administration of individual analgesics (Kehlet&Dahl, 1993). It also refers to concurrent application of analgesic pharmacotherapy in combination with regional analgesia (Elvir Lazo&White, 2010).

This chapter's aim is to overview on the topic of multimodal analgesia for postoperative pain management and to provide an update on the drugs and techniques used for this approach.

2. Consequences of postoperative pain

When an appropriate analgesic treatment is not given for postoperative pain, various adverse effects might occur in the respiratory, cardiovascular, gastrointestinal, urinary, endocrinological systems, as well as in patient's metabolisms and mentality. These changes were relievable with application of appropriate types of analgesic regimens.

Postoperative pain, especially when poorly controlled, may produce a range of detrimental acute (i.e., adverse physiologic responses) (Vadivelu et al, 2010) and chronic effects (i.e., delayed long-term recovery and chronic pain) (Perkins&Kehlet, 2000). Good pain control after surgery is important to prevent negative outcomes such as tachycardia, hypertension, myocardial ischemia, decrease in alveolar ventilation, immobility, deep venous thrombosis and poor wound healing (Vadivelu et al, 2010; Nett, 2010).

Pathophysiology of acute pain, includes of changes in neuroendocrine, respiratory and renal function, gastrointestinal activity, circulatory and autonomic nervous system activity.

Unsufficient pain management can cause acute and chronic effects:

2.1 Acute effects
- Emotional and physical suffering for the patient
- Sleep disturbance (with negative impact on mood and mobilisation)
- Respiratory system side effects (leading to atelectasis, retention of secretions and pneumonia)
  - Decreased respiratory motion
  - Inhibition of cough and sputum excretion
- Cardiovascular side effects (such as hypertension and arrhythmias)

- Increased oxygen consumption (with negative impact in the case of coronary artery disease, leading to coronary ischemia and myocardial infarction)
- Impaired gastrointestinal motility (while opioids induce constipation or nausea, untreated pain may also be an important cause of impaired bowel movement or postoperative nausea and vomiting-PONV)
- Delays mobilisation and promotes thromboembolism (postoperative pain is one of the major causes for delayed mobilisation)
- Increased sympathetic activity
  - increased release of catecholamines (resulting increase in systemic vascular resistance, cardiac work and myocardial oxygen consumption associated negative effects in patients with coronary artery diseases)
  - reduced blood flow in lower extremities (resulting a higher risk of deep vein thrombosis)

2.2 Chronic effects
- Severe acute pain is a risk factor for the development of chronic pain
- Sleep disturbance (with negative impact on mood and mobilisation)
- Risk of behavioural changes (frequently in children for a prolonged period after surgical pain)
- Poor wound healing
- Delay in long-term recovery

Chronic pain is a potential adverse outcome from surgery. It is costly to society in terms of suffering and disability. For humanitarian and economic reasons, the problem of chronic pain after surgery should be addressed. In a review of Perkins et al. (Perkins&Kehlet, 2000) they showed there was a significant variability in the incidence of chronic pain among surgical procedures (i.e. 3-56% for cholecystectomy, 0-37% for inguinal hernia surgery, 11-57% for breast surgery). They concluded that chronic pain after surgery was common as that has been confirmed with another review (Camann, 1998). Another conclusion of this study is; the intensity of acute postoperative pain was one of the most striking predictive factor for chronic pain, especially following breast surgery (Elia, 2005), thorasic surgery (Carli F,2002; Viscusi, 2004) and hernia repair (Birnbach, 1989).

3. Multimodal approach to postoperative pain

Advances in the knowledge of molecular mechanisms have led to the development of multimodal analgesia and new pharmaceutical products to treat postoperative pain.

Postoperative pain treatment may not be enough to provide major improvements in some outcomes because it is unlikely that a unimodal intervention can be effective in addressing a complex problem such as perioperative outcomes (Boisseau, 2001; Kehlet&Nolte, 2001). The analgesic benefits of controlling postoperative pain are generally maximized when a multimodal strategy to facilitate the patient's convalescence is implemented (Kehlet, 1997). Pain involves multiple mechanisms that ideally require treatment using a multimodal (or 'balanced') analgesic technique (White&Kehlet, 2010) Principles of a multimodal strategy include control of postoperative pain to allow early mobilization, early enteral nutrition, education, and attenuation of the perioperative stress response through the use of regional anesthetic techniques and a combination of analgesic agents (i.e., multimodal analgesia).

The concept of multimodal analgesia was introduced more than a decade ago as a technique to improve analgesia and reduce the incidence of opioid-related adverse events. Multimodal analgesia is achieved by combining different analgesics that act by different mechanisms at different sites in the nervous system, reducing the incidence of side effects owing to the lower doses of the individual drugs (Buvanendran&Kroin 2009). For example, epidural opioids can be administered in combination with epidural local anesthetics; intravenous opioids can be administered in combination with Nonsteroidal Antiinflammatory Drug (NSAID)s, which have a dose sparing effect for systemically administered opioids. It also refers to concurrent application of analgesic pharmacotherapy in combination with regional analgesia (Elvir Lazo&White, 2010; Rawal).

In the literature some different definitions of multimodal analgesia exists. In some contexts, multimodal analgesia refers to systemic administration of analgesic drugs with different mechanisms of action, whereas in other situations it refers to concurrent application of analgesic pharmacotherapy in combination with regional analgesia. Multimodal analgesia is based on to choice paracetamol and NSAIDs for low intensity pain with opioid analgesics and/or local analgesia techniques being used for moderate and high intensity pain as indicated. (Elvir Lazo&White, 2010; Rawal) (Table 1)

Mild intensity pain	Moderate intensity pain	Severe intensity pain
For example: Inguinal hernia Varices Laparoscopy	*For example:* Hip replacement Hysterectomy Jaw surgery	*For example:* Thoracotomy Upper abdominal surgery Aortic surgery Knee replacement
		(i) Paracetamol and wound infiltration with local anesthetic (ii) NSAIDs (unless contraindicated) and (iii) Epidural local analgesia or major peripheral nerve or plexus block or opioid injection (IV PCA)
	(i) Paracetamol and wound infiltration with local anesthetic (ii) NSAIDs (unless contraindicated) and (iii) Peripheral nerve block (single shot or continuous infusion) or opioid injection (IV PCA)	
(i) Paracetamol and wound infiltration with local anesthetic (ii) NSAIDs (unless contraindicated) and (iii) Regional block analgesia Add weak opioid or rescue analgesia with small increments of intravenous strong opioid if necessary		

Table 1. Treatment options in relation to magnitude of postoperative pain expected following different types of surgery (by permission from Publisher AstraZeneca)

A better incidence of adverse effects and improved analgesia has been demonstrated with multimodal analgesia techniques, which may provide for shorter hospitalization times, improved recovery and function, and possibly decreased healthcare costs (Buvanendran & Kroin, 2009).

To achieve a maximum short-term and long-term benefits from multimodal analgesic therapies, the pain management would be initiated as a preventive in the preoperative period continued in the early postoperative period and extended into the postcharge period for 3-7 days (Bisgaard, 2006; White et al, 2007). A deficiency in the design of many of the published studies involving multimodal analgesic therapies is that the drug regimens were not continued into the postdischarge period (Ma, 2004). For example, only immediate pre- and postoperative administration of the cyclooxygenase 2 (COX-2) inhibitor rofecoxib as part of a multimodal analgesic regimen in outpatients undergoing inguinal hernia repair provided limited benefits beyond the early postoperative period (White&Kehlet, 2007). However, when the COX-2 inhibitors are administered for 3 to 5 days after ambulatory surgery, (Gan, 2004; Joshi, 2004) the greater benefits were achieved with respect to clinically relevant patient outcomes (eg, resumption of normal activities) and improvements in pain control. Bisgaard et al (Bisgaard, 2006) concluded that a multimodal analgesic regimen consisting of a preoperative single dose of dexamethasone, incisional local anesthetics (at the beginning and/or end of surgery), and continuous treatment with NSAIDs (or COX-2 inhibitors) during the first 3 to 4 days provided the best clinical outcome. Moreover, recent clinical studies suggest that when classical NSAIDs or more selective COX-2 inhibiting drugs were administered for 3–5 days after ambulatory surgery, a significant benefit was achieved with respect to clinically relevant patient outcomes (e.g., resumption of normal activities) and improvements in short-term pain control (Gan, 2004; White, 2007).

A multimodal analgesic regimen should be adjusted to meet the needs of the individual patient by taking into consideration their pre-existing medical conditions, types of surgery, and previous experiences related to both acute and chronic pain management. Critical multimodal protocols must be designed based on surgical procedures and structural organization to warrant improved outcome including having minimum side effects related to the treatment and rapid returning to social life and daily activities (Fanelli, 2008).

Several multimodal approaches have been advocated based on different combinations of anti-inflammatory drugs, and regional anesthesia (epidural, peripheral nerve blocks, paravertebral blocks, and local injection/infusion of local anesthetics) (Buvanendran, 2010; Mathiesen, 2009). Although each of these drugs and/or techniques has been demonstrated as being effective in reducing the need for postoperative intravenous opioids alone, the evidence supporting specific combinations of drugs and/or regional techniques is still limited.

3.1 Multidisciplinary approach

Faster recovery, reduced hospital stay, and decreased length of convalescence can occur if multimodal analgesia is combined with a rehabilitation program that is multidisciplinary and multimodal (Gajraj&Joshi, 2005).

Treatment of postoperative pain requires good multi-disciplinary and multi-professional co-operation. Multidisciplinary team consists of the anesthesiologist himself has overall responsibility, pain nurse and specialist surgeon, sometimes pharmacist. In the ward the patient's physician and nurse, physiotherapist when needed are responsible for all care, in partnership with the pain team. The nurse is responsible to report the patient's intensity of pain to the physician and to treat the pain within the defined rules of the local guidelines. Also should pay attention to the effects and side effects of the pain treatment. The pain team nurse is the first point of contact while the anesthesiologist and pharmacist are available to provide specialist advice (Rawal).

All staff involved in the treatment of postoperative pain require regularly updated training emphasising the importance of team-working and co-operation. In this training programme the main headings should be included as; a. Physiology and pathophysiology of pain, b. Pharmacology of analgesics, c. Locally available treatment methods d. Monitoring routines with regard to treatment of pain and e. Local document for treatment and assessment of pain (Rawal).

It is important to understand of the postoperative pain experience from a patient's perspective, if health care professionals are to identify ways to improve care. In Apfelbaum et al study (Apfelbaum et al, 2003); when asked about attitudes regarding pain and pain medications, 75% of patients believed that it was necessary to experience some pain after surgery, and 8% of patients had postponed surgery because they were worried about the possibility of experiencing pain. Although most patients claimed to receive preoperative education on postoperative pain management, that study's findings suggested that a patient's real concern is not adequately addressed.

The patient himself and family members are also to be undertaken as the members of the multidisciplinary team. Education is an important role in this point. Patients are unlikely to be aware of postoperative pain treatment techniques and as the success of pain relief is influenced by their knowledge and beliefs, it is helpful to give patients (and parents in case of cognitively impaired, severely emotionally disturbed, children) detailed information about postoperative pain and pain treatment. Adequate information gives the patient realistic expectations of the care that can be provided (pain relief, not a "pain free status"). Patients who do not speak the local language, and patients whose level of education or cultural background differs significantly from that of their health care team need special concern. A preoperative discussion with the patient and relatives can be helpful about an effective postoperative pain management (Rawal).

It is important to emphasize the need for collaboration between the various health care providers involved in the patient's perioperative care (eg, anesthesiologists, surgeons, nurses, and physiotherapists) to integrate improved perioperative pain management strategies with the recently described fast-track recovery paradigms (White, 2007). This type of multi-disciplinary approach has been documented to improve the quality of the recovery process and reduce the hospital stay and postoperative morbidity, leading to a shorter period of convalescence after surgery (White&Kehlet, 2010).

3.2 Pre-emptive – Preventive analgesia

The concept of pre-emptive analgesia has its origins in the idea that painful stimuli, if not prevented by administration of preoperative analgesic drugs, could lead to spinal sensitization and neuroplasticity processes, resulting in increased pain intensity and duration after surgery. Many authors have studied the effects of different timing of administration of single drugs (e.g., pre-, intra- or postoperative) and have reported no differences in efficacy (Moiniche, 2002).

This approach does not seem to offer any clinically significant advantages over so-called preventative multimodal analgesic regimens when an effective pro-active approach to pain management is initiated in the early postoperative period and extended into the postdischarge period (Sun, 2008). Starting with intensive pain therapy at the beginning and analgesia must be continued, using step-down techniques that involve a change in drugs or route of administration (*i.e.*, from the epidural and intravenous routes to *per os* administration) (Fanelli, 2008).

The main goals of preventive analgesia are: to decrease pain after tissue injury, to prevent spinal sensitization and to reduce the incidence of inflammatory or chronic pain (Senturk, 2002).

4. Drugs in postoperative pain management

Multimodal (or balanced) analgesia represents an increasingly popular approach to preventing postoperative pain. The approach involves administering a combination of opioid and nonopioid analgesics (and adjuvant agents) that act at different sites within the central and peripheral nervous systems in an effort to improve pain control, with fewer opioid-related side effects mainly sedation, nausea, vomiting pruritis, constipation (Elvir Lazo&White, 2010; Vadivelu, 2010).

The development of newer agents available for postoperative pain control opens up possibilities for newer combinations in multimodal analgesia. Multi-pharmacological therapy based on synergistic effects of two or more drugs gives better results than a mono-pharmacologic approach (Vadivelu, 2010).

4.1 Opioids

Opioid analgesics continue to play an important role in the acute treatment of moderate-to-severe pain in the early postoperative period. The problem about these drugs is the variety of perioperative complications eg, drowsiness and sedation, PONV, pruritus, urinary retention, ileus, constipation, ventilatory depression of them. These opioid-related adverse effects inhibit rapid recovery and rehabilitation (Buvanendran&Kroin, 2009; Vadivelu, 2010). Their effects can be summarized as hyperpolarization of first- and second-order sensory neurons, with inhibition of synaptic transmission. They act by binding to μ receptors, which initially results in increased G protein activity; this, in turn, leads to K+ efflux and inhibition of Ca2+ influx into the cell. Opioids also stimulate the supraspinal descending inhibitory system, which further increases the hyperpolarization of second-order neurons by releasing 5-HT and glycine. Opioid receptors have been demonstrated *in vitro* in peripheral nerve terminals, but they are unable to influence the inflammatory reaction, resulting lack of effectiveness on postoperative pain during movement (Christie, 2000).

Opioids can be used in different ways; i.e intravenous, intramuscular, subcutaneous, transmucosal, epidural, intrathecal, transdermal. The most common route of postoperative systemic opioid analgesic administration is intravenous. When the most important source of nociceptive stimuli is visceral pain, good results may be achieved by intrathecal administration of small doses of opioids (Rathmell, 2005).

Patient controlled analgesia (PCA) optimizes delivery of analgesic opioids and minimizes the effects of pharmacokinetic and pharmacodynamics variability in individual patients. It can be programmed for several variables: demand (bolus) dose, lockout interval, continuous or basal infusion, and 4 h limit (Table 2). PCA provides superior postoperative analgesia and improves patient satisfaction when compared with traditional PRN analgesic regimens.

Drug *- Concentration	Bolus dose	Lockout interval (min)	Basal-Continuous infusion **
Morphine (1 mg/ml)	0.5-2 mg	5-10	0-2 mg/h
Fentanyl (0.01 mg/ml)	10-20 µg	5-10	0-60 µg/h
Alfentanil (0.1 mg/ml)	0.1-0.2 mg	5-8	
Sufentanil (0.002 mg/ml)	2-5 µg	4-10	0-8 µg/h
Meperidine (10 mg/ml)	5-25 mg	5-10	0-20 mg/h
Tramadol (4-5 mg/ml)	10-20 mg	6-10	0-20 mg/ml

* Individual patient requirements vary widely. Titrated loading doses can be used if necessary to establish initial analgesia.
** Continuous infusions are not initially recommended for opioid-naive adult patients

Table 2. Intravenous PCA Regimens

Opioid analgesics will likely remain the primary treatment option for patients who require rescue analgesic therapy in the postoperative period until more potent and rapid-acting nonopioid analgesics become available for routine clinical use.

4.1.1 Controlled-release opiods
Controlled-release opioids are not traditionally considered useful in the immediate postoperative period, but some studies have demonstrated that controlled-release oxycodone may be used for postoperative pain control when remifentanil is used for maintenance of anesthesia. Its preoperative administration leads to adequate plasma concentrations for postoperative analgesia and hyperalgesia treatment following short surgery (1-2 h) (Nishimori, 2006). In addition, controlled-release opioids are an optimal choice for step-down analgesia in the late postoperative and rehabilitation periods following orthopedic surgical procedures (de Beer J de, 2005).

4.1.2 Tramadol
Tramadol enhances inhibitory effects on pain transmission at the spinal level blocking nociceptive signal transduction both by opioid and monoaminergic mechanisms. Its opioid and nonopioid modes of action appear to act synergistically. The drug is available in formulations suitable for oral, rectal and parenteral administration. Tramadol has been shown to provide effective analgesia after intravenous and oral (in a few of newer clinical studies) administration for postoperative pain management. The main advantage of tramadol in postoperative analgesia is a relative lack of respiratory depression. The potential of abuse is also negligible.

4.2 Nonopioids
Opioid analgesics, once considered the standard approach to preventing acute postoperative pain, are being replaced by a combination of nonopioid analgesic drugs with diverse modes of action as part of a multimodal approach to preventing pain after ambulatory surgery.
Nonopioid analgesics are increasingly being used before, during, and after surgery to facilitate the recovery process especially after ambulatory surgery because of their anesthetic-and analgesic-sparing effects and their ability to reduce postoperative pain (with movement), opioid analgesic requirement, and side effects, thereby shortening the duration of the hospital

play. Nonopioid analgesics will likely assume a greater role as preventive analgesics in the future as the number of minimally invasive (keyhole) surgery cases continues to expand.

Recent studies have confirmed that a rational combination of different nonopioid analgesics when given as part of multimodal analgesia reduces postoperative pain. The use of traditional NSAIDs, COX-2 inhibitors, acetaminophen, ketamine, dexmedetomidine, dextromethorphan, alpha2-agonists, gabapentin, pregabalin, and glucocorticoid steroids can provide beneficial effects when administered in appropriate doses as part of a multimodal analgesic regimen in the perioperative setting (Elvir Lazo&White, 2010).

Nonopioid drugs used in postoperative pain management can be classified as:

1. NSAIDs and COX-2 inhibitors
2. Acetaminophen
3. Paracetamol
4. Adjuvants
    a. Alpha-2 adrenergic agonists
        i.   Clonidine
        ii. Dexmedetomidine
    b. N-methyl-D-aspartate antagonists (Antihyperalgesic drugs)
        i.   Ketamine
        ii. Dextramethorphan
        iii. Magnesium
    c. Gabapentin-type drugs
        i.   Gabapentin
        ii. Pregabalin
    d. Glucocorticoids
        i.   Dexamethasone
    e. Newer drugs
        i.   Capsaicin
        ii. Glyceryl trinitrate
        iii. Cholinergic drugs
                Nicotine
5. Local Anesthetics

4.2.1 NSAIDs and cyclooxygenase-2-selective inhibitors

NSAIDs are known to achieve pain relief by their effect on COX-1 and 2 with the various NSAIDs differing in the proportion to which they inhibit COX-1 and COX-2. They are acid compounds with analgesic, antipyretic and anti-inflammatory properties via inhibition of prostaglandin (PG) synthesis. Prostaglandins, including PG-E2, are responsible for reducing the pain threshold at the site of injury, resulting in central sensitization and a lower pain threshold in the surrounding uninjured tissue. The primary site of action of NSAIDs is believed to be in the periphery though recent research indicates that central inhibition of COX-2 may also play an important role in modulating nociception. NSAIDs inhibit the synthesis of prostaglandins both in the spinal cord and at the periphery, thus diminishing the hyperalgesic state after surgical trauma (Buvanendran&Kroin, 2009; Fanelli, 2008; McClane, 2010).

NSAIDs are administered orally, parenterally or by the rectal route.

NSAIDs are useful as the sole analgesic after minor surgical procedures. They provide moderate postoperative analgesia and thereby have a significant opioid-sparing effect of 20-

30% after major surgery (Power, 1999). This may be of clinical importance as NSAIDs may reduce the incidence of opioid-related side-effects (respiratory depression, sedation, nausea and vomiting, ileus, urinary bladder dysfunction and possibly sleep disturbances). Since the COX-2 enzyme, the primary target of NSAIDs, is inducible, it is not found in damaged tissues until a few hours following the onset of a noxious stimulus. This could explain the lack of efficacy of preemptive administration of these drugs (Ness, 2001).

NSAID use is not appropriate in all patients because of their age or renal or hematological status or because of previous dyspeptic symptoms (McClane, 2010). COX-2-selective inhibitors (celecoxib, etoricoxib, rofecoxib- is no longer in use due to adverse cardiovascular events-) have the advantage over NSAIDs in the perioperative setting of not increasing the risk of bleeding (Buvanendran&Kroin, 2009).

Many patients now receive a NSAID as a routine part of their postoperative analgesic management. Recent practice guidelines for acute pain management in the perioperative setting specifically state 'unless contraindicated, all patients should receive around-the-clock regimen of NSAIDs, COX-2 inhibitors, or acetaminophen' (Ashburn, et al, 2004).

4.2.2 Acetaminophen

Acetaminophen is antipyretic and analgesic but has little, if any, anti-inflammatory action. Its analgesic efficacy is not more than that of traditional analgesics; however, it has fewer side effects. Preparation of intravenous acetaminophen recently has been released in Europe. A 100 ml solution is presented as 10 mg/ml for administration over a period of 15 minutes. The onset of action is within five to 10 minutes, with the peak at one to two hours. Optimal analgesia for moderate to severe postoperative pain cannot be achieved using a single agent alone, but a balanced approach in combination with non-steroidal agents can result in up to a 40 to 50 percent reduction in opioid requirements (Vadivelu, 2010).

4.2.3 Paracetamol

Paracetamol has antipyretic and analgesic properties, but it is devoid of anti-inflammatory effects. It has an inhibitory action on central COX-2 and COX-3 enzymes, which would explain its antipyretic activity. The analgesic effect seems to be due to activation of descending serotonergic inhibitory pathways as well as inhibition of central NO synthases (Graham&Scott, 2005). Similar to other analgesic drugs, paracetamol shows differential properties in terms of pain control. Paracetamol may be more effective in treating episiotomy or abdominal pain rather than pain following orthopedic surgery or tooth extraction (Gray, et al, 2005; macario&Lipman, 2001). The different relative roles of peripheral COX enzymes in postoperative pain may explain these differing efficacies.

When paracetamol and NSAIDs are administered by an intravenous route, they show sparing effects on opioid consumption (about 25% and 30%, respectively); this effect begins 4 h after their first administration and is synergistic (Elia et al, 2005; Mirande, 2006).

4.2.4 Adjuvants

Adjuvant drugs are defined as substances that may improve pain treatment and pain control, but they are not commonly defined as analgesics. Adjuvants are compounds, which by themselves have undesirable side effects or low potency but in combination with opioids allow a reduction of narcotic dosing for postoperative pain control. Thus they can provide beneficial effects when administered in appropriate doses as part of a multimodal analgesic regimen in the perioperative setting (Fanelli et al, 2008; Vadivelu et al, 2010).

Multimodal analgesia incorporates the use of analgesic adjuncts with different mechanisms of action to enhance postoperative pain management. Adjuvants are important in postoperative pain management due to side effects of opioid analgesics, which hinder recovery, especially in the increasingly utilized ambulatory surgical procedures (Buvanendran&Kroin, 2007). Multiple adjuvants recently have been developed for the control of pain.

4.2.4.1 Alpha-2 adrenergic agonists

Alpha-2 adrenergic activation represents an intrinsic pain control network of the central nervous system. The alpha-2 adrenergic receptor has high density in the substantia gelatinosa of the dorsal horn in humans and that is believed to be the primary site of action by which alpha-2 adrenergic agonists can reduce pain (Buvanendran&Kroin, 2007).

4.2.4.1.1 Clonidine

Clonidine is originally classified as an anti-hypertensive drug with negative chronotropic activity, but has antinociceptive properties as well. In the spinal cord, clonidine acts at alpha-2 adrenergic receptors to stimulate acetylcholine release, which acts at both muscarinic and nicotinic receptor subtypes with analgesic effects (Fanelli et al, 2008).

Clonidine can be administered orally, intravenously, neuraxially or perineurally in combination with local anesthetics. However, the side effects could be significant. The most important ones are hypotension, bradycardia and sedation (Rawal). Data about the systemic administration of clonidine could support the usefulness of low-dose IV administration. Nonetheless due to the many side effects of systemic clonidine administration, the spinal route is preferred.

Low doses of clonidine proved to be a useful adjunct analgesic when given neuraxially and in combination with peripheral nerve blocks (Habib et al, 2005). Significant results in terms of block duration were obtained when clonidine was added to local anesthetics for epidural or perineural analgesia. At low doses (2 µg/kg), it was shown to increase the duration of perineural blockade. Animal studies suggest that the mechanism of clonidine's potentiation of lidocaine nerve block is inhibition of the hyperpolarization-activated cation current, not via its binding to alpha-2 adrenergic receptors (Jurna, 1995).

4.2.4.1.2 Dexmedetomidine

Dexmedetomidine is a relatively new, highly selective central alpha-2 agonist. Dexmedetomidine, when used as an adjunct, can reduce postoperative morphine consumption in various surgical settings using various routes such as intravenous (Dholakia et al, 2007; Gurbet et al, 2006; Lin et al, 2009). In a recent study the authors found that; the addition of dexmedetomidine to intravenous PCA morphine resulted in superior analgesia, significant morphine sparing, and less morphine-induced nausea,while it was devoid of additional sedation and untoward hemodynamic changes (Dholakia et al, 2007).

4.2.4.2 N-methyl-D-aspartate antagonists (Antihyperalgesic drugs)

With the discovery of the N-methyl-D-aspartate (NMDA) receptor and its links to nociceptive pain transmission and central sensitization, there has been renewed interest in utilizing noncompetitive NMDA receptor antagonists, such as ketamine, dextromethorphan, magnesium ions as potential antihyperalgesic agents.

4.2.4.2.1 Ketamine

Ketamine has been a well known general anesthetic and analgesic for the past 3 decades. There is evidence that low-dose ketamine may play an important role in postoperative pain management when used as an adjunct to opioids, local anesthetics, and other analgesic agents.

Ketamine, is the most commonly used antihyperalgesic drug. There is a definite role of ketamine in preventing opioid-induced hyperalgesia in patients receiving high doses of opioid for their postoperative pain relief (Mitra, 2008). It acts as an antagonist of NMDA receptors and may reduce the intensity of hyperalgesia following rapid μ opioid receptor stimulation by short-acting agonists such as remifentanil and, to a lesser extent, sufentanil and fentanyl. Perioperative administration of 2-10 μg/kg/min following a loading dose of 0.5 mg/kg decreases hyperalgesia and allodynia after thoracic and abdominal surgery (Bilgin et al, 2005; Joly et al, 2005), although doses may vary depending on the overall duration and amount of exposure to short-acting opioids.

Routes of administration include oral, intravenous, intramuscular, subcutaneous, epidural, transdermal, and intra-articular.

Clinical use of ketamine can be limited due to psychotomimetic adverse effects such as hallucinations, excessive sedation and bad dreams. Other common adverse effects are dizziness, blurred vision, and nausea and vomiting (Bell et al, 2006). Although high doses of ketamine have been implicated in causing psychomimetic effects, subanesthetic or low doses of ketamine have demonstrated significant analgesic efficacy without these side effects (Buvanendran&Kroin, 2009). It can be used in sub-anesthetic doses as an adjunct to provide postoperative pain relief in opioid-dependent patients (Mitra et al, 2004).

4.2.4.2.2 Dextramethorphan

Dextromethorphan has a similar mechanism of action with a lower affinity for the NMDA receptor. Following oral administration, it is rapidly absorbed from the gut and crosses the blood-brain barrier. A systematic review of perioperative dextromethorphan treatment for acute post-surgical pain concluded that the drug was a safe potential adjunct to classical opioid-based analgesia, but the results were inconsistent (Duedahl et al, 2006).

4.2.4.2.3 Magnesium

The magnesium ion was the first agent discovered to be an NMDA channel blocker. Similarly to ketamine and dextromethorphan, magnesium ions act by blocking the NMDA receptor pore. Since magnesium crosses the blood-brain barrier with difficulty in humans, it is not clear whether its therapeutic effects are related to NMDA antagonism in the central nervous system.

Several clinical studies have shown that magnesium increases postoperative analgesia, but the best dosage regimen remains to be determined (Lysakowski et al, 2007). At very high doses, perioperative intravenous magnesium sulfate has been reported to reduce postoperative morphine consumption but not postoperative pain scores (Koinig et al, 1998; Tramer et al, 1996).

4.2.4.3 Gabapentin-type drugs

Pregabalin and gabapentin bind to voltage-gated calcium channels in the spinal cord and brain. Both drugs are used for seizures and neuropathic pain. One advantage of pregabalin in clinical use is that it has higher bioavailability than gabapentin and linear pharmocokination. The supplementional compounds have been used as part of multimodal analgesic in the postoperative period. Earlier clinical trials with gabapentin for early postsurgical pain have recently been reviewed (Buvanendran&Kroin, 2009).

4.2.4.3.1 Gabapentin

Gabapentin, a third-generation anti-epileptic drug, is a structural analogue of Gaba Aminobutyric Acid (GABA), an important neurotransmitter in the central nervous system. Its main action, however, is to inhibit the alpha2δ subunit of Ca2+ channels with a resultant decrease in neuronal hyperexcitability. During the immediate postoperative period, however, its activation of descending inhibitory pathways may be more relevant and might explain its synergistic effect with opioids (Hurley et al, 2006).

Most of the reviews and meta-analyses concur that perioperative gabapentin helps to produce a significant opioid-sparing effect and probably also improves postoperative pain score relative to the control group (Hartrick et al, 2009; Tiipana et al, 2007).

4.2.4.3.2 Pregabalin

Pregabalin a structural analog of GABA and a derivative of gabapentin (S+ 3-isobutyl GABA). It is a novel drug with a heightened research interest in the analgesic, sedative, anxiolytic, and opioid-sparing effects, in various pain settings, including postoperative pain.

Its main advantages may be faster onset and reduced adverse side effects. Some studies suggest pregabalin to have effective sedative and opioid-sparing effects (Hartrick et al, 2009; Mathiesen et al, 2008), useful characteristics for the control of acute pain. Research on its established role as an analgesic adjuvant as a part of multimodal analgesia for acute pain control is ongoing.

4.2.4.4 Glucocorticoids

Glucocorticoids, including dexamethasone, have been used to reduce inflammation and postoperative pain in surgical procedures (Salerno et al, 2006). Glucocorticoid steroids can provide beneficial effects when administered in appropriate doses as part of a multimodal analgesic regimen in the perioperative setting (White, 2005, 2007).

4.2.4.4.1 Dexamethasone

Dexamethasone is a synthetic glucocorticoid with high potency and a long duration of action (half-life: 2 days), and has low mineralocorticoid activity. Although dexamethasone reduces PG synthesis, its possible analgesic effects have not yet been demonstrated.

In patients undergoing total hip arthroplasty under spinal anesthesia with propofol sedation a single preoperative intravenous dose of dexamethasone decreased the pain upon standing at 24 h compared to placebo (Kardash et al, 2008). In a recent study, it did not reduce postoperative pain scores and analgesic requirements after laparoscopic cholecystectomy. The main advantage of postoperative dexamethasone is its ability to reduce postoperative nausea and vomiting (Feo et al, 2006).

4.2.4.5 Newer drugs

4.2.4.5.1 Capcaisin

Capsaicin (8-methyl-N-vanillyl-6-nonenamide) is a non narcotic and acts peripherally. It can be used as a cream and also as an injectable analgesic.

Capsaicin cream is usually combined with narcotic analgesics and NSAIDs to relieve a variety of painful ailments such as back pain, arthritic joint pains, and strains and sprains. Injectable capsaicin is used for the control of post operative pain, such as after total knee replacement, total hip replacement, hernia repair, shoulder arthroscopy, and bunionectomy (Aasvang et al, 2008). Pre-administration of neural blockade before injection of capsaicin may greatly decrease the burning discomfort.

Capsaicin appears to be a relatively safe drug. In the elderly who are sensitive to respiratory depression that can occur with opioids, capsaicin can be particularly beneficial as an adjuvant. The only absolute contraindication being patient hypersensitivity. Relative contraindications include age less than 2 years, patients with elevated liver enzymes, patients on ACE inhibitors, and patients showing signs of septic arthritis and joint infections (Vadivelu et al, 2010).

4.2.4.5.2 Glyceryl trinitrate

The organic nitrates, such as glyceryl trinitrate (GTN), act as nitric oxide donors.

High dose nitroglyserin patches, such as 30 mg daily, are hyperalgesic, whereas doses less than 6 mg per day are analgesic under different circumstances. Previously it has been observed that patients with past histories of angina who had spinal block, in which the nitroglycerin transdermal patch was applied prophylactically, required fewer analgesic after operation (Lauretti et al, 1999).

4.2.4.5.3 Cholinergic drugs

Acetylcholine may cause analgesia through direct action on spinal cholinergic muscarinic receptors M1 and M3 and nicotinic receptors subtypes.

4.2.4.5.3.1 Nicotine

In a study in nonsmoker patients having radical retropubic prostatectomy under general anesthesia, the application of a 7 mg nicotine patch 30–60 min before surgery for postoperative 24 hrs, resulted with lower cumulative PCA morphine consumption versus placebo group. But the intensity of nausea was greater in the nicotine group (Habib et al, 2008).

Table 3 summarizes the doses and routes of administration of frequently used drugs.

	Administration	**Dosage**
OPIOIDS		
Morphine	(i) Intravenous. (ii) Subcutaneous by continuous infusion or intermittent boluses via indwelling cannula. (iii) Intramuscular (not recommended due to incidence of pain. 5-10 mg 3-4 hourly).	IV PCA Bolus: 1-2 mg, lockout: 5-15 min (usually 7-8 min), no background infusion. Subcutaneous 0.1-0.15 mg/kg 4-6 hourly, adapted in relation to pain score, sedation and respiratory rate.
Codeine	Oral	3 mg/kg/day combined with paracetamol. A minimum of 30 mg codeine/tablet is required

	Administration	Dosage
OPIOIDS		
Tramadol	(i) Intravenous: inject slowly (risk of high incidence of nausea and vomiting). (ii) Intramuscular. (iii) Oral administration as soon as possible.	0.75-1.0 mg/kg 50-100 mg 6 hourly.
NONOPIOIDS		
Paracetamol	Oral	4 x 1 g paracetamol/day (2 g propacetamol/day). Dose to be reduced (e.g. 3 x 1 g/day) in case of hepatic insufficiency.
Combination of paracetamol and codeine	Oral	Paracetamol 500 mg + codeine 30 mg. 4 x 1 g paracetamol/day.
NSAIDs	(i) Intravenous administration should start at least 30-60 min before end of surgery. (ii) Oral administration should start as soon as possible. Duration: 3-5 days. (iii) Rectal	Ketorolac: 3 x 30-40 mg/day (only IV form) Diclofenac: 2 x 75 mg/day Ketoprofen: 4 x 50 mg/day (ii) Selective NSAIDs include: Meloxicam 15 mg once daily Celecoxib: 200 mg/day.
Acetaminophen	Intravenous	100 ml solution (10 mg/ml) administration over a period of 15 minutes.
ADJUVANTS		
Clonidine	(i) Oral (ii) Intravenous (iii) Combined with local anesthetics-neuraxially or perineurally	3- 5 µg/kg (oral) 1 µg/kg (intravenous) 1-2 µg/kg (epidural) or 75-100 µg (intrathecal)
Ketamine	Intravenous	Loading dose of 0.5 mg/kg followed by 2-10 µg/kg/min

* The doses and routes of administration of drugs described above are general examples and each patient should be assessed individually before prescribing

Table 3. The doses and routes of administration of frequently used drugs * (modified table by permission from Publisher AstraZeneca)

4.2.5 Local anesthetics

Sodium channel blocking drugs are usually used in the management of both acute and chronic pain. When dealing with postoperative pain, local anesthetics such as lidocaine and bupivacaine mostly preferred (McCleane, 2010).

Local anesthetics block sodium channels, thereby, preventing transmission of nerve impulse along the axonal fibre. This is a local effect at the site of injection. Tissue anesthesia occurs after the injection of the local anesthetics into tissue at appropriate concentration, but it lasts after the duration of the drug ended. However, local anesthetics are also absorbed into the systemic circulation from the site of injection and, depending on the dose and rate of absorption, may have systemic analgesic effects (Gupta,2010; McCleane, 2010).

Local anesthetic solutions delivered through an epidural or perineural route are the most important treatments for decreasing incident pain, hormonal stress and sympathetic responses during and after surgery (Chelly, 2001; Liu, 2007). Generally, higher doses are used intraoperatively and then reduced to reach differential motor-sensory block in the postoperative period. The best results are achieved when local anesthetic solutions are infused neuraxially with lipophilic opioids, such as sufentanil and fentanyl at adequate concentrations (George, 2006; de-Leon-Casaola&Lema, 1996).

In some studies the effectiveness of the intravenous infusion of lidocaine in reducing postoperative pain and facilitating the recovery process have been demonstrated (Kaba et al, 2007; Lauwick et al, 2008). Yardeni and colleagues (Yardeni et al, 2009) suggested that, perioperative administration of intravenous lidocaine could improve early postoperative pain control and reduce surgery-induced immune alterations. The injection of local anesthetic around wound edges has been proven to reduce postoperative pain, but only for the duration of that local anesthetic (Moinichi et al, 1998). Several concerns about these drugs have been expressed in the literature including the risk of infection, chondrolysis and systemic local anesthetics toxicity when they used locally.

The maximum doses for local anesthetics are summarized in Table 4.

Local anesthetic	Maximum total dosage
Prokain	400 mg
Chlorprocaine	800 mg
Lidocaine	4 mg/kg (without epinephrine) 7 mg/kg(with epinephrine) **or** 300 mg
Prilocaine	6 mg/kg (without epinephrine) 9 mg/kg(with epinephrine) **or** 500 mg
Bupivacaine	2 mg/kg (without epinephrine) 2.5 mg/kg(with epinephrine) **or** 150 mg
Levobupivacaine	2.5-3 mg/kg (insufficient data) **or** 150 mg
Ropivacaine	3-4 mg/kg (without or with epinephrine)

Table 4. Maximum doses of frequently used local anesthetics

5. Techniques in postoperative pain management

One approach for multimodal analgesia is the use of regional anesthesia and analgesia to inhibit the neural conduction from the surgical site to the spinal cord and decrease spinal cord sensitization (Buvanendran&Kroin, 2009). A variety of neuraxial and peripheral regional analgesic techniques can provide analgesia superior to that with systemic opioids and may even result in improvement in various outcomes. However, there are some risks associated with the use of such techniques. The clinician should evaluate the risks and benefits of these techniques on an individual basis in determining the appropriateness of neuraxial or

variable and is given for techniques for most patients, especially in light of some of the controversies
about the use of these techniques in the presence of various anticoagulants.

Neuraxial (primarily epidural) and peripheral regional analgesic techniques (e.g., brachial
plexus, lumbar plexus, femoral, sciatic-popliteal, and scalp nerve blocks), also a variety of
wound infiltration techniques may be used for the effective treatment of postoperative pain.
In general, the analgesia provided by epidural and peripheral techniques (particularly when
local anesthetics are used) is superior to that with systemic opioids, (i.e., superior analgesia
and decreased opioid-related side effects) and use of these techniques may even reduce
morbidity and mortality (Wu&Fleisher 2000).

Techniques used in postopetaive pain management are:
1. Neuraxial Techniques
2. Peripheral Regional Analgesia Techniques
3. Infiltration Techniques
    a. Wound Infiltration
    b. Topical Application
    c. Local Infiltration Analgesia
4. Other – Nonpharmacological Techniques

5.1 Neuraxial techniques

Spinal or epidural analgesia techniques in single or continuous forms can be used in
postoperative pain management. The use of epidural anesthesia and analgesia is an integral
part of the multimodal approach because of the superior analgesia and physiologic benefits
conferred by epidural analgesia.

Among the most commonly used pain-relieving techniques, there is evidence that the
epidural local anesthetic or local anesthetic-opioid techniques are the most effective on
providing dynamic pain relief after major surgical procedures (Kehlet et al, 1999). Epidural
local anesthetic application comes in as the major component of multimodal analgesia.

Postoperative epidural analgesia is usually accomplished with a combination of a long-
acting local anesthetic and an opioid, in dilute concentrations (Table 5). Long-acting local
anesthetics are preferred because they are associated with less tachyphylaxis. Thoracic
epidural analgesia with local anesthetics and opioids for abdominal, thoracic and vascular
surgery improves bowel recovery times while decreasing the risks of cardiovascular
adverse events and of developing persistent pain (Liu, 2004; Nishimori et al, 2006;). In an
unpublished study of ours (Sivrikaya et al, 2000), preemptive analgesia with epidural
tramadol has supressed the peroperative stress response and also reduced the pain
intensity in the early postoperative period in patients had abdominal hysterectomy under
general anesthesia.

Maintenance techniques in epidural analgesia include:

Continuous Infusion: An easy technique that requires little intervention. The cumulative
dose of local anesthetic is likely to be higher and side effects are more likely than with the
other two techniques.

Intermittent Top-up: Results in benefits due to frequent patient/staff contact but can
produce a high staff workload and patients may have to wait for treatment.

Patient-Controlled Epidural Analgesia (PCEA): This technique produces high patient
satisfaction and reduced dose requirements compared with continuous infusion. However,
sophisticated pumps are required and accurate catheter position is important for optimal
efficacy (Rawal).

Local anesthetics / opioids	Ropivacaine 2% (2 mg/ml) or Levobupivacaine or Bupivacaine 0.1-0.2% (1-2 mg/ml)	Sufentanil 0.5-1 µg/ml or Fentanyl 2-4 µg/ml or Morphine 0.05-0.1 mg/ml or Clonidine 5-20 µg/ml (clinical application is limited by its side effects) or Epinephrine 2- 5 µg/ml
Dosage for continuous infusion (thoracic or lumbar level)	6-12 ml/h	
Dosage for patient controlled infusion (thorasic or lumbar level) **	Background: 4-6 ml/h Bolus dose: 2 ml (2-4 ml) Minimum lockout interval 10 min (10-30 min) Recommended maximum hourly dose (bolus + background): 12 ml	

* The tip of the catheter should be placed as close as possible to the surgical dermatomes: T_6-T_{10} for major intra-abdominal surgery, and L_2-L_4 for lower limb surgery.
** There are many possible variations in local anesthetic/opioid concentration yielding good results, the examples given here should be taken as a guideline; higher concentrations than the ones mentioned here are sometimes required but cannot be recommended as a routine for postoperative pain relief.

Table 5. Examples of local anesthetics and opioids and doses in epidural analgesia *
(by permission from Publisher AstraZeneca)

Continuous central neuraxial blockade is one of the most effective forms of postoperative analgesia, but it is also one of the most invasive. However, this technique remains the first choice for a number of indications, such as abdominal, thoracic, and major orthopedic surgery, where adequate pain relief cannot be achieved with other analgesia techniques alone. Continuous central neuraxial blockade can be achieved via two routes: Continuous epidural analgesia - the recommended first choice and continuous spinal analgesia - should be limited to selected cases only, as there is less experience with this technique.

5.2 Peripheral regional analgesia techniques
It is clear that local anesthetic techniques, particularly peripheral nerve blockade, will be one of the cornerstones of postoperative pain management. A variety of peripheral regional analgesic techniques (e.g. brachial plexus, lumbar plexus, femoral, paravertebral nerve blocks) as a single injection or continuous infusion can be used to enhance postoperative analgesia. Peripheral regional techniques may have several advantages over systemic opioids (i.e., superior analgesia and decreased opioid-related side effects). Also

the side effects associated with central neuraxial blockade, such as hypotension and wide motor blockade with reduced mobility and proprioception, and complications such as epidural Hematoma, epidural abscess and paraparesis can be avoided (Liu&Salinas, 2003).

Continuous peripheral nerve blocks are being increasingly used since they may provide more selective but still excellent postoperative analgesia with reduced need for opioids over an extended period (Table 6). The vailability of disposable local anesthetic infusion systems and the encouraging results from these early studies have led to the increasing popularity of these techniques for pain control in the postdischarge period (Elvir Lazo&White, 2010). This technique has become increasingly popular due to its ability to control moderate to severe pain and accelerate recovery especially after orthopedic surgery procedures (Capdevila et al, 2005; Ilfeld&Enneking, 2005; White, 2003).

Patient controlled regional analgesia (PCRA) can also be used to maintain peripheral nerve block. A low basal infusion rate (e.g. 3-5 ml/h) associated with small PCA boluses (e.g. 2.5-5 ml - lockout: 30-60 min) is the preferred technique (Rawal).

Site of catheter	Local anesthetics and dosage*
	Ropivacaine 0.2%-0.375% Bupivacaine 0.1-0.125% Levobupivacaine 0.1-0.2%
Interscalene	5-9 ml/h
Infraclavicular	5-9 ml/h
Axillary	5-10 ml/h
Femoral	7-10 ml/h
Popliteal	3-7 ml/h
Patient controlled regional analgesia	Background: 3-5 ml/h Bolus dose: 2,5-5 ml Lockout interval: 30-60 min

*Sometimes, higher concentrations are required in individual patients. As a standard, starting with a low concentration/dose is recommended to avoid sensory loss or motor block.

Table 6. Examples of local anesthetics and doses in continuous peripheral nerve analgesia and PCA (modified table after using by permission from Publisher AstraZeneca)

5.2.1 Paravertebral blocks

The evidence suggests that the use of paravertebral blocks provide effective postoperative pain control following breast and thoracic surgery as well as for inguinal hernia repair (Greengrass et al, 1996; Karmakar, 2011; Pusch et al, 1999). On their own, paravertebral blocks have been demonstrated to provide effective postoperative analgesia lasting up to 24 hrs (Chelly et al, 2011).

Chelly et al showed in their study that; a multimodal approach, including paravertebral blocks (prior to surgery), celecoxib (pre and post surgey), and ketamine (immediately prior to surgery), provides better postoperative pain control than PCA morphine alone in patients undergoing open radical retropubic prostatectomy. This approach also allows a reduction in the postoperative need for opioids, lessens the related side effects (e.g., PONV, constipation, and bladder spasm), and facilitates earlier patient recovery which can be connoted that it fascilitates the patient's early recovery (Chelly et al, 2011).

5.3 Infiltration techniques

Local anesthetics can be administered for perioperative pain management via different routes (Table 7). It is crucial for improving the perioperative outcomes especially after day-case surgery (White&Kehlet, 2010).

	Local anesthetic	Volume	Additives
Intraarticular instillation			
Knee arthroscopy	0.75% Ropivacaine	20 ml	Morphine 1-2 mg
	0.5% Bupivacaine	20 ml	Morphine 1-2 mg
Shoulder arthroscopy	0.75% Ropivacaine	10-20 ml	
Intraperitoneal instillation			
Gynecological	0.75% Ropivacaine	20 ml	
Cholecystectomy	0.25% Ropivacaine	40-60 ml	
Wound infiltration			
Inguinal hernia	0.25-0.5% Ropivacaine	30-40 ml	
Perianal surgery	0.25-0.5% Levobupivacaine	30-40 ml	
	0.25-0.5% Bupivacaine	Up to 30 ml	
Thyroid surgery	0.25-0.5% Ropivacaine	10-20 ml	
	0.25-0.5% Levobupivacaine	10-20 ml	
	0.25-0.5% Bupivacaine	Up to 20 ml	

Table 7. Local anesthetic infiltration (by permission from Publisher AstraZeneca)

There are a few techniques for the delivery of the drugs locally into the tissues: intermittent injection, continuous infusion or a combination of two: Intermittent injections (also sometimes referred to as patient-controlled regional analgesia) have the advantage that pain relief can be timed in order to achieve maximal effect during the painful periods such as during mobilization. However, the disadvantage is that sleep quality may be disturbed, as patients sometimes wake up at night due to severe pain, which may be annoying and can also be a cause of patient dissatisfaction. Continuous local anesthetic administration has its advantage in that the patient has adequate pain relief most of the time. However, during periods of activity, the pain could be more severe, which may hamper mobilization. Methods using pumps that have a dual function with low-dose continuous infusion combined with self-administered bolus doses during mobilization are ideal. Several such pumps are available in the market today, including mechanical (elastometric) and electronic (Gupta, 2010).

5.3.1 Wound infiltration

Infiltrating local anesthetics into the skin and subcutaneous tissue prior to making an incision may be the simplest approach to analgesia. It is a safe procedure with few side effects and low risk for toxicity. Particularly, local anesthetic toxicity, wound infection and healing do not appear to be major problems (Buvanendran&Kroin, 2009).

Although the benefit of local wound infiltration has been documented (Barr-Dayan et al, 2004; Legeby et al, 2009; Park et al, 2002), controversy exists as to the appropriate timing of administering local anesthesia for surgery. A single injection of local anesthetics into the wound is unlikely to have long-lasting effects. Therefore, new techniques for wound infiltration have evolved during the last 10 years and several of them are today used routinely during ambulatory surgery and even in the inpatient setting. One such technique is the use of catheters inserted into incision, fascia, intra-articularly and intraabdominally for the intermittent injection or continuous infusion of local anesthetics and adjuvants for pain management (Gupta, 2010).

Continuous wound infusion of local anesthetics, which is mainly used in general surgery and orthopedics, is an interesting technique in postoperative pain therapy. Continuous wound infusion of local anesthetics is able to reduce postoperative opioid requirements and results in decreased pain scores (Gupta et al, 2004; Rasmussen et al, 2004). Recent studies indicate that rehabilitation seems to be enhanced and postoperative hospital stay may be shorter. Continuous wound infusion is an effective analgesic technique, which is simple to perform. Comparisons with other analgesic techniques, such as peripheral nerve blocks, epidural analgesia and other multimodal analgesic concepts are still required.

Hollmann and Durieux (Hollmann&Durieux, 2000) found that there was a reduction in ileus and hospital stay when lidocaine was given intravenously following major abdominal surgery. Therefore, when administered in larger doses during wound infiltration analgesia, it is possible that some of the analgesic effect seen is via systemic absorption and anti-inflammation.

Wound infiltration with local anesthetics is a simple, effective and inexpensive way of regimen which can be used in a multimodal analgesic regime without major complications. Nonetheless this technique still open some questions to be answered as; to the site of catheter placement, catheter type to be placed, the drugs and concentrations recommended, the technique of administration and side-effects of the technique, including toxicity of local anesthetics. Also it remains unclear as to whether this technique is useful in all types of surgery or should preferably be used for specific operations (Gupta, 2000).

5.3.2 Topical application

5.3.2.1 Local anesthetics

Lidocaine patches were applied to the wound area in the next two studies, and the evidence shows that these are particularly effective for wound pain when the patient coughes and they reduce the postoperative pain score at discharge (Habib et al, 2009; Saber et al, 2009). To place lidocaine patches over or at least close to the wound is suggested as a safe and promising modality to consider in the management of postoperative pain control.

5.3.2.2 Clonidine

Clonidine is an alpha adrenoreceptor agonist and these receptors are known to be located centrally. In a volunteer study (Pratab et al, 2007) clonidine had a significant peripheral action in enhancing duration of local anesthesia on superficial co-infiltration with lidocaine. Hence an opportunity with this co-administration to prolong the duration of pain relief apparent after postoperative wound infiltration could be possible.

5.3.2.3 Nonsteroidal anti-inflammatory drugs

The topical application of NSAIDs could produce significant pain relief as the systemic levels achieved by transdermal application. Topically use of NSAIDs has become popular in the ophthalmic field, in which it has been shown that topically applied NSAIDs can reduce postoperative pain and inflammation (Cho, 2009; Jones&Francis, 2009). In a study, the use of a topical diclofenac patch resulted with reduced wound pain and analgesic requirement in patients who have undergone laparoscopic gynecologic surgery (Alessandri et al, 2006). As a result NSAID patch formulations, to be placed directly over the wound, would have a useful pain-relieving effect. But there is still some studies needed to compare this application with systemic administration of the same drug and what the side effect frequency might be with such application (McCleane, 2010).

5.3.2.4 Glyceryl trinitrate

Experimental data suggest that the production of endogenous nitric oxide is necessary for tonic cholinergic inhibition of spinal pain transmission. In a study; transdermal nitroglycerin and the central cholinergic agent neostigmine have enhanced each other's antinociceptive effects at the dose studied (Lauretti et al, 2010). In two recent more studies transdermal nitroglycerin enhanced the analgesic effect of intrathecal neostigmine following abdominal hysterectomy (Ahmed et al, 2010) and intrathecal fentanyl with bupivacaine following gynecological surgery (Gang et al, 2010).

5.3.3 Local infiltration analgesia

The administration of large volumes of local anesthetics with or without adjuvants into different tissue planes perioperatively is called local infiltration analgesia (LIA) (Gupta, 2010).

It is a multimodal technique developed by Kerr et al. (Kerr at al, 2008) for the control of pain following knee and hip surgery. In their study it was based on systematic infiltration of a mixture of a long acting local anesthetics (ropivacaine), a NSAID (ketorolac), and adrenaline into the tissues around the surgical field (periarticularly intraoperatively and via an intra-articular catheter postoperatively) to achieve satisfactory pain control with little physiological disturbance. The technique allows virtually immediate mobilization and earlier discharge from hospital. A recent study by Essving et al (Essving et al, 2009) on unicompartmental knee arthroplasty performed with minimal invasive technique, using the LIA technique found significantly shorter hospital stay, lower morphine consumption and pain intensity compared with placebo.

5.4 Other – Nonpharmacological techniques

A number of non-pharmacological methods of pain management may be used in conjunction with pharmacological methods in the postoperative setting. These nonpharmacological techniques, such as transcutaneous electrical nerve stimulation, acupuncture, psychological approaches (cold) and relaxing therapy and distraction, can be used in an attempt to alleviate postoperative pain.

5.4.1 Transcutaneous electrical nerve stimulation (TENS)
The use of TENS at paravertebral dermatomes corresponding to the surgical incision and/or acupoints has also been reported to improve postoperative pain management (Chen et al, 1998). Because this technique cause few if any adverse effects, its use as an adjunct to conventional pharmaceutical approaches should be considered as part of multimodal analgesic regimens in the future, particularly for patients in whom conventional analgesic techniques fail and/or are accompanied by severe medication-related adverse events (Chen et al, 1998; Usichenko, 2007; Wang et al, 1997).

5.4.2 Acupuncture
The term acupuncture describes a family of procedures involving the stimulation of anatomical points on the body using a variety of techniques. Acupuncture theory is based on two conditions: "yin," which is considered feminine, passive, dark, and cold, and "yang," which is masculine, aggressive, bright, and hot, as well as "qi," which is considered the vital energy that flows and cycles throughout the body. The acupuncture theory is to harmonize any imbalance in yin-yang and qi in a human body to restore the body to a healthy condition. Acupuncture is thought to unblock any obstruction to the flow of qi and, thereby, relieves pain.
Usichenko et al. (Usichenko, 2008) focused on randomized controlled trials of only auricular acupuncture (a popular method in which needles are placed in various parts of the earlobe) for postoperative pain control. They identified nine studies of acceptable quality (though none of the best quality), and concluded that the evidence that auricular acupuncture controls postoperative pain is promising but not compelling. Sun et al. (Sun et al, 2008) conducted a systematic review to quantitatively evaluate the efficacy of acupuncture and related techniques as adjunct analgesics for acute postoperative pain management. The authors concluded that perioperative acupuncture might be a useful adjunct for acute postoperative pain management. However, there are issues with applicability and generalizability of the procedure (Lee&Chan, 2006).

5.4.3 Cold
Iced-water or continuous flow cold therapy is used in orthopedic surgery after knee-surgery (Barber et al, 2000). It can be used both at hospital and at home. There are commercial systems, which are easy to use. The use of iced-water in other kinds of surgery needs further investigation.

5.4.4 Relaxing therapy and distraction
Music, or imagery, or hypnosis may have a positive effect in individual cases. There are commercial music CDs available for relaxation (Rawal).

6 Special aspects

6.1 Ambulatory procedures
The percentage of surgical procedures being performed on an outpatient basis continues to rise. Many more complex and potentially painful procedures in comorbid conditions of the

surgical outpatients are being routinely performed in the ambulatory setting (White & Kehlet, 2010).

Postoperative pain management have some disadvantages in this population; a. pain after minor surgery or in ambulatory patients is more difficult to treat because many of the aforementioned techniques are not available or are too risky. b. The increasing number and complexity of elective operations that are being performed on an ambulatory (or short-stay) basis in which the use of conventional opioid-based intravenous patient controlled analgesia and central neuraxial (spinal and epidural) analgesia techniques are simply not practical for acute pain management. c. The pressure to discharge patients after surgery could limit the pain medications health care professionals are willing to prescribe and it may explain the inadequate management of acute pain after surgery.

Most common medical causes of delayed discharge after ambulatory surgery are; pain, drowsiness and nausea/vomiting (Vadivelu et al, 2010). Although many factors, in addition to pain, must be carefully controlled to minimize postoperative morbidity and facilitate the recovery process after elective surgery, the adequacy of pain control should remain a major focus of health care providers, caring for patients undergoing ambulatory surgical procedures (Elvir Lazo&White, 2010). Many patients undergoing ambulatory surgery continue to experience unacceptably high levels of pain after their operation. A survey by McGrath et al. showed that 30% of patients suffer moderate-to-severe pain following minor surgical procedures (McGrath et al, 2004).

To have a qualified postoperative pain control after ambulatory surgery, it is required that patient discharge is not delayed and that pain control remains effective once the patient is at home. It is important to avoid to use of long acting analgesics and to use regional anesthesia techniques for the anesthesia. Regional analgesia techniques offer a number of advantages for day case surgery patients such as: flexible duration of analgesia (with single shot techniques and/or with catheter infusions), flexible intensity of blockade (according to the type, concentration and volume of local anesthetic) and reduced need for opioids. Wound infiltration, intraperitoneal instillation, peripheral nerve blocks e.g. brachial plexus, paravertebral, femoral nerve blocks can be used in ambulatory surgery patients.

The adaptation of multimodal (or balanced) analgesic techniques as the standard approach for the prevention of pain in the ambulatory setting is one of the keys to improving the recovery process after day-case surgery (McGrath et al, 2004; White, 2007). Early studies evaluating approaches to facilitating the recovery process have demonstrated that the use of multimodal analgesic techniques can improve early recovery as well as other clinically meaningful outcomes after ambulatory surgery. These benefits have been confirmed in more recent studies (Elvir Lazo&White, 2010).

An aggressive multimodal perioperative analgesic regimen that provides effective pain relief, has minimal side-effects, is intrinsically safe, and can be managed by the patient and their family members away from a hospital or surgical center is the ideal one. Current evidence suggests that these improvements in patient outcome related to pain control can best be achieved by using a combination of preventive analgesic techniques involving both centrally and peripherally acting analgesic drugs, as well as novel approaches to administering drugs in locations remote from the hospital setting (White&Kehlet, 2010).

Nonopioid analgesics are increasingly being used as adjuvant before, during, and after surgery to facilitate the recovery process after ambulatory surgery because of their anesthetic and analgesic-sparing effects, their ability to reduce postoperative pain (with movement), and their opioid related side-effects (e.g., gastrointestinal and bladder dysfunction), thereby shortening the duration of the hospital stay and the convalescence period (White&Kehlet, 2010).

Patient-controlled regional analgesia (PCRA) encompasses a variety of techniques that provide effective postoperative pain relief without systemic exposure to opioids. Using PCRA, patients control the application of pre-programmed doses of local anesthetics, most frequently ropivacaine or bupivacaine (occasionally in combination with an opioid), via an indwelling catheter, which can be placed in different regions of the body depending upon the type of surgery. It is important to use suitable local anesthetics in low concentration and to inform patient adequately to avoid the risk of local anesthetic toxicity (Rawal, Vadivelu et al, 2010).

6.2 Stress response

Many detrimental pathophysiologic effects occur in the perioperative period and are associated with activation of nociceptors and the stress response. Uncontrolled pain may result in activation of the sympathetic nervous system, which can cause a variety of potentially harmful physiologic responses that may adversely influence the extent of morbidity and mortality (Vadivelu et al, 2010).

As afferent neural stimuli and activation of the autonomic nervous system and other reflexes by pain may serve as a major release mechanism of the endocrine metabolic responses and thus contribute to various organ dysfunctions, pain relief may be a powerful technique to modify surgical stress responses.

Systemic opioids (PCA or intermittent), NSAID, epidural opiod, lumbar and thorasic epidural local anesthetics are analgesic techniques are mostly used to supress the postoperative surgical stress responces but there is a pronounced differential effect of these various techniques on surgical stress responses (Kehlet&Holte, 2001). Any treatment with opioids, being epidural or PCA opioids, has very little effect on surgical stress responses and organ dysfunctions. Same applies to clonidine and also NSAIDs. Epidural anesthesia has the most profound inhibitory effect on surgical stress responses.

Several studies investigating lower extremity surgery have shown continuous lumbar epidural local anesthetic techniques to be most effective, probably because of a more effective afferent blockade. In abdominal procedures, there is a somewhat smaller efficacy of thoracic epidural local anesthetic techniques in modulating endocrine-metabolic responses, probably due to insufficient afferent blockade as well as the presence of other release mechanisms in eliciting the surgical stress response.

The neuraxial application of local anesthetics and opioids combined to general anesthesia (especially in patients undergoing major abdominal or thoracic procedures) as a multimodal strategy can provide superior pain relief, reduced hormonal and metabolic stress, enhanced normalization of gastrointestinal function, and thus a shortened postoperative recovery time, facilitating mobilization and physiotherapy (Schug&Chong, 2009). In a study by Sivrikaya et al (Sivrikaya et al, 2008) general anesthesia combined lumbar epidural analgesia can only partially attenuate the peroperative stress response and has some limited effects on recovery of gastrointestinal functions, nevertheless provided a better postoperative analgesia compared to general anesthesia alone. Epidural opioid techniques are less effective on the stress response, and are comparable with systemic opioid techniques and the use of NSAIDs. More data on the use of multimodal analgesic techniques with combinations of different analgesics are needed on this issue.

7. Conclusion

Postoperative pain is a complication of surgery, which, in turn, complicates recovery with functional impairment and drug-related adverse effects. Despite an increased focus on pain management programs and the development of new standards for pain management, many patients continue to experience intense pain after surgery.

Many factors must be considered before deciding on the type of pain therapy to be provided to the surgical patient. These include the patients' co-morbid conditions, psychological status, exposure to analgesic therapies, and the type of surgical procedure.

The multimodal approach may potentially decrease perioperative morbidity, reduce the length of hospital stay, and improve patient satisfaction without compromising safety. However, widespread implementation of these programs requires multidisciplinary collaboration, change in the traditional principles of postoperative care, additional resources, and expansion of the traditional acute pain service. Although a multi-pharmacologic approach may be universally recommended, drugs and their route of administration must be changed according to the type of surgery and hospital resources, and of course to the patient needs.

8. References

Aasvang E, Hansen J, Malmstrøm J, Asmussen T, *et al* (2008). The effect of wound instillation of a novel purified capsaicin formulation on postherniotomy pain: a double-blind, randomized, placebo-controlled study. *AnesthAnalg*, Vol.107, No.1(Jul), pp.282-91, ISSN 0003-2999.

Acute pain management: operative or medical procedures and trauma, part 1 (1992). Agency for Health Care Policy and Research. *Clin Pharm* , Vol.11, No.4(Apr), pp.309-31. ISSN 0278-2677.

Ahmed F, Garg A, Chawla V, Khandelwal M (2010). Transdermal nitroglycerine enhances postoperative analgesia of intrathecal neostigmine following abdominal hysterectomies. *Indian J Anaesth*, Vol.54, No. 1(Jan), pp.24-8, ISSN 0019-5049.

Alessandri F, Lijoi D, Mistrangelo E, Nicoletti a, *et al* (2006). Topical diclofenac patch for postoperative wound pain in laparoscopic gynaecologic surgery: a randomized study. *J Minim Invasive Gynecol*, Vol.13, No.3(May-June), pp.195-200, ISSN 1553-4650.

American Pain Society Quality of Care Committee. Quality improvement guidelines for the treatment of acute pain and cancer pain (1995). *JAMA* , Vol.274, No.23(Dec), pp.1874-80, ISSN 0098-7484.

American Society of Anesthesiologists Task Force on Acute Pain Management (2004). Practice guidelines for acute pain management in the perioperative setting. An updated report by the American Society of Anesthesiologists task force on acute pain management. *Anesthesiology*, Vol.100, No.6(June), pp.1573-81, ISSN 0003-3022.

Apfelbaum J, Chen C,Mehta S, Gan T (2003). Postoperative pain experience: results from a national survey suggest postoperative pain continues to be undermanaged. *Anesth Analg*, Vol.97, No.2(Aug), pp.534-40, ISSN 0003-2999.

Barber FA. A comparison of crushed ice and continuous flow cold therapy (2000). *Am J Knee Surg*, Vol.13, No.2(Spring), pp.97-101, ISSN 0899-7403.

Bar-Dayan A, Natour M, Bar-Zakai B, Zmora O, *et al* (2004). Preperitoneal bupivacaine attenuates pain following laparoscopic inguinal hernia repair. *Surg Endosc*, Vol.18, No.7(Jul), pp.1079-81, ISSN 0930-2794.

Bell R, Dahl J, Moore R, Kalso E. Perioperative ketamine for acute postoperative pain (2006). *Cochrane Database Syst Rev*, Vol.25, No.1(Jan), CD004603, ISSN 1469-493X(Electronic).

Bilgin H, Ozcan B, Bilgin T, Kerimoglu B, *et al* (2005). The influence of timing of systemic ketamine administration on postoperative morphine consumption. *J Clin Anesth*, Vol.17, No.8(Dec), pp.592-7, ISSN 0952-8180.

Birnbach DJ, Johnson MD, Arcario T, Datta S, *et al* (1989). Effect of diluent volume on analgesia produced by epidural fentanyl. *Anesth Analg*, Vol.68, No.6(Jun), pp.808-10, ISSN 0003-2999.

Bisgaard T (2006). Analgesic treatment after laparoscopic cholecystectomy: a critical assessment of the evidence. *Anesthesiology*, Vol.104, No.4(Apr), pp.835-46, ISSN 0003-3022.

Boisseau N, Rabary O, Padovani B, Staccini P, *et al* (2001). Improvement of 'dynamic analgesia' does not decrease atelectasis after thoracotomy. *Br J Anaesth*, Vol.87, No.4(Oct), pp.564-9, ISSN 0007-0912.

Buvanendran A, Kroin J (2007). Useful adjuvants for postoperative pain management. *Best Pract Res Clin Anaesthesiol*, Vol.21, No.1(Mar), pp.31-49, ISSN 1521-6896.

Buvanendran A, Kroin JS (2009). Multimodal analgesia for controlling acute postoperative pain. *Curr Opin Anaesthesiol*, Vol.22, No.5(Oct), pp.588-93, Review, ISSN 0952-7907.

Buvanendran A, Kroin JS, Della Valle CJ, Kari M, *et al* (2010). Perioperative oral pregabalin reduces chronic pain after total knee arthroplasty: a prospective, randomized, controlled trial. *Anesth Analg*, Vol.110, No.1(Jan), pp.199-207, ISSN 0003-2999.

Camann W, Abouleish A, Eisenach J, Hood D, *et al* (1998). Intrathecal sufentanil and epidural bupivacaine for labor analgesia: dose-response of individual agents and in combination. *Reg Anesth Pain Med*, Vol.23, No.5(Sep-Oct), pp.457-62, ISSN 0952-7907.

Capdevila X, Pirat P, Bringuier S, Gaertner R, *et al* (2005). Continuous peripheral nerve blocks in hospital wards after orthopedic surgery: a multicenter prospective analysis of the quality of postoperative analgesia and complications in 1,416 patients. *Anesthesiology*, Vol.103, No.5(Nov), pp.1035-45, ISSN 0003-3022.

Carli F, Mayo N, Klubien K, Schricker T, *et al* (2002). Epidural analgesia enhances functional exercise capacity and health-related quality of life after colonic surgery: results of a randomized trial. *Anesthesiology*, Vol.97, No.3(Sep), pp.540-9, ISSN 0003-3022.

Carr DB, Goudas LC (1999). Acute pain. *Lancet*, Vol.353(9169), No.12(Jun), pp.2051-8, Review, ISSN 0140-6736.

Chelly JE (2001). General concepts and indications. In: Chelly JE, Casati A, Fanelli G, editors. Continuous peripheral nerve block techniques. London: Mosby, pp.11-21.

Chelly JE, Ploskanych T, Dai F, Nelson JB (2011). Multimodal analgesic approach incorporating paravertebral blocks for open radical retropubic prostatectomy: a randomized double-blind placebo-controlled study. *Can J Anaesth*, Vol.58, No.4(Apr), pp.371-8, ISSN 0832-610X.

Chen L, Tang J, White PF, Sloninsky A, *et al* (1998). The effect of location of transcutaneous electrical nerve stimulation on postoperative opioid analgesic requirement: acupoint versus nonacupoint stimulation. *Anesth Analg*, Vol.87, No.5(Nov), pp.1129-34, ISSN 0003-2999.

Cho H, Wolf KJ, Wolf EJ (2009). Management of ocular inflammation and pain following cataract surgery: focus on bromfenac ophthalmic solution. *Clin Ophthalmol*, Vol.3, pp.199-210, ISSN 1177-5467.

Christie MJ, Connor M, Vaughan CW, Ingram SL, *et al* (2000). Cellular actions of opioids and other analgesics: implications for synergism in pain relief. *Clin Exp Pharmacol Physiol*, Vol.27, No.7(Jul), pp.520-3, ISSN 0305-1870.

de Beer Jde V, Winemaker MJ, Donnelly GA, Miceli PC, *et al* (2005). Efficacy and safety of controlled release oxycodone and standard therapies for postoperative pain after knee or hip replacement. *Can J Surg*, Vol.48, No.4(Aug), pp.277-83, ISSN 0008-428X.

de Leon-Casasola OA, Lema MJ (1996). Postoperative epidural opioid analgesia: what are the choices? *Anesth Analg*, Vol.83, No.4(Oct), pp.867-75, ISSN 0003-2999.

Dholakia C, Beverstein G, Garren M, Nemergut C, *et al* (2007). The impact of perioperative dexmedetomidine infusion on postoperative narcotic use and duration of stay after laparoscopic bariatric surgery. *J Gastrointest Surg*, Vol.11, No.11(Nov), pp.1556-9, ISSN 1091-255X.

Dolin SJ, Cashman JN, Bland JM (2009). Effectiveness of acute postoperative pain management: I. Evidence from published data. *Br J Anaesth*, Vol.89, No.3(Sep), pp.409-23, ISSN 0007-0912.

Duedahl TH, Romsing J, Moiniche S, Dahl JB (2006). A qualitative systematic review of peri-operative dextromethorphan in post-operative pain. *Acta Anaesthesiol Scand*, Vol.50, No.1(Jan), pp.1-13, ISSN 0001-5172.

Eccleston C (2001). Role of psychology in pain management. *Br J Anaesth*, Vol.87, No.1(Jul), pp.144-52, Review, ISSN 0007-0912.

Elia N, Lysakowski C, Tramèr MR (2005). Does multimodal analgesia with acetaminophen, nonsteroidal antiinflammatory drugs, or selective cyclooxygenase-2 inhibitors and patient-controlled analgesia morphine offer advantages over morphine alone? Meta-analyses of randomized trials. *Anesthesiology*, Vol.103, No.6(Dec), pp.1296-304, ISSN 0003-3022.

Elvir-Lazo OL, White PF (2010). Postoperative pain management after ambulatory surgery: role of multimodal analgesia. *Anesthesiol Clin*, Vol.28, No.2(Jun), pp.217-24, ISSN 1932-2275.

Essving P, Axelsson K, Kjellberg J, Wallgren O, *et al* (2009). Reduced hospital stay, morphine consumption, and pain intensity with local infiltration analgesia after unicompartmental knee arthroplasty. *Acta Orthop*, Vol.80, No.2(Apr), pp.213-9, ISSN 1745-3674.

Fanelli G, Berti M, Baciarello M (2008). Updating postoperative pain management: from multimodal to context-sensitive treatment. *Minerva Anestesiol*, Vol.74, No.9, pp 489-500, ISSN 0375-9393.

Feo CV, Sortini D, Ragazzi R, De Palma M, *et al* (2006). Randomized clinical trial of the effect of preoperative dexamethasone on nausea and vomiting after laparoscopic cholecystectomy. *Br J Surg*, Vol.93, No.3(Mar), pp.295-9, ISSN 0007-1323.

Gajraj N, Joshi G (2005). Role of cyclooxygenase-2 inhibitors in postoperative pain management. *Anesthesiol Clin North America*, Vol.23, No.1(Mar), pp.49-72, ISSN 0889-8537.

Gan TJ, Joshi GP, Viscusi E, Cheung RY, *et al* (2004). Preoperative parenteral parecoxib and follow-up oral valdecoxib reduce length of stay and improve quality of patient recovery after laparoscopic cholecystectomy surgery. *Anesth Analg*, Vol.98, No.6(Jun), pp.1665-73, ISSN 0889-8537.

Garg A, Ahmed F, Khandelwal M, Chawla V, *et al* (2010). The effect of transdermal nitroglycerine on intrathecal fentanyl with bupivacaine for postoperative analgesia following gynaecological surgery. *Anaesth Intensive Care*, Vol.38, No.2(Mar), pp.285-90, ISSN 0310-057X.

George MJ (2006). The site of action of epidurally administered opioids and its relevance to postoperative pain management. *Anaesthesia*, Vol.61, No.1(Jul), pp.659-64, ISSN 0003-2409.

Graham GG, Scott KF (2005). Mechanism of action of paracetamol. *Am J Ther*, Vol.12, No.1(Jan-Feb), pp.46-55, ISSN 1075-2765.

Gray A, Kehlet H, Bonnet F, Rawal N (2005). Predicting postoperative analgesia outcomes: NNT league tables or procedure-specific evidence? *Br J Anaesth*, Vol.94, No.6(Jun), pp.710-4, ISSN 0007-0912.

Greengrass R, O'Brien F, Lyerly K, Hardman D, *et al* (1996). Paravertebral block for breast cancer surgery. *Can J Anaesth*, Vol.43, No.8(Aug), pp.858-61, ISSN 0832-610X.

Gupta A, Perniola A, Axelsson K, Thörn SE, *et al* (2004). Postoperative pain after abdominal hysterectomy: a double-blind comparison between placebo and local anesthetic infused intraperitoneally. *Anesth Analg*, Vol.99, No.4(Oct), pp.1173-9, ISSN 0003-2999.

Gupta A (2010). Wound infiltration with local anaesthetics in ambulatory surgery. *Curr Opin Anaesthesiol*, Vol.23, No.6(dec), pp.708-13, Review, ISSN 0952-7907.

Gurbet A, Basagan-Mogol E, Turker G, Ugun F, *et al* (2006). Intraoperative infusion of dexmedetomidine reduces perioperative analgesic requirements. *Can J Anaesth*, Vol.53, No.7(Jul), pp.646-52, ISSN 0832-610X.

Habib A, Gan T (2005). Role of analgesic adjuncts in postoperative pain management. *Anesthesiol Clin North America*, Vol.23, No.1(Mar), pp.85-107, ISSN 0889-8537.

Habib AS, White WD, El Gasim MA, Saleh G, *et al* (2008). Transdermal nicotine for analgesia after radical retropubic prostatectomy. *Anesth Analg*, Vol.107, No.3(Sep), pp.999-1004, ISSN 0003-2999.

Habib AS, Polascik TJ, Weizer AZ, White WD, *et al* (2009). Lidocaine patch for postoperative analgesia after radical retropubic prostatectomy. *Anesth Analg*, Vol.108, No.6(Jun), pp.1950-53, ISSN 0003-2999.

Hartrick C, Van Hove I, Stegmann J, Oh C, *et al* (2009). Efficacy and tolerability of tapentadol immediate release and oxycodone HCl immediate release in patients awaiting primary joint replacement surgery for end-stage joint disease: a 10-day, phase III, randomized, double-blind, active- and placebo-controlled study. *Clin Ther*, Vol.31, No.2(Feb), pp.260-71, ISSN 0149-2918.

Hollmann MW, Durieux ME (2000). Local anesthetics and the inflammatory response: a new therapeutic indication? *Anesthesiology*, Vol.93, No.3(Sep), pp.858-75, ISSN 0003-3022.

Hurley RW, Cohen SP, Williams KA, Rowlingson AJ, *et al* (2006). The analgesic effects of perioperative gabapentin on postoperative pain: a meta-analysis. *Reg Anesth Pain Med*, Vol.31, No.3(May-Jun), pp.237-47, ISSN 1098-7339.

Ilfeld BM, Enneking FK (2005). Continuous peripheral nerve blocks at home: a review. *Anesth Analg*, Vol.100, No.6(Jun), pp.1822-33, Review, ISSN 0003-2999.

Joly V, Richebe P, Guignard B, Fletcher D, *et al* (2005). Remifentanil-induced postoperative hyperalgesia and its prevention with small-dose ketamine. *Anesthesiology*, Vol.103, No.1(Jul), pp.147-55, ISSN 0003-3022.

Jones J, Francis P (2009). Ophthalmic utility of topical bromfenac, a twice-daily nonsteroidal anti-inflammatory agent. *Expert Opin Pharmacother*, Vol.10, No.14(Oct), pp.2379-85, ISSN 1465-6566.

Joshi GP, Viscusi ER, Gan TJ, Minkowitz H, *et al* (2004). Effective treatment of laparoscopic cholecystectomy pain with intravenous followed by oral COX-2 specific inhibitor. *Anesth Analg*, Vol.98, No.2(Feb), pp.336-42, ISSN 0003-2999.

Jurna I (1995). [Antinociceptive effects of alpha(2)-adrenoceptor agonists ("analgesic" actions in animal experiments)agonists ("analgesic" actions in animal experiments).]. *Schmerz*, Vol.9, No.6(Nov), pp.286-92, ISSN 0932-433X.

Kaba A, Laurent SR, Detroz BJ, Sessler DI, *et al* (2007). Intravenous lidocaine infusion facilitates acute rehabilitation after laparoscopic colectomy. *Anesthesiology*, Vol.106, No.1(Jan), pp.11-8, ISSN 0003-3022.

Kardash KJ, Sarrazin F, Tessler MJ, Velly AM (2008). Single-dose dexamethasone reduces dynamic pain after total hip arthroplasty. *Anesth Analg*, Vol.106, No.4(Apr), pp.1253-57, ISSN 0003-2999.

Karmakar MK (2001). Thoracic paravertebral block. *Anesthesiology*, Vol.95, No.3(Sep), pp.771-80, Review, ISSN 0003-3022.

Kehlet H, Dahl JB (1993). The value of multimodal or balanced analgesia in the postoperative pain treatment. *Anesth Analg*, Vol.77, No.5(Nov), pp. 1048-56, Review, ISSN 0003-2999.

Kehlet H (1997). Multimodal approach to control postoperative pathophysiology and rehabilitation. *Br J Anaesth*, Vol.78, No.5(May), pp.606-17, ISSN 0007-0912.

Kehlet H, Werner M, Perkins F (1999). Balanced analgesia: what is it and what are its advantages in postoperative pain? *Drugs*, Vol.58, No.5(Nov), pp.793-7, ISSN 0012-6667.

Kehlet H, Holte K (2001). Effect of postoperative analgesia on surgical outcome. *Br J Anaesth*, Vol.87, No.1(Jul), pp.62-72, Review, ISSN 0007-0912.

Kerr DR, Kohan L (2008). Local infiltration analgesia: a technique for the control of acute postoperative pain following knee and hip surgery: a case study of 325 patients. *Acta Orthop*, Vol.79, No.2(Apr), pp.174-83, ISSN 1745-3674.

Koinig H, Wallner T, Marhofer P, Andel H, et al (1998). Magnesium sulfate reduces intra- and postoperative analgesic requirements. *Anesth Analg*, Vol.87, No.1(Jul), pp.206-10, ISSN 0003-2999.

Lauretti GR, de Oliveira R, Reis MP, Mattos AL, et al (1999). Transdermal nitroglycerine enhances spinal sufentanil postoperative analgesia following orthopedic surgery. *Anesthesiology*, Vol.90, No.3(Mar), pp.734-9, ISSN 0003-3022.

Lauretti GR, Oliveira AP, Julião MC, Reis MP, et al (2000). Transdermal nitroglycerine enhances spinal neostigmine postoperative analgesia following gynecological surgery. *Anesthesiology*, Vol.93, No.4(Oct), pp.943-6, ISSN 0003-3022.

Lauwick S, Kim DJ, Michelagnoli G, Mistraletti G, et al (2008). Intraoperative infusion of lidocaine reduces postoperative fentanyl requirements in patients undergoing laparoscopic cholecystectomy. *Can J Anaesth*, Vol.55, No.11(Nov), pp.754-60, ISSN 0832-610X.

Lee A, Chan S (2006). Acupuncture and anaesthesia. *Best Pract Res Clin Anaesthesiol*, Vol.20, No.2(Jun), pp.303-14, ISSN 1521-6896.

Legeby M, Jurell G, Beausang-Linder M, Olofsson C (2009). Placebo-controlled trial of local anaesthesia for treatment of pain after breast reconstruction. *Scand J Plast Reconstr Surg Hand Surg*, Vol.43, No.6, pp.315-9. ISSN 0284-4311.

Lin TF, Yeh YC, Lin FS, Wang YP, et al (2009). Effect of combining dexmedetomidine and morphine for intravenous patient-controlled analgesia. *Br J Anaesth*, Vol.102, Vol.1(Jan), pp. 117-22, ISSN 0007-0912.

Liu SS, Salinas FV (2003). Continuous plexus and peripheral nerve blocks for postoperative analgesia. *Anesth Analg*, Vol.96, No.1(Jan), pp. 263-72, Review, ISSN 0003-2999.

Liu SS (2004). Anesthesia and analgesia for colon surgery. *Reg Anesth Pain Med*, Vol.29, No.1(Jan-Feb), pp.52-7, ISSN 1098-7339.

Liu SS, Wu CL (2007). Effect of postoperative analgesia on major postoperative complications: a systematic update of the evidence. *Anesth Analg*, Vol.104, No.3(Mar), pp.689-702, ISSN 0003-2999.

Lysakowski C, Dumont L, Czarnetzki C, Tramer MR (2007). Magnesium as an adjuvant to postoperative analgesia: a systematic review of randomized trials. *Anesth Analg*, Vol.104, No.6(Jun), pp.1532-9, ISSN 0003-2999.

Ma H, Tang J, White PF, Zaentz A, et al (2004). Perioperative rofecoxib improves early recovery after outpatient herniorrhaphy. *Anesth Analg*, Vol.98, No.4(Apr), pp.970-5, ISSN 0003-2999.

Macario A, Lipman AG (2001). Ketorolac in the era of cyclo-oxygenase-2 selective nonsteroidal anti-inflammatory drugs: a systematic review of efficacy, side effects, and regulatory issues. *Pain Med*, Vol.2, No.4(Dec), pp.336-51, ISSN 1526-2375.

Mathiesen O, Møiniche S, Dahl J (2007). Gabapentin and postoperative pain: a qualitative and quantitative systematic review, with focus on procedure. *BMC Anesthesiol*, Vol.7, No.7(Jul), pp.6, ISSN 1471-2253.

Mathiesen O, Jacobsen L, Holm H, Randall S, et al (2008). Pregabalin and dexamethasone for postoperative pain control: a randomized controlled study in hip arthroplasty. *Br J Anaesth*, Vol.101, No.4(Oct), pp.535-41, ISSN 0007-0912.

Mathiesen O, Rasmussen ML, Dierking G, Leck H, et al (2009). Pregabalin and dexamethasone in combination with paracetamol for postoperative pain control after abdominal hysterectomy. A randomized clinical trial. *Acta Anaesthesiol Scand*, Vol.53, No.2(Feb), pp.227-35, ISSN 0001-5172.

McCleane G (2010). Topical application of analgesics: a clinical option in day case anaesthesia? *Curr Opin Anaesthesiol*, Vol.23, No.6(Dec), pp.704-7, ISSN 0952-7907.

McGrath B, Elgendy H, Chung F, Kamming D, *et al* (2004). Thirty percent of patients have moderate to severe pain 24 hr after ambulatory surgery: a survey of 5,703 patients. *Can J Anaesth*, Vol.51, No.9(Nov), 886-91, ISSN 0832-610X.

Miranda HF, Puig MM, Prieto JC, Pinardi G (2006). Synergism between paracetamol and nonsteroidal anti-inflammatory drugs in experimental acute pain. *Pain*, Vol.121, No.1-2(Mar), pp.22-8, ISSN 0304-3959.

Mitra S, Sinatra R (2004). Perioperative management of acute pain in the opioid-dependent patient. *Anesthesiology*, Vol.101, No.1(Jul), pp.212-27, ISSN 0003-3022.

Mitra S (2008). Opioid-induced hyperalgesia: pathophysiology and clinical implications. *J Opioid Manag*, Vol.4, No.3(May-Jun), pp. 123-30, ISSN 1551-7489.

Møiniche S, Mikkelsen S, Wetterslev J, Dahl JB (1998). A qualitative systematic review of incisional local anaesthesia for postoperative pain relief after abdominal operations. *Br J Anaesth*, Vol. 81, No.3(Sep), pp.377-83, ISSN 0007-0912.

Moiniche S, Kehlet H, Dahl JB (2002). A qualitative and quantitative systematic review of preemptive analgesia for postoperative pain relief: the role of timing of analgesia. *Anesthesiology*, Vol.96, No.3(Mar), pp.725-41, ISSN 0003-3022.

Ness TJ (2001). Pharmacology of peripheral analgesia. *Pain Pract*, Vol.1, No.3(Sep), pp.243-54, ISSN 1530-7085.

Nett MP (2010). Postoperative pain management. *Orthopedics*, Vol.33, No.9 Suppl(Sep), pp.23-6, ISSN 0147-7447.

Nishimori M, Ballantyne JC, Low JH (2006). Epidural pain relief *versus* systemic opioid-based pain relief for abdominal aortic surgery. *Cochrane Database Syst Rev*, Vol.19, No.3(Jul), CD005059, ISSN 1469-493X(Electronic).

Park JY, Lee GW, Kim Y, Yoo MJ (2002). The efficacy of continuous intrabursal infusion with morphine and bupivacaine for postoperative analgesia after subacromial arthroscopy. *Reg Anesth Pain Med*, Vol.27, No.2(Mar-Apr), pp.145-9, ISSN 1098-7339.

Perkins FM, Kehlet H (2000). Chronic pain as an outcome of surgery. A review of predictive factors. *Anesthesiology*, Vol.93, No.4(Oct), pp.1123-33; ISSN 0003-3022.

Power I, Barratt S. Analgesic agents for the postoperative period. Nonopioids (1999). *Surg Clin N Am*, Vol.79, No.2(Apr), pp.275-95, ISSN 0039-6109.

Practice guidelines for acute pain management in the perioperative setting: a report by the American Society of Anesthesiologists Task Force on Pain Management, Acute Pain Section (1995). *Anesthesiology*, Vol.82, No.4(Apr), pp.1071-81, ISSN 0003-3022.

Pratap JN, Shankar RK, Goroszeniuk T (2007). Co-injection of clonidine prolongs the anesthetic effect of lidocaine skin infiltration by a peripheral action. *Anesth Analg*, Vol.104, No.4(Apr), pp.982-3, ISSN 0003-2999.

Pusch F, Freitag H, Weinstabl C, Obwegeser R, *et al* (1999). Single-injection paravertebral block compared to general anesthesia in breast surgery. *Acta Anaesthesiol Scand*, Vol.43, No.7(Aug), pp.770-4, ISSN 0001-5172.

Rasmussen S, Kramhøft MU, Sperling KP, Pedersen JH.(2004) Increased flexion and reduced hospital stay with continuous intraarticular morphine and ropivacaine after

ꞏꞏꞏꞏ ꞏꞏꞏꞏ ꞏꞏꞏꞏ ꞏꞏꞏꞏ ꞏꞏꞏꞏ ꞏꞏꞏꞏ ꞏꞏꞏꞏ upon intervention study of efficacy and safety in 154 patients. *Acta Orthop Scand*, Vol.75, No.5(Oct), pp.606-9, ISSN 0001-6470.

Rathmell JP, Lair TR, Nauman B (2005). The role of intrathecal drugs in the treatment of acute pain. *Anesth Analg*, Vol.101, No.5 Suppl(Nov), pp.S30-43, ISSN 0003-2999.

Rawal N (Co-Ordinator) Postoperative Pain Management – Good Clinical Practice, General recommendations and principles for succesful pain management. http://www.esraeurope.org/PostoperativePain Management.pdf

Saber AA, Elgamal AH, Rao AJ, Itawi EA, et al (2009). Early experience with lidocaine patch for postoperative pain control after laparoscopic ventral hernia repair. *Int J Surg*, Vol.7, No.1(Feb), pp.36-8, ISSN 1743-9191.

Salerno A, Hermann R (2006). Efficacy and safety of steroid use for postoperative pain relief. Update and review of the medical literature. *J Bone Joint Surg Am*, Vol.88, No.6(June), pp.1361-72, ISSN 0021-9355.

Schug S, Chong C (2009). Pain management after ambulatory surgery. *Curr Opin Anaesthesiol*, Vol.22, No.6(Dec), pp.738-43, ISSN 0952-7907.

Senturk M, Ozcan PE, Talu GK, Kiyan E, et al (2002). The effects of three different analgesia techniques on long-term postthoracotomy pain. *Anesth Analg*, Vol.94, No.1(Jan), pp.11-5, ISSN 0003-2999.

Sivrikaya GU, Eksioglu B, Basgul A, Enhos H, et al (2000). The effects of preemptive epidural tramadol on peroperative stress response and postoperative analgesia (Oral communication), 19th Annual ESRA Congress, 20–23 November 2000, Rome, Italy. *The International Monitor (IMRAPT)*, Vol.12, No.3, pp.65.

Sivrikaya GU, Koc Bekil EH, Hanci A, Kilinc LT, et al (2008). The effect of combined epidural-general anaesthesia on intraoperative stress response and postoperative analgesic consumption and gastrointestinal function in lower abdominal surgery. *J Turk Anaesth Int Care*, Vol.36, No.6(Nov-Dec), pp.358-65, ISSN 1304-0871.

Sun T, Sacan O, White PF, Coleman J, et al (2008). Perioperative vs postoperative celecoxib on patient outcome after major plastic surgery procedures. *Anesth Analg*, Vol.106, No.3(Mar), pp.950-8, ISSN 0003-2999.

Sun Y, Gan T, Dubose J, Habib A (2008). Acupuncture and related techniques for postoperative pain: a systematic review of randomized controlled trials. *Br J Anaesth* Vol.101, No.2(Aug), pp.151-60, ISSN 0007-0912.

Tiippana E, Hamunen K, Kontinen V, Kalso E (2007). Do surgical patients benefit from perioperative gabapentin/pregabalin? A systematic review of efficacy and safety. *Anesth Analg*, Vol.104, No.6(Jun), pp.1545-56, ISSN 0003-2999.

Tramer MR, Schneider J, Marti R-A, Rifat K (1996). Role of magnesium sulfate in postoperative analgesia. *Anesthesiology*, Vol.84, No.2(Feb), pp.340-7, ISSN 0003-3022.

Usichenko TI, Kuchling S, Witstruck T, Pavlovic D, et al (2007). Auricular acupuncture for pain relief after ambulatory knee surgery: a randomized trial. *CMAJ*, Vol.176, No.2(Jan), pp.179-83, ISSN 1488-2329.

Usichenko T, Lehmann C, Ernst E (2008). Auricular acupuncture for postoperative pain control: a systematic review of randomised clinical trials. *Anaesthesia*, Vol.63, Vol.12(Dec), pp.1343-8, ISSN 0003-2409.

Vadivelu N, Mitra S, Narayan D (2010). Recent advances in postoperative pain management. *Yale J Biol Med*, Vol.83, No.1(Mar), pp.11-25, Review, ISSN 0044-0086.

Viscusi ER, Reynolds L, Chung F, Atkinson LE, et al (2004). Patient-controlled transdermal fentanyl hydrochloride vs intravenous morphine pump for postoperative pain: a randomized controlled trial. *JAMA*, Vol.17, No.11(Mar), pp.1333-41, ISSN 0098-7484.

Wang B, Tang J, White PF, Naruse R, et al (1997). Effect of the intensity of transcutaneous acupoint electrical stimulation on the postoperative analgesic requirement. *Anesth Analg*, Vol.85, No.2(Aug), pp.406-13, ISSN 0003-2999.

Warfield CA, Kahn CH (1995). Acute pain management: programs in U.S. hospitals and experiences and attitudes among U.S adults. *Anesthesiology*Vol.83, No.5(Nov), pp.1090-4, ISSN 0003-3022.

White PF, Issioui T, Skrivanek GD, Early JS, et al (2003). Use of a continuous popliteal sciatic nerve block for the management of pain after major podiatric surgery: does it improve quality of recovery? *Anesth Analg*, Vol.97, No.5(Nov), pp.1303-9, ISSN 0003-2999.

White PF (2005). The changing role of nonopioid analgesic techniques in the management of postoperative pain. *Anesth Analg*, Vol.101, No.5 Suppl(Nov), pp.S5-22, ISSN 0003-2999.

White PF (2007). Multimodal pain management: the future is now! *Curr Opin Investig Drugs*, Vol.8, No.7(Jul), pp.517-8, ISSN 1472-4472.

White PF, Sacan O, Tufanogullari B, Eng M, et al (2007). Effect of short-term postoperative celecoxib administration on patient outcome after outpatient laparoscopic surgery. *Can J Anaesth*, Vol.54, No.5(May), pp.342-8, ISSN 0832-610X.

White PF, Kehlet H (2007). Postoperative pain management and patient outcome: time to return to work! [editorial]. *Anesth Analg*, Vol.104, No.3(Mar), pp.487–90, ISSN 0003-2999.

White PF, Kehlet H, Neal JM, Schricker T, et al (2007). Role of the anesthesiologist in fast-track surgery: from multimodal analgesia to perioperative medical care. *Anesth Analg*, Vol.104, No.6(Jun), pp.1380-96, ISSN 0003-2999.

White PF, Kehlet H (2010). Improving postoperative pain management: what are the unresolved issues? *Anesthesiology*, Vol.112, No.1(Jan), pp.220-5, ISSN 0003-3022.

Wu CL, Fleisher LA (2000). Outcomes research in regional anesthesia and analgesia. *Anesth Analg*, Vol.91, No.5(Nov), pp.1232-42, ISSN 0003-2999.

Yardeni IZ, Beilin B, Mayburd E, Levinson Y, et al (2009). The effect of perioperative intravenous lidocaine on postoperative pain and immune function. *Anesth Analg*, Vol.109, No.5(Nov), 1464-9, ISSN 0003-2999.

10

Regional Anesthesia for the Trauma Patient

Stephen D. Lucas, Linda Le-Wendling and F. Kayser Enneking
Department of Anesthesiology,
University of Florida College of Medicine, Gainesville, Florida,
USA

1. Introduction

Trauma is the sixth most common cause of death globally [WHO, 2011]. In the United States, almost 30 million patients receive medical care for trauma every year [CDC, 2011], and trauma results in 30% of intensive care unit (ICU) admissions in the United States [Mackenzie et al., 2007]. In the Emergency Department, 91% of trauma patients are in pain [Berben et al., 2008], and two-thirds of those patients are discharged from the Emergency Department with moderate to severe pain [Berben et al., 2008]. Regional anesthesia (RA) can reduce pain in many of these patients. In this chapter, common problems with managing trauma patients that can be addressed with RA, and data suggesting that regional anesthesia can improve outcomes will be presented, as well as the different challenges to using RA in this patient population. We will also look into new and controversial areas of inquiry in this field.

2. Patients with traumatic injuries who can benefit from regional anesthesia

2.1 Thoracic trauma and rib fractures

Thoracic injury accounts for 25% of deaths among trauma patients. It is second only to head injury as a cause of trauma-related deaths in the United States [Trunkey & Lewis, 1980]. Rib fractures are common, and morbidity and mortality are directly correlated with the number of rib fractures [Flagel et al., 2005].Elderly patients have a particularly high incidence of rib fractures, with a higher rate of morbidity and mortality from these fractures than younger patients [Bulger et al., 2000; Shorr et al., 1989]. Improved analgesia, by various methods, has been shown to improve pulmonary function, including peak expiratory flow, maximum inspiratory force, tidal volume, and oxygen saturation [Luchette et al., 1994; Moon et al., 1999; Osinowo et al., 2004].

Thoracic epidural analgesia (TEA) has been shown to improve outcome after multiple rib fractures [Bulger et al., 2004;Flagel et al., 2005; Moon et al., 1999; Wisner, 1990].As early as 1990, a retrospective regression analysis of a trauma database revealed decreased pulmonary complications and decreased mortality in elderly patients with rib fractures that were treated with TEA as compared to parenteral opiates [Wisner, 1990].Moon et al showed improved pulmonary mechanics and decreased levels of the proinflammatory chemoattractant, interleukin 8, in a prospective, randomized trial that compared TEA with parenteral opioids in patients with thoracic trauma [Moon et al., 1999]. Another prospective study comparing TEA and parenteral opioid analgesia for patients with rib fractures showed decreased rates of nosocomial pneumonia and a shorter duration of mechanical ventilation in the TEA group [Bulger et al., 2004].However, one frequently cited meta-analysis is noteworthy to illustrate its limitations. Carrier et al reported that there was no significant difference when using epidural analgesia over other methods in terms of mortality, ICU length of stay, and duration of mechanical ventilation [Carrier et al., 2009]. Their analysis is of limited utility, however, because they included two studies using lumbar epidural catheters and three studies using only opiate medications with the epidural infusions; these are significant departures from recommended practices. Flagel et al performed a thorough analysis of a large, sophisticated trauma database [Flagel et al., 2005].They showed that TEA was associated with a reduction in mortality for all patients who sustained rib fractures, particularly those having more than four fractures. These findings have resulted in the recommendation that TEA be included in a widely proliferated pain management guideline for blunt thoracic trauma [Simon et al., 2005].

Despite all of the enthusiasm for epidural analgesia in patients with blunt thoracic trauma, there are considerable limitations to this approach. In the previously mentioned study by Bulger et al [Bulger et al., 2004], 282 patients of 408 admitted to the hospital had to be excluded for a variety of reasons. Thoracic epidural analgesia is contraindicated in patients on anticoagulants or those who have developed a coagulopathy [Horlocker et al., 2010].Brain or spinal injuries represent, at minimum, relative contraindications to the use of TEA, as most practitioners are uncomfortable placing epidurals in the face of elevated intracranial pressure. Possible spinal cord injury, even remote from the proposed insertion site, presents a dilemma, as an epidural may obscure or alter the neurologic examination. Spinal bone injuries may also make epidural placement more technically challenging. The hypotension caused by epidurals can frequently be a significant deterrent in critically ill patients who are already hemodynamically unstable from other causes.

Thoracic paravertebral catheterization (TPVC) has emerged as an enticing answer to some, if not all of the above mentioned concerns. A small pilot study showed comparable outcomes between TEA and TPVC when they were used in patients with unilateral rib fractures [Mohta et al., 2009].These findings are bolstered by similar results in the analogous case of analgesia after thoracotomy [Davies et al., 2006; Pintaric et al., 2011; Powell et al., 2011]. Davies et al presented a systematic review and meta-analysis of 10 randomized clinical trials comparing TPVC and TEA for thoracic surgery. They found no difference in pain scores, but did note a lower incidence of pulmonary complications, urinary retention, nausea and vomiting, and hypotension in the TPVC groups [Davies et al., 2006]. A large, prospective multicenter study of pneumonectomy in the United Kingdom found that TEA was associated with a higher incidence of major complications compared to TPVC [Powell et al., 2011]. A recent prospective randomized study comparing TEA and TPVC, with a primary endpoint of hemodynamic stability, found that TPVC was associated with similar analgesia levels to TEA, but with greater hemodynamic stability [Pintaric et al., 2011].

Should TPVC supplant TEA as the primary modality for providing analgesia for blunt thoracic trauma? A few caveats are in order. Epidural spread has been reported with thoracic paravertebral block [Purcell-Jones et al., 1989]. The authors have also experienced and reported the unintended placement of a catheter in the epidural space during TPVC placement [Lucas et al., 2011, Epub ahead of print]. Considerable controversy exists regarding the relative safety of paravertebral blocks vs. epidurals in the face of anticoagulation and coagulopathy, which will be discussed later in the chapter. Frequently, bilateral rib fractures or other injuries, such as an exploratory laparotomy incision, require bilateral blockade. Although studies on the use of TPVC are still quite undeveloped, findings by Richardson et al, in a literature review on bilateral paravertebral blocks, found a favorable side effect profile. The high local anesthetic load associated with bilateral TPVC is a worthwhile consideration for analgesia in thoracic trauma patients [Richardson et al., 2011].

The clinician is faced with a number of questions about how to proceed with regional analgesia techniques for blunt thoracic trauma. Does the patient need a catheter or not? The literature supports using either TEA or TPVC for more than three rib fractures, and in the elderly. The timing of catheter placement should be as early as *practicable*, although sometimes a short delay may be prudent to allow the anticoagulant effects to dissipate. Patients with very severe injuries may not benefit from early catheter placement, as the improvement in analgesia from RA may not likely alter the length of ventilator management. However, continuous and close monitoring in close consultation with Trauma Surgery and Critical Care Medicine can be used to determine when a patient will benefit from TPVC. Should TEA or bilateral TPVC be used? Extensive bilateral pathology is considered an indication for using thoracic epidural catheters over thoracic paravertebral catheters because of the extensive amount of local anesthetic required for multiple bilateral TPVC; however, there is scant literature to address this question. Another area of practical practice management in question is in regard to the number of catheters to place. Studies have shown loss of pinprick sensation in one to 13 dermatomes after a single-shot paravertebral block [Cheema et al., 1995; Saito et al., 2001]. Richardson et al measured somatosensory evoked potentials of the intercostal nerves and reliably ablated one, but only occasionally two or three nerve potentials [Richardson et al., 1998]. Most patients appear to reliably experience analgesia in approximately five dermatomes; therefore we recommend placing a second unilateral catheter for greater than four fractured ribs. This will provide some margin for error. As the process of adequately positioning and sedating these types of patients can be quite challenging, this seems to be a prudent approach. Figure 1 provides a simplified algorithm for managing these patients.

A number of different techniques have been reported for TPVC. When advancing a predetermined, fixed distance (1.0-1.5 cm) beyond the transverse process, loss of resistance, peripheral nerve stimulation(PNS), and various ultrasound-guided techniques have been described [Ben-Ari et al., 2009; Eason & Wyatt, 1979; Luyet et al., 2009; Naja et al., 2006]. Although any of these techniques can be used in different situations, it should be noted that ultrasound guidance and peripheral nerve stimulation can be technically limited in these patients, as they often have subcutaneous emphysema and hematomas. Measuring the depth of the transverse process and the parietal pleura on CT scan provides definitive information that can be used to guide the depth of needle insertion, thereby improving the safety margin and significantly expediting catheter placement. A CT scan also helps to determine the most severely injured ribs and flail segments.

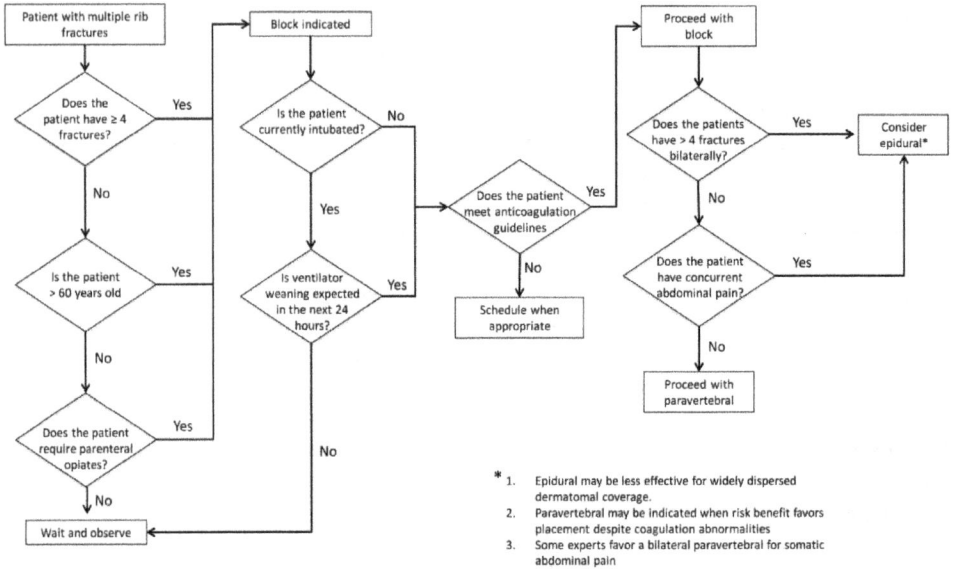

Fig. 1. Algorithm for managing analgesia in patients with multiple rib fractures.

2.2 Long bone fractures

Long bones are composed of a diaphysis, or hollow shaft, connected to the physis, or growth plate, at each end via the metaphysis. Long bones in the body include the humerus, radius, ulna, femur, tibia, fibula, and phalanges. Long bone fractures can result in significant pain, especially prior to stabilization, due to the significant number of nerve endings located in the periosteum and mineralized bone [Mach et al., 2002]. While sclerotome maps have been created to assist in the understanding of innervation to the bones, little evidence exists to confirm their accuracy. Classic studies, including those by Inman and Saunders in 1944 [Inman & Saunders, 1944], provide some evidence for the skeletal innervation [Ivanusic, 2007]. We will review anatomical considerations of the most common fractures and suggest strategies for analgesic management (Table 1).

Fracture	Innervation	Recommended Nerve Block for Analgesia	Considerations
Proximal femur	Femoral nerve Sciatic nerve Obturator nerve	-Single injection or continuous -Femoral nerve block, fascia iliaca block, or lumbar plexus block -Obturator nerve block	For surgical anesthesia, neuraxial anesthesia may decrease incidence of postoperative confusion

Midshaft and distal femur	Femoral nerve Sciatic nerve	-Single injection or continuous -Femoral nerve block -Sciatic nerve block	Greater predominance of sciatic nerve innervation
Proximal and midhumerus	-Brachial plexus, predominantly C5-C6 roots	-Single injection or continuous -Interscalene block, cervical paravertebral block, or supraclavicular block	Radial nerve injury may occur with midshaft humeral fractures
Distal humerus	-Brachial plexus, predominantly C6-C7-roots	-Single injection vs continuous -Interscalene block, cervical paravertebral, supraclavicular, or infraclavicular block	
Clavicle (distal)	Brachial plexus, predominantly C5-C6 roots	-Single injection vs continuous -Interscalene or cervical paravertebral	Possibility of brachial plexus injury due to surgical fixation
Clavicle (proximal)	Brachial plexus, predominantly C4, C5, C6 roots	-Single injection -Cervical paravertebral or deep cervical plexus	Skin overlying clavicle is innervated by supraclavicular nerves, which may be injured during surgery
Radius/Ulna	Brachial plexus, C5-T1	-Single injection -Supraclavicular block, infraclavicular block, or axillary block	
Tibia/Fibula	Sciatic nerve predominantly Possibly femoral nerve in proximal fractures such as tibial plateau	-Single injection or continuous -Sciatic nerve block (Labat or subgluteal or popliteal) -Femoral nerve block for more proximal fractures or to provide for skin sensation to medial lower extremity below knee	Compartment syndrome may occur, especially with young males in high-velocity accidents

Table 1. Regional Anesthesia Considerations for Common Long Bone Fractures

2.2.1 Femur fractures

Femur fractures represent a majority of the patients who suffer from long bone fractures, with one-third of these eventually undergoing surgical stabilization. Regional anesthesia for lower extremity fractures, including femur and hip fractures, has been extensively studied in the literature. Meta-analyses suggest that regional anesthesia, specifically neuraxial anesthesia, decreases the incidence of DVT and pulmonary embolism as well as the incidence of postoperative confusion, in addition to reducing the risk of postoperative pneumonia in patients who require surgical stabilization. Whether regional anesthesia affects mortality in the patient with a femur fracture has yet to be determined [Luger et al., 2010; Parker et al., 2004]. Evidence does suggest that analgesia is improved, and systemic analgesics are spared, when regional anesthesia techniques, such as perineural nerve blocks, are used to help manage pain in patients with hip fractures [Parker, 2002]. Femoral nerve blocks have also been shown to optimize patient positioning for performance of a neuraxial block [Sia et al., 2004; Yun, 2009].

Analgesia for proximal femur fractures may be obtained by blocking the femoral nerve, whether via a single injection or continuous block technique. Although the femur has innervations from multiple nerves, proximally, the femur is predominantly innervated by the femoral nerve, with contributions from the sciatic nerve and an articular branch of the obturator nerve [Locher et al., 2008].

There are a variety of methods available for performance of femoral nerve blocks. The femoral nerve can be anesthetized using stimulation, ultrasound [Beaudoin et al., 2010; Marhofer et al., 1998], or a fascial-pop technique [Candal-Couto et al., 2005; Dalens et al., 1989; Haddad et al., 1995]

Nerve stimulation approaches to the femoral nerve block are common but may cause significant discomfort in a patient with a fracture. The use of ultrasound has been popularized in the past decade for its various benefits. The femoral nerve can be easily visualized at the inguinal crease lateral to the femoral artery, below the fascia lata and iliaca, on the anteromedial aspect of the iliopsoas muscle as it attaches to the proximal femur. The needle can be readily identified since the femoral nerve is typically superficial in nature, and local anesthetic spread is obvious on ultrasound as it encircles the nerve.

In the absence of available ultrasound machines or nerve stimulators, the fascia iliaca compartment block can be easily performed using a simple blunt needle and local anesthetic. This technique has been successfully used in the emergency department setting [Foss et al., 2007; Monzon et al., 2007; Wathen et al., 2007]. The proceduralist draws a line connecting the pubic bone to the anterior superior iliac spine, and divides this line into thirds. At the marking between the distal third (near the anterior superior iliac spine) and middle third, a blunt needle is advanced one centimeter below this point until two pops are felt, the first as the needle punctures the fascia lata and the second as the needle punctures the fascia iliaca. Local anesthetic volumes similar to those used for stimulation-based approaches (20 mL) have been used successfully with the fascia iliaca block with good efficacy [Lopez et al., 2003]; however, weight-based dosing (0.3 mL/kg) [Monzon et al., 2007; Mouzopoulos et al., 2009] and higher doses may be considered to improve local anesthetic delivery [Candal-Couto et al., 2005]. As with any block performed with high volume, confirmation that no intravascular injection has occurred is necessary.

Sciatic nerve blocks become more important in more distal femur fractures and fractures of the leg and ankle. Various approaches to the sciatic nerve are utilized. For femur fractures, more proximal approaches, such as the classic Labat technique or the subgluteal approach [Di Benedetto et al, 2002; Franco et al., 2006], are appropriate. For leg and ankle fractures, a more distal approach, such as a popliteal catheter, may be more suitable, as sparing of the hamstring musculature is important for ambulation.

The subgluteal approach can be achieved with stimulation or ultrasound. Using the stimulation technique, the proceduralist elicits appropriate motor twitches, such as plantar/dorsiflexion and gastrocnemius twitches. When employing ultrasound [Danelli et al., 2009; Karmaker et al., 2007], a low frequency ultrasound probe allows visualization of the proximal femur and ischial tuberosity, as well as the sciatic nerve between these two bones. Confirmation of the nerve location on ultrasound can be done by tracing the nerve distally to the popliteal crease as the nerve divides into its two terminal branches: the common perineal and posterior tibial nerve [Bruhn et al., 2008].

2.2.2 Humerus and clavicle fractures

Proximal humerus fractures are the third, most common fracture in the elderly patient (4-5% of all fractures) after femur fractures and radial fractures [Court-Brown et al., 2001]. The most common mechanism of proximal humeral fractures in the elderly are falls [Chu et al., 2004]. Midhumeral fractures occur in 1-2% of patients, with the mechanism of this injury usually resulting from a direct blow to the arm or application of a bending force to the humeral shaft. This type of fracture typically occurs in the young, physically active patient [Ogawa et al., 1998]. Documentation of any radial nerve injury is important prior to proceeding with a regional anesthetic technique, especially with midhumeral shaft fractures in which the radial nerve may be injured from the trauma as it courses posteriorly alongside the humerus in the spiral groove [Ekholm et al., 2006]. Clavicle fractures also occur in the younger population and are usually related to direct or indirect trauma to the clavicle, commonly due to traffic accidents or a sports-related injury [Pecci et al., 2008; Postacchini et al., 2002; Robinson et al., 1998].

The humerus receives its innervation from the brachial plexus. Like the femur, multiple nerves are involved in providing sensation to the bone. Derivations of the C5 and C6 nerve root predominantly innervate the humerus. As the fracture becomes more distal, the innervation emanates from derivations of the C7 nerve root, and a regional anesthetic technique should be targeted accordingly.

Single injections may be performed using a cervical paravertebral, interscalene, or supraclavicular block. However, fractures of the humerus are painful, even after surgical stabilization, and a continuous approach is recommended for prolonged analgesia. Both stimulation and ultrasound-guided approaches have been utilized successfully. If using stimulation, biceps and deltoids are elicited as endpoints for a proximal humerus fracture and triceps stimulation for distal humeral fractures. As with femur fractures, use of stimulation may result in severe pain, and short but intense systemic analgesia may be needed for patient comfort. Ultrasound allows visualization of the brachial plexus from the root all the way to the terminal nerve, and can assist in minimizing needle attempts. By using ultrasound, nerves can be traced to their origin where they exit the intervertebral foramen as they convene in the interscalene groove, and further down as they become situated posterolateral to the subclavian artery in the supraclavicular approach.

The clavicle is innervated from nerve roots that are more cephalad in origin [Choi et al., 2005]. While distal clavicle fractures can be anesthetized with a C5/C6 block, more medial fractures, which are more common, may be anesthetized as well by depositing local anesthetic near the C4 nerve root, which can be blocked and confirmed by ultrasound. The physician should be aware that numbness across the shoulder and upper chest wall may occur from surgical fixation due to injury to the supraclavicular nerve [Wang et al., 2010]. Furthermore, the brachial plexus lies between the first rib and clavicle as it courses to the upper extremity, and may be at risk for injury due to its proximity to a clavicle fracture.

2.2.3 Radial/ulnar fractures

Repair of radial and ulnar fractures are typically carried out in an outpatient setting, and analgesia prior to surgery is usually provided using oral systemic analgesics. Reduction of a dislocated fracture, however, is extremely painful and may be alleviated by either potent and short-acting anesthetics or a regional anesthetic technique [McManus et al., 2008]. Pain from the surgery itself is typically not severe beyond the initial perioperative phase [Chung et al., 2010], and single-injection brachial plexus blocks using a supraclavicular, infraclavicular [Chin et al., 2010], or axillary approach usually results in adequate intraoperative anesthesia and postoperative analgesia. Ultrasound guidance allows for minimal needle passes, sparing of volumes of local anesthetics, and faster onset [Liu et al., 2010; McCartney et al., 2010; Neal et al., 2010]. Because the radius and ulna are innervated by the entire brachial plexus, all branches of the brachial plexus should be considered when providing surgical anesthesia in the operating room; at the trunk level (supraclavicular), this includes the superior, middle and lower trunk, and at the cord level (infraclavicular), the lateral, posterior and medical cord should be covered. At the axillary level, all terminal nerves should be blocked, which includes the median, ulnar, radial, musculocutaneous, and medial cutaneous nerve of the forearm.

2.2.4 Tibia/fibula fractures

Fractures of the tibia and fibula may occur due to indirect (torsional injuries) or direct impact [Johner et al., 2000]. Open tibia and fibula fracture injuries occur due to high-velocity trauma, such as motor vehicle accidents [Ivarsson et al., 2008], while closed injuries occur due to falls or a sports-related injury. Isolated fibula fractures without concurrent tibial fractures are rare and usually require nonoperative treatment.

The tibia and fibula are predominantly innervated by the sciatic nerve. More proximally, the bones may receive innervation from the femoral nerve. For proximal tibia and fibula fractures, a combined femoral and sciatic nerve block is needed for more complete analgesia, especially if regional anesthesia is utilized for surgical repair Continuous blockade is the technique typically employed for proximal fractures, as many of these patients continue to have severe pain after surgical stabilization. Continuous blockade will also allow monitoring for severe pain out of proportion to what is deemed an appropriate analgesic regimen, as this may signify a developing compartment syndrome. It is important to be aware that patients with tibial fractures are at a particularly high risk of developing compartment syndrome [Park et al., 2009] (discussed in more detail below). Distal tibia and fibula fractures, if uncomplicated, normally do not require more than a single-injection sciatic nerve block, with or without a saphenous nerve block depending on the medial cutaneous involvement of the injury or location of the surgical incision.

3. Challenges and opportunities

The anesthesiologist who performs RA for trauma patients has several challenges that must be addressed, and, thus, it is imperative to have a solid understanding of the complexities of compartment syndrome and coagulation issues in the trauma patient. Included in this chapter is a discussion on a number of technical challenges that frequently arise in trauma patients will be discussed, along with various solutions to these challenges. There are presently exciting opportunities in the field of RA for the trauma patient, one of which will be elucidated: the provision of RA in the prehospital or early hospital period.

3.1 Compartment syndrome

Compartment syndrome has been defined as a condition in which increased pressure within a closed compartment is compromising the circulation and function of the tissues within that space [Matsen, 1975].

In the setting of patients who have experienced trauma, we are primarily concerned with acute compartment syndrome (ACS). The most common sites of ACS are the forearm or leg, although it can occur in any closed compartment. Over 200,000 patients are diagnosed with ACS in the United States every year [Konstanantakos et al., 2007];fractures and various soft tissue injuries are the most common causes (Table 2) [McQueen et al., 2000] .Men are at a substantially greater risk than women, as are patients <35 years old [McQueen et al., 2000].

Tibial diaphyseal fracture
Soft tissue injury
Distal radius fracture
Crush syndrome
Diaphyseal fracture of the radius or ulna

Table 2. Most Common Causes of Acute Compartment Syndrome

The sine qua non of ACS management is early diagnosis and treatment, with extensive fasciotomy [Kashuk et al., 2009].Classically, the diagnosis of ACS is made by recognition of the 6 P's (Table 3) [Elliott & Johnstone, 2003].Of these, pulselessness and paralysis occur too late to effectively provide an intervention, and palpation abnormalities are difficult to discern in the traumatized patient. The other signs and symptoms all involve the need for the patient to sense the pain or parasthesia. For this reason, the use of RA in patients at risk for developing compartment syndrome is controversial [Davis et al., 2005; Thonse et al., 2004].

Pain out of proportion to injury
Parasthesia
Pain with forced dorsiflexion
Palpation (tense)
Paralysis
Pulselessness

Table 3. The 6 P's: Signs and Symptoms of Acute Compartment Syndrome

There are no randomized controlled trials comparing outcomes in patients at risk for ACS who had local anesthetic-based analgesia versus opioid-based analgesia. Clinical practice and recommendations have been founded on case reports and retrospective case series [Mar et al., 2009]; Clark's recent excellent editorial pointed out the usefulness of these case reports [Clark, 2011]. However, it is imperative that we carefully review these reports and not over-interpret their significance. It would seem an archaic practice to simply allow all patients at risk for ACS to suffer. Alternatives to RA, such as patient-controlled analgesia, have also been implicated as obscuring an ACS diagnosis [Richards et al., 2004].The literature on these topics will be briefly reviewed, and several recommendations for reasonable practices will be offered.

Recommendations against RA in patients at risk for ACS are based on the premise that any degree of sensory blockade will block the ischemic pain the patient is experiencing in a compromised compartment. Little distinction is made between a limb in which a patient has analgesia but still can sense a pinprick exam, and one that is completely insensate. A recent case report by Cometa illustrated a scenario of a patient with an initially good analgesic block who experienced increasing pain as he developed ACS [Cometa et al., 2011].Because of the prompt recognition of this increasing pain by the anesthesiologists involved, the patient underwent a timely and limb-saving fasciotomy. Although no clear-cut evidence exists to support it, most experts suspect that somewhere on a continuum of density of nerve blockade lies the "danger zone" of sensory blockade in which we are at risk of masking the symptoms of ACS. For this reason, prolonged duration of a dense blockade, such as with a long-acting, potent neuraxial block, are to be discouraged. Intraoperatively and immediately postoperatively, these patients will not be able to report the pain of ACS, so RA and general anesthesia (GA) represent a similar risk. If, however, a dense sensory block persists long after the operative period, then the choice of RA may place the patient at increased risk. For that reason, intraoperative RA - whether neuraxial, single shot peripheral nerve block, or dosing of a continuous perineural catheter - should be limited to short-acting local anesthetic regimens. A much more controversial question is whether a continuous regional anesthetic technique, aimed at providing analgesia but avoiding the "danger zone", should be offered to these patients. Epidural infusions have been implicated in delayed diagnosis of lower extremity ACS [Mar et al., 2009].Unfortunately, in this review of 35 cases, the infusion drugs and concentrations were not reported in the majority of the patients. Of those that were reported, some involved infusates that are much more concentrated than current practices. Eighteen of the 35 patients had symptoms of ACS while the epidural infusions were running. Interestingly, there is a paucity of reports of ACS diagnosis delay in peripheral nerve blockade (PNB), in either single-shot or continuous infusions. Upper limb nerve block has not been associated with delayed ACS diagnosis, but lower limb PNB has been reported in two cases, but the validity of that attribution is extremely doubtful [Mar et al., 2009].In one report, a femoral nerve block was cited for masking a lower leg ACS; as discussed previously, it is obvious that the femoral nerve supplies only cutaneous innervation of the medial lower leg via the saphenous nerve and a small portion of the proximal tibia anteriorly. It cannot block ischemic pain coming from lower leg muscles, all of which are innervated by the sciatic nerve. In the other case, an ankle block was presumed to mask an ACS in the foot, but although severe pain was reported, it was ignored.

There are no reported cases of delayed ACS diagnosis attributed to continuous perineural infusions. The absence of reports certainly does not imply that RA poses no risk to these patients, but may represent a number of factors, such as failure to report complications or avoidance of RA in these patients. Conversely, the literature certainly does not support a wholesale abandonment of RA in patients at risk. We would recommend avoiding long-lasting dense blockade, using minimally effective infusions, and promptly addressing insensate limbs by withholding infusions until pinprick sensation returns. Perhaps even more importantly is a high level of vigilance as was exhibited by Cometa et al [Cometa et al., 2011] and close cooperation between the orthopedic surgeons and anesthesiologists involved. Using RA in these patients should only be considered in centers with a willingness to dedicate resources to the close monitoring of these patients and with caregivers who are acutely aware of the risks involved.

Despite all the attention to the subjective symptoms of ACS, they have actually been found to be quite unreliable [Ulmer, 2002]. A reliable objective measure to diagnose ACS would drastically improve care. Most of the attention in the past has been centered on direct, invasive measurement of intracompartmental pressures [Al-Dadah et al., 2008; Harris, et al., 2006].These techniques have, to date, been somewhat limited by technical problems. The most promising use of this approach would appear to be the series reported by McQueen and Court-Brown, who suggest that maintaining a differential pressure between the diastolic blood pressure and an intracompartmental pressure greater than 30 mm Hg is protective [McQueen et al., 1996].Much more exciting is the prospect of a noninvasive modality, such as near-infrared spectroscopy or laser Doppler flowmetry capable of diagnosing ACS [Elliott & Johnstone, 2003]. Evidently, further research is needed in this area.

3.2 Regional anesthesia and anticoagulation

The trauma patient, depending on the injury, may be at risk for bleeding or clotting. Patients with a high volume blood loss and massive resuscitation can end up with a dilutional coagulopathy, while patients with lower extremity fractures, intracranial injuries, and immobility may be at risk for thromboembolic complications necessitating aggressive anticoagulation strategies. An increasing number of patients present with anticoagulants as part of their home medicine regimen (e.g. Plavix for patients with coronary stents). Close vigilance of the patient's coagulation status, whether hyper- or hypocoagulable, is important prior to initiation of a regional technique.

3.2.1 Venous thromboembolism risk in the trauma patient

Venous thromboembolism can lead to pulmonary embolism, the most common preventable cause of hospital death. In patients with major trauma who are not receiving thromboprophylaxis, rates of DVT can range anywhere between 40 and 80% [Geerts et al., 2008], with rates of pulmonary embolism between 1 and 2% depending on severity of the injury [Schuerer et al., 2005]. Pulmonary embolism is the 3rd leading cause of death for patients who survive beyond the first day [Geerts et al., 2008]. Independent predictors of DVT include spinal cord injury, lower extremity or pelvic fracture, surgery, increasing age, prolonged immobility, and delay in institution of thromboprophylaxis [Geerts et al., 2008].

The American College of Chest Physicians published their updated guidelines on antithrombotic and thrombolytic therapy in 2008 [Geerts et al., 2008]. Low-dose unfractionated heparin alone appears to be insufficient as thromboprophylaxis in trauma patients. The recommendation for patients with major trauma is the use of low molecular weight heparin (LMWH) thromboprophylaxis in the absence of major contraindications. If active bleeding or high risk for clinically significant bleeding is a contraindication for LMWH, mechanical thromboprophylaxis is appropriate. In the patient with hip fracture awaiting surgery, the recommendations include routine use of thromboprophylaxis with fondaparinux, LMWH, adjusted dose of a vitamin K antagonist, or low-dose unfractionated heparin if not at high risk for bleeding. Based on evidence and expert opinion, all these recommendations were grade 1 recommendations, indicating that the benefits of thromboprophylaxis outweigh the risks, burden, and costs of implementation. The panel did recognize that, for patients undergoing neuraxial procedures and deep peripheral blocks, the physician should exercise caution when selecting anticoagulant thromboprophylaxis [Geerts et al., 2008].

The EAST Practice Parameter Workgroup for DVT Prophylaxis also published guidelines on anticoagulation focusing on the trauma patient [Simon et al., EAST Practice Management Guidelines Work Group, 2005]. This group states that, while there is inadequate class I evidence for the general use of LMWH in venous thromboembolism prophylaxis, they do recommend that LMWH be standard for thromboprophylaxis in patients with complex pelvic, lower extremity, and spinal cord injuries who are not at risk for significant bleeding. These authors acknowledge that appropriate selection of the subset of patients to administer LMWH without increasing the risk of significant bleeding may be challenging.

3.2.2 American Society of Regional Anesthesia and Pain Medicine (ASRA) guidelines

The American Society of Regional Anesthesia and Pain Medicine (ASRA) convened a 3rd Consensus Conference on anticoagulation and published the guidelines in 2010 [Horlocker et al., 2010] .Recommendations were made with regard to optimal timing and placement of regional anesthetic techniques when patients have received anticoagulants. The guidelines focus on the appropriate timing of needle placement and catheter manipulation until the patient achieves a reasonable state of coagulation in order to avoid significant bleeding complications associated with needle and catheter placement (spinal hematomas, retroperitoneal hemorrhage). These recommendations were made for patients in the inpatient and outpatient setting, including patients in the intensive care unit who are to receive neuraxial, plexus, or deep peripheral blockade. Little mention is made of the trauma or ICU patient, and much of the literature presented was focused on the patient receiving a regional anesthetic technique in the perioperative setting.

The authors of the ASRA guidelines did acknowledge that fewer recommendations were being presented to allow for "flexibility and individuality in patient management", but stressed proper vigilance when managing a patient with a regional anesthetic and anticoagulation [Horlocker et al., 2010]. The guidelines represent a conservative but safe way to practice regional anesthesia in the anticoagulated patient, and are based on the pharmacologic activity of anticoagulants and large case series reported over a 20-year period. Recently, Chelly et al [Chelly & Schilling, 2008] described a series of orthopedic patients undergoing lumbar paravertebral and perineural blocks placed prior to the administration of thromboprophylaxis. The catheters were maintained during routine use of prophylactic dosing and withdrawn regardless of timing of the anticoagulant. The authors noted no significant hematomas.In another study, Buckenmeier described no bleeding complications in a series of 187 patients receiving continuous nerve blocks and LMWH [Buckenmaier et al., 2006]. These series might suggest that, with a high amount of vigilance and a great deal of technical skill, the ASRA guidelines (Table 4) [Horlocker et al., 2010] may represent too conservative an approach to the use of peripheral nerve blocks. However, neither series was powered to detect serious bleeding complications, and, thus, judgment about safety is not warranted.

Anticoagulant	Recommendations prior to block placement or catheter removal	Time from block placement to resuming anticoagulant	Time from catheter removal to resume anticoagulant
Subcutaneous unfractionated heparin (5000 U twice daily)	-Check platelet count for heparin-induced thrombocytopenia if patient on UFH for more than 4 days -No contraindication, may reduce bleeding by delaying dose until after block	No contraindication	No contraindication
Subcutaneous unfractionated heparin (>5000 U twice daily)	-Check platelet count for heparin-induced thrombocytopenia if patient on UFH for more than 4 days -No current recommendations	-Consider enhanced neurologic monitoring or -Consider switching to twice daily dosing	
Prophylactic LMWH	-12 hours -Anti-Xa level not predictive of bleeding	-If bloody catheter placement, consider postponement of dose for 24 hours -If not difficult placement, 6-8 hours	-2 hours
Therapeutic LMWH	-24 hours	Regardless of technique, postponement of LMWH for 24 hours -Contraindicated while catheter in situ	-2 hours

Warfarin	-Discontinue 4-5 d prior to procedure -INR < 1.5 Consider reversal agent to normalize INR	-INR < 1.5 ideal -Caution in INR 1.5-3 -Contraindicated INR >3	-INR < 1.5
Nonsteroidal antiinflammatory agents	No contraindication	No contraindication	No contraindication
Antiplatelet agents Plavix

Ticlpidine | -7 days -if 5-7 days (for high risk patients) documentation of normalization of platelet function recommended -14 days | -Likely Contraindicated while continuous catheter in situ | No recommendation |
Thrombolytic therapy	-No recommendation on length of time -Neuraxial techniques should be avoided if possible	Contraindicated	Avoidance for 10days after puncture of noncompressible vessels
Platelet GPIIb/IIIa inhibitors	-Abciximab 24-48 hours -Eptifibatide and tirofiban 4-8 hours -Document normal platelet function	Contraindicated	No recommendation
Fondiparinux (Arixtra)	Recommendations are to follow strict conditions in 2 studies	Contraindicated while continuous catheter in situ	-Follow strict conditions in 2 studies --or -Consider switching to alternative anticoagulant
Thrombin inhibitors	Contraindication	Contraindication	Contraindication
Herbals	No contraindication	No contraindication	No contraindication

*Note these recommendations are for single drug therapy and may not apply if patient receives concomitant anticoagulation with other agents

Table 4. ASRA guidelines for common anticoagulant management in the patient receiving a neuraxial, plexus or deep peripheral nerve block[Horlocker et al., 2010].*

3.2.3 Risks versus benefits

In the trauma patient, the risks of bleeding must be weighed against the benefits of regional anesthesia - for instance, the risk of bleeding from TPVC or thoracic epidural catheterization in a patient on LMWH versus the benefit of improved pulmonary function due to improved analgesia with minimal sedative effects, resulting in decreased incidence of hospital-acquired pneumonia [Bulger et al., 2004; Flagel et al., 2005; Karmakor et al, 2003].

When comparing a central neuraxial technique to a more peripheral technique (TEA versus TPVC or lumbar plexus block versus a lumbar epidural), one must always consider the closed nature of the spinal column. With a central neuraxial technique, compression of the epidural space may lead to devastating neurologic injury, including paraplegia, compared to a more peripheral technique in which bleeding into the paravertebral space may lead to extensive blood loss or compression neuropraxia but not paraplegia. The choice of a paravertebral block may be more appropriate in a patient on thromboprophylaxis therapy. Perineural blocks are usually performed at the terminal branches of the nerve (e.g. sciatic nerve block, popliteal nerve block, femoral nerve block, saphenous nerve block, axillary nerve block), and, while bleeding may result in neuropraxia and hematoma formation, the severity of the complications is less than that involving neuraxial or deep plexus blocks.

The decision to proceed should be based on a careful review of the patient's medical record. Informed consent for the patient and/or their family should include a review of the risks and benefits of the procedure, and their input into medical decision-making should be sought. While normal coagulation status would be preferable prior to the placement of a continuous catheter, this may not be possible or desirable. This decision requires astute clinical judgment on the part of the physician and a careful consideration of the risks versus benefits.

Even if the physician and patient both agree to maintain continuous epidural or paravertebral block with thromboprophylactic doses of anticoagulants, waiting until after the peak effect of a potent anticoagulant is prudent in order to avoid further bleeding complications in the already injured patient. Once a neuraxial technique or deep paraneuraxial or perineural technique is performed, maintenance on a prophylactic dose of a potent anticoagulant is reasonable to allow the patient to not only have improved analgesic but effective deep vein thrombosis prophylaxis as well. However, extreme vigilance is required, particularly during the high risk period that occurs when the catheter is removed.

4. Technical considerations

Anatomy can be distorted due to the patient's injuries. Swelling and subcutaneous emphysema may result in a difference in the standard sensations felt as the needle is advanced. If a loss of resistance approach is utilized, this may result in an indistinct or false sensation of loss. Even the use of ultrasound may not be helpful in the patient with subcutaneous emphysema, as the image is altered by the air underneath the skin. The use of CT scans to gauge the depth of the epidural space and paravertebral space is very important in allowing the physician to have an intelligent "guesstimate" of the depth of the targeted space.

Stimulating catheters may be utilized to guide catheters based on the motor response elicited via the catheter. While this provides an extra endpoint for confirmation of catheter placement, motor stimulation may result in further worsening of the patient's pain by stimulating muscle movement around a fractured bone. This, in turn, may produce increased analgesic requirements for block placement and an increase in time needed to thread a stimulating catheter.

In the patient placed in the lateral decubitus position on an ICU bed with an inflatable mattress, the spinal curvature may be altered and dependent on the patient's body habitus. Rotation of the spine or lateral displacement of the spine may lead to inaccurate placement of continuous blocks and difficulties in determining midline.

4.1 Confirmation of analgesic effects of the continuous block

In the nonobtunded and nonintubated patient, the efficacy of a continuous regional analgesic technique is simple to assess. Unfortunately, this is not the case in the intubated patient receiving sedatives. While there are many reasons for altered mental status and agitation in the intensive care unit, it is important to rule out severe pain as the cause.

In the patient who received an epidural catheter, accurate placement may be confirmed with a sympathectomy, which can be pronounced, and routinely requires management with fluids or pressors. While the sympathectomy confirms placement in the epidural space, it does not confirm which nerve roots are affected by the local anesthetic spreads, and analgesia may still be inadequate if the nerve roots to the fractured or injured site are spared.

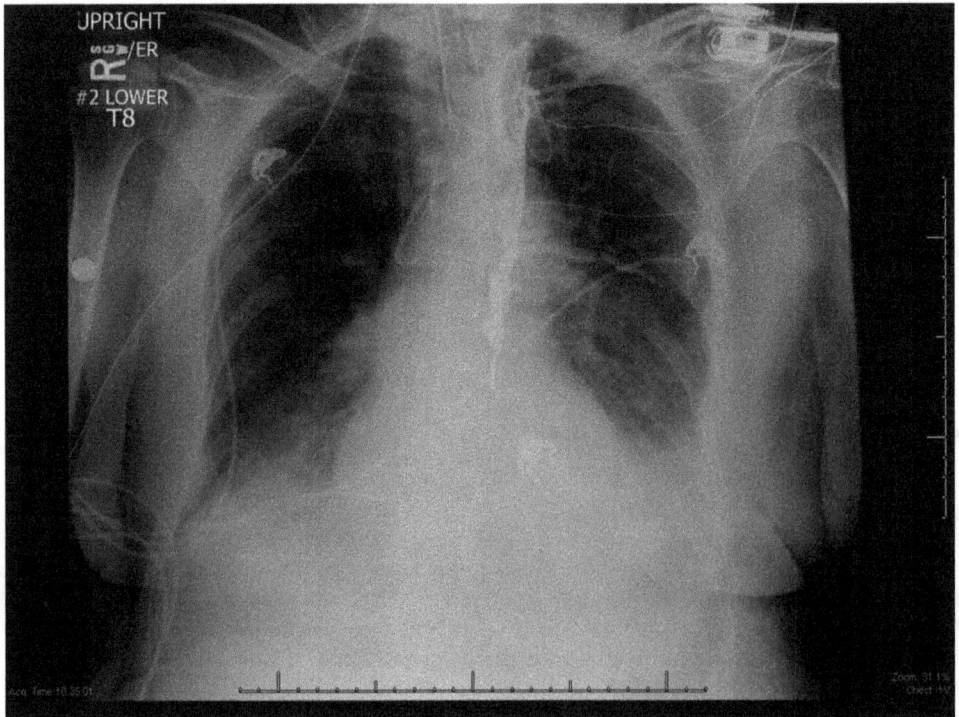

Fig. 2. Dye injection through paravertebral catheter and confirmation of spread of solution.

In the patient with minimal catheters, spread of local anesthetic, while not resulting in hemodynamic effects, can be visualized using ultrasound guidance, as these structures are superficial and can be visualized readily with this mode. In patients with paravertebral continuous blocks, the spread of local anesthetic is difficult to assess and may be inconsistent in its distribution. Therefore, dye injection through the catheter and visualization under fluoroscopy can be used as an alternative gauge of local anesthetic spread, assuming that the patient has no contraindications to contrast dye (Figure 2).

Nursing staff spend the most amount of time with these patients, and can provide important information concerning their perception of whether the patient demonstrates signs of improved or adequate comfort.

4.2 Early management with regional anesthesia

As previously noted, trauma patients often suffer moderate to severe pain in the Emergency Department [Berben et al., 2008]. In Europe, emergency response teams are frequently physician-based. Regional anesthesia performed in the field, prior to hospital admission, has been described for patients with femoral fractures [Lopez et al., 2003; Schiferer et al., 2007]. A simple fascia iliaca block and a nerve stimulator-guided femoral nerve block have been described. Both studies showed reasonably high success rates, with Schiferer reporting a 90% success rate in the RA group [Schiferer et al., 2007].Pain and anxiety scores were much lower in the RA group, as was heart rate. A mean treatment time of seven minutes in the RA group did delay transport time, which is of concern in this setting. While this paradigm will probably not take hold in the rest of the world, including the United States, it surely represents a call to action, to set up processes to provide earlier RA in the hospital setting.

5. Conclusion

Trauma patients represent a significant proportion of current surgical volume and of patients being cared for ICUs. Estimates suggest that this proportion will increase [Lopez et al., 2006]. These patients present many challenges and require extreme vigilance on the part of the health care team. An in-depth understanding of anatomy, physiology, and pharmacology is important when dealing with the trauma patient. Flexibility on the part of the physician to respond to the myriad challenges by adapting to different approaches and modalities is key. Clearly, RA can safely decrease suffering and improve outcomes in these patients when applied judiciously.

6. References

Al-Dadah, O.Q., Darrah, C., Cooper, A., Donell, S.T. & Patel, A.D. (2008). Continuous compartment pressure monitoring vs. clinical monitoring in tibial diaphysial fractures. *Injury* Oct; Vol. 39(No. 10): 1204-1209.

Beaudoin, F.L., Nagdev, A., Merchant, R.C. & Becker, B.M. (2010). Ultrasound-guided femoral nerve block in elderly patients with hip fractures. *American Journal of Emergency Medicine* Jan; Vol. 28(No. 1): 76-81.

Ben-Ari, A., Moreno, M., Chelly, J.E. & Bigeleisen, P.E. (2009). Ultrasound-guided paravertebral block using an intercostal approach. *Anesthesia & Analgesia* Nov; Vol. 109(No. 5): 1691-1694.

Berben, S.A., Meijs, T.H., van Dongen, R.T., van Vugt, A.B., Vloet, L.C., Mintjes-de Groot, J.J. & van Achterberg, T. (2008). Pain prevalence and pain relief in trauma patients in the Accident & Emergency department. *Injury* May; Vol. 39(No. 5): 578-85.

Bjurholm A., Kreicbergs, A., Brodin, E. & Schultzberg, M. (1988). Substance P – and CGRP-immunoreactive nerves in bone. *Peptides* Jan-Feb; Vol. 9(No. 1): 165-171.

Bruhn, J., Van Geffen, G.J., Gielen, M.J. & Scheffer, G.J. (2008). Visualization of the course of the sciatic nerve in adult volunteers by ultrasonography. *Acta Anaesthesiologica Scandinavica* Oct; Vol. 52(No. 9): 1298-1302.

Buckenmaier, C.C. 3rd, Shields, C.H., Auton, A.A., Evans, S.L., Croll, S.M., Bleckner, L.L., Brown, D.S. & Stojadinovic, A. (2006). Continuous peripheral nerve block in combat casualties receiving low-molecular weight heparin. *British Journal of Anaesthesia* Dec; Vol. 97(No. 6): 874-877.

Bulger, E.M., Arneson, M.A., Mock, C.N. & Jurkovich, G.J. (2000). Rib fractures in the elderly. *J Trauma* Feb; Vol. 48(No. 2): 1040-1046.

Bulger, E.M., Edwards, T., Klotz, P. & Jurkovich, G.J. (2004). Epidural analgesia improves outcome after multiple rib fractures. *Surgery* Aug; Vol. 136(No. 2): 426-430.

Candal-Couto, J.J., McVie, J.L., Haslam, N., Innes, A.R. & Rushmer, J. (2005). Pre-operative analgesia for patients with femoral neck fractures using a modified fascia iliaca block technique. *Injury* Apr; Vol. 36(No. 4): 505-510.

Carrier, F.M., Turgeon, A.F., Nicole, P.C., Trepanier, C.A., Fergusson, D.A., Thauvette, D. & Lessard, M.R. (2009). Effect of epidural analgesia in patients with traumatic rib fractures: a systematic review and meta-analysis of randomized controlled trials. *Can J Anesth* Mar; Vol. 56(No. 3): 230-242.

Centers for Disease Control and Prevention. (Last updated February 24, 2011). *Web-based injury statistics query and reporting system,* Accessed July 11, 2011, Available from:www.cdc.gov/injury/wisqars/index.html.

Cheema, S.P., Ilsley, D., Richardson, J. & Sabanathan, S. (1995). A thermographic study of paravertebral analgesia. *Anaesthesia* Feb; Vol. 50(No. 2): 118-1121.

Chelly, J.E. & Schilling, D. (2008). Thromboprophylaxis and peripheral nerve blocks in patients undergoing joint arthroplasty. *Journal of Arthroplasty* Apr; Vol. 23(No. 3): 350-354.

Chin, K.J., Singh, M., Velayutham, V. & Chee, V. (2010). Infraclavicular brachial plexus block for regional anaesthesia of the lower arm. *Cochrane Database of Systematic Reviews* Feb 17; (2): CD 005487.

Chu, S.P., Kelsey, J.L., Keegan, T.H., Sternfeld, B., Prill M., Quesenberry, C.P. & Sidney, S. Risk factors for proximal humerus fracture. (2004). *American Journal of Epidemiology* Aug; Vol. 160(No. 4): 360-367.

Chung, M.S., Roh, Y.H., Baek, G.H., Lee, Y.H., Rhee, S.H. & Gong, H.S. (2010). Evaluation of early postoperative pain and the effectiveness of perifracture site injections following volar plating for distal radius fractures. *Journal of Hand Surgery Am* Nov; Vol. 35(No. 11): 1787-1794.

Clark, L.L. (2011). The value of the case report in the age of evidence–based medicine. *Pain Med* May; Vol. 12(No. 5): 692-694.

Cometa, M.A., Esch, A.T. & Boezaart, A.P. (2011). Did continuous femoral and sciatic nerve block obscure the diagnosis or delay the treatment of acute lower leg compartment syndrome? A case report. *Pain Medicine* Vol. 12(No. 5): 823-828.

Court-Brown, C.M., Garg, A. & McQueen, M.M. (2001). The epidemiology of proximal humeral fractures. *Acta Orthopaedica Scandinavica* Aug; Vol. 72(No. 4): 365-371.

Choi DS, Atchabahian A, Brown AR. (2005). *Anesthesia and Analgesia* May; Vol. 100(No. 5): 1542-1543.

Dalens, B., Vanneuville, G. & Tanquy, A. (1989). Comparison of the fascia iliaca compartment block with the 3-in-1 block in children. *Anesthesia and Analgesia* Dec; Vol. 69(No. 6): 705-713.

Danelli, G., Ghisi, D., Fanelli, A., Ortu, A., Moschini, E., Berti, M., Ziegler, S. & Fanelli, G. (2009). The effects of ultrasound guidance and neurostimulation on the minimum effective anesthetic volume of mepivacaine 1.5% required to block the sciatic nerve using the subgluteal approach. *Anesthesia and Analgesia* Nov; Vol. 109(No. 5): 1674-1678.

Davies, R.G., Myles, P.S. & Graham, J.M. (2006). A comparison of the analgesic efficacy and side-effects of paravertebral vs. epidural blockade for thoracotomy - a systematic review and met-analysis of randomized controlled trials. *Br J Anaesth* Apr; Vol. 96(No. 4):418-426.

Davis, ET, Harris, A, Keene, D, Porter, K, Manji, M. (2005). The use of regional anaesthesia in patients at risk of acute compartment syndrome. Injury 2006; Vol. 37(No. 3): 128-133.

Di Benedetto, P., Casati, A., Bertini, L. & Fanelli, G. (2002). Posterior subgluteal approach to block the sciatic nerve: description of the technique and initial clinical experiences. *European Journal of Anaesthesiology* Sep; Vol. 19(No. 9): 682-686.

Eason, M.J. & Wyatt, R. (1979). Paravertebral thoracic block - a reappraisal. *Anaesthesia* Jul; Vol. 34(No. 7): 638-642.

Ekholm, R., Adami, J., Tidermark, J., Hansson, K., Tornkvis, H. & Ponzer, S. (2006). Fractures of the shaft of the humerus. An epidemiological study of 401 fractures. *Journal of Bone and Joint Surgery British* Nov; Vol. 88(No. 11): 1469-1473.

Elliott, K.G. & Johnstone, A.J. (2003). Diagnosing acute compartment syndrome. *Journal of Bone and Joint Surgery British* Jul; Vol. 85(No. 5): 625-632.

Flagel, B.T., Luchette, F.A., Reed, L., Esposito, T.J., Davis, K.A., Santaniello, J.M. & Gamelli, R.L. (2005). Half-a-dozen ribs: the breakpoint for mortality. *Surgery* Oct; Vol. 138(No. 4): 717-725.]

Foss, N.B., Kristensen, B.B., Bundgaard, M., Bak, M., Heiring, C., Virkelyst, C., Hougaard, S. & Kehlet, H. (2007). *Anesthesiology* Apr; Vol. 106(No. 4): 773-778.

Franco, C.D., Choksi, N., Rahman, A., Voronov, G. & Almachnouk, M.H. (2006). A subgluteal approach to the sciatic nerve in adults at 10 cm from the midline. *Regional Anesthesia and Pain Medicine* May-Jun; Vol. 31(No. 3): 215-220.

Geerts, W.H., Bergqvist, D., Pineo, G.F., Heit, J.A., Samama, C.M., Lassen, M.R. & Colwell, C.W.; American College of Chest Physicians. (2008). Prevention of venous thromboembolism: American College of Chest Physicians Evidence-Based Clinical Practice Guidelines (8th Edition). *Chest* Jun; Vol. 133(6 Suppl); 381S-453S.

Haddad, F.S. & Williams, R.L. (1995). Femoral nerve block in extracapsular femoral neck fractures. *Journal of Bone and Joint SurgeryBr* Nov; Vol. 77(No. 6): 922-923.

Harris, I.A., Kadir, A. & Donald, G. (2006). Continuous compartment pressure monitoring for tibia fractures: does it influence outcomes? *Journal of Trauma* Jun; Vol. 60(No. 6): 1330-1335.

Horlocker, T.T., Wedel, D.J., Rowlingson, J.C., Enneking, F.K., Kopp, S.L., Benzon, H.T., Brown, D.L., Heit, J.A., Mulroy, M.F., Rosenquist, R.W., Tryba, M., & Yuan, C.S. (2010). Regional anesthesia in the patient receiving antithrombotic or thrombolytic therapy: American Society of Regional Anesthesia and Pain Medicine Evidence-Based Guidelines (Third Edition). *Regional Anesthesia and Pain Medicine* Jan; Vol. 35(No. 1): 64-101.

Inman, V. & Saunders, J. Referred pain from skeletal structures. *Journal of Nervous and Mental Disease* 1944; 99: 660-667.

Ivanusic, J. The evidence for the spinal segmental innervation of bone. *Clinical Anatomy* 2007; Nov; Vol. 20(No. 8): 956-960.

Ivanusic, JJ. (2007). The evidence for the spinal segmental innervation of bone. *Clinical Anatomy* Nov; Vol. 20(No. 8): 956-960.

Ivarsson, B.J., Manaswi, A., Genovese, D., Crandall, J.R., Hurwitz, S.R., Burke, C. & Fakhry, S. (2008). Site, type, and local mechanism of tibial shaft fracture in drivers in frontal automobile crashes. *Forensic Science International* Mar; Vol. 175(No. 2-3): 186-192.

Johner, R., Staubli, H.U., Gunst, M. & Cordey, J. (2000). The point of view of the clinician: a prospective study of the mechanism of accidents and the morphology of tibial and fibular shaft structures. *Injury* Sep; Vol. 31 (Suppl 3): C45-49.

Karmakar, M.J., Critchley, L.A., Ho, A.M., Gin, T., Lee, T.W. & Yim, A.P. (2003). Continuous thoracic paravertebral infusion of bupivacaine for pain management in patients with multiple fractured ribs. *Chest* Feb; Vol. 123(No. 2): 424-431.

Karmakar, M.K., Kwok, W.H., Ho, A.M., Tsang, K., Chui, P.T. & Gin, T. (2007). Ultrasound-guided sciatic nerve block: description of a new approach at the subgluteal space. *British Journal of Anaesthesia* Mar; Vol. 98(No. 3): 390-395.

Kashuk, JL, Moore, EE, Pinski, S, Johnson, JL, Moore, JB, Morgan, S, Cothren, CC, Smith, W. (2009). Lower extremity compartment syndrome in the acute care surgery paradigm: safety lessons learned. Patient Safety in Surgery 2009; Vol. 3(No. 1): 11.

Konstantakos, E.K., Dalstrom, D.J., Nelles, M.E., Laughlin, R.T. & Prayson, M.J. (2007). Diagnosis and management of extremity compartment syndrome: an orthopedic perspective. *American Surgeon* Dec; Vol. 73(No. 12): 1199-1209.

Liu, S.S., Ngeow, J. & John, R.S.. (2010). Evidence basis for ultrasound-guided block characteristics: onset, quality, and duration. *Regional Anesthesia and Pain Medicine* Mar-Apr; Vol. 35(2 Suppl): S26-35.

Locher, S., Burmeister, H., Bohlen, T., Eichenberger, U., Stoupis, C., Moriggl, B., Siebenrock, K. & Curatolo, M. (2008). Radiological anatomy of the obturator nerve and its articular branches: basis to develop a method of radiofrequency denervation for hip joint pain. *Pain Medicine* Apr; Vol. 9(No. 3): 291-298.

Lopez, S., Gros, T., Bernard, N., Plasse, C. & Capdevila, X. (2003). Fascia iliaca compartment block for femoral bone fractures in prehospital care. *Regional Anesthesia and Pain Medicine* May-Jun; Vol. 28(No. 3): 203-207.

Lopez, A.D., Mathers, C.D., Ezzati, M., Jamison, D.T. & Murray, C.J.L. (Eds.). (2006). *Global Burden of Disease and Risk Factors*. Oxford University Press and the World Bank, New York, NY.

Lucas, S.D., Higdon, T.A. & Boezaart, A.P. (2011). Unintended epidural placement of a thoracic paravertebral catheter in a patient with severe chest trauma. *Pain Medicine* Jun 30; doi: 10.1111/j.1526-4637.2011.01180.x. [Epub ahead of print]

Luchette, F.A., Radafshar, S.M., Kaiser, R., Flynn, W. & Hassett, J.M. (1994). Prospective evaluation of epidural versus intrapleural catheters for analgesia in chest wall trauma. *Journal of Trauma* Jun; Vol. 36(No. 6): 865-869.

Luger, T.J., Kammerlander, C., Gosch, M., Luger, M.F., Kammerlander-Knauer, U., Roth, T. & Kreutziger, J. (2010). Neuroaxial versus general anaesthesia in geriatric patients for hip fracture surgery: does it matter? *Osteoporos International* Dec; Vol. 21(No. 4): S555-572.

Luyet, C., Eichenberger, U., Greif, R., Vogt, A., Szucs Farkas, Z. & Moriggl, B. (2009). Ultrasound-guided paravertebral puncture and placement of catheters in human cadavers: an imaging study. *British Journal of Anaesthesia* Apr; Vol. 102(No. 4): 534-539.

Mach, D.B., Rogers, S.D., Sabino, M.C., Luger, N.M., Schwei, M.J., Pomonis, J.D., Keyser, C.P., Clohisy, D.R., Adams, D.J., O'Leary, P. & Mantyh, P.W. (2002). Origins of skeletal pain: sensory and sympathetic innervation of the mouse femur. *Neuroscience* Vol. 113(No. 1): 155-156.

Mackenzie, E.J., Rivara, F.P., Jurkovich, G.J., Nathens, A.B., Frey, K.P., Egleston, B.L., Salkever, D.S., Weir, S. & Scharfstein, D.O. (2007). The National Study on Costs and Outcomes of Trauma. *J Trauma* Dec; Vol. 63(6 Suppl): S54-67.

Mar, G.J., Barrington, M.J. & McGuirk, B.R. (2009). Acute compartment syndrome of the lower limb and the effect of postoperative analgesia on diagnosis. *British Journal of Anaesthesia* Jan; Vol. 102(No. 1): 3-11.

Marhofer, P., Schrogendorfer, K., Wallner, T., Konig, H., Mayer, N. & Kapral, S. (1998). Ultrasonographic guidance reduces the amount of local anesthetic for 3-in-1 blocks. *Regional Anesthesia and Pain Medicine* Nov-Dec; Vol. 23(No. 6): 584-588.

Matsen, F.A. 3rd. (1975). Compartment syndrome. A unified concept. *Clinical Orthopaedics and Related Research* Nov-Dec; Vol. 113: 8-14.

McCartney, C.J., Lin, L. & Shastri, U. (2010). Evidence basis for the use of ultrasound for upper-extremity blocks. *Regional Anesthesia and Pain Medicine* Mar-Apr; Vol. 35(2 Suppl): S10-15.

McQueen, M.M. & Court-Brown, C.M. (1996). Compartment monitoring in tibial fractures. The pressure threshold for decompression. *Journal of Bone and Joint Surgery British* Jan; Vol. 78(No. 1): 99-104.

McQueen, M.M., Gaston, P. & Court-Brown, C.M. (2000). Acute compartment syndrome. Who is at risk? *Journal of Bone and Joint Surgery British* Mar; Vol. 82(No. 2): 200-203.

McManus, J.G., Morton, M.J., Crystal, C.S., McArthur, T.J., Helphenstine, J.S., Masneri, D.A., Young, S.E. & Miller, M.A. (2008). Use of ultrasound to assess acute fracture reduction in emergency care settings. *American Journal of Disaster Medicine* Jul-Aug; Vol. 3(No. 4): 241-247.

Mohta, M., Verma, P., Saxena, A.K., Sethi, A.K., Tyagi, A. & Girotra, G. (2009). Prospective, randomized comparison of continuous thoracic epidural and thoracic paravertebral infusion in patients with unilateral multiple fractured ribs-a pilot study. *Journal of Trauma* Apr; Vol. 66(No. 4): 1096-1101.

Monzon, D.G., Iserson, K.V. & Vazquez, J.A. (2007). Single fascia iliaca compartment block for post-hip fracture pain relief. *Journal of Emergency Medicine* Apr; Vol. 32(No. 3): 257-262.

Moon, M.R., Luchette, F.A., Gibson, S.W., Crews, J., Sudarshan, G., Hurst, J.M., Davis, K. Jr, Johannigman, J.A., Frame, S.B. & Fischer, J.E. (1999). Prospective, randomized comparison of epidural versus parenteral opioid analgesia in thoracic trauma. *Annals of Surgery* May; Vol. 229(No. 5): 684-691.

Mouzopoulos, G., Vasiliadis, G., Lasanianos, N., Nikolaras, G., Morakis, E. & Kaminaris, M. (2009). Fascia iliaca block prophylaxis for hip fracture patients at risk for delirium: a randomized placebo-controlled study. *Journal of Orthopaedics and Traumatology* Sep; Vol. 10(No. 3): 127-133.

Naja, Z.M., El-Rajab, M., Al-Tannir, M.A., Ziade, F.M., Tayara, K., Younes, F. & Lonnqvist, P.A. (2006). Thoracic paravertebral block: influence of the number of injections. *Regional Anesthesia and Pain Medicine* May-Jun; Vol. 31(No. 3): 196-201.

Neal, J.M., Brull, R., Chan, V.W., Grant, S.A., Horn, J.L., Liu, S.S., McCartney, C.J., Narouze, S.N., Perlas, A., Salinas, F.V., Sites, B.D. & Tsui, B.C. (2010). *Regional Anesthesia and Pain Medicine* Mar-Apr; Vol. 35(2 Suppl): S1-9.

Ogawa, K. & Yoshida, A. (1998). Throwing fracture of the humeral shaft. An analysis of 90 patients. *American Journal of Sports Medicine* Mar-Apr; Vol. 26(No. 2): 242-246.

Osinowo, O.A., Zahrani, M. & Softah, A. (2004). Effect of intercostal nerve block with 0.5% bupivacaine on peak expiratory flow rate and arterial oxygen saturation in rib fractures. *Journal of Trauma* ;Feb; Vol. 56(No. 2): 345-347.

Powell, E.S., Cook, D., Pearce, A.C., Davies, P., Bowler, G.M., Naidu, B. & Gao, F.; UKPOS Investigators. (2011). A prospective, multicentre, observational cohort study of analgesia and outcome after pneumonectomy. *Br J Anaesth* Mar; Vol. 106(No. 3): 364-370.

Park, S., Ahn, J., Gee, A.O., Kuntz, A.F. & Esterhai, J.L. (2009). Compartment syndrome in tibial fractures. *Journal of Orthopaedic Trauma* Aug; Vol. 23(No. 7): 514-518.

Parker, M.J., Griffiths, R. & Appadu, B.N. (2002). Nerve blocks (subcostal, lateral cutaneous, femoral, triple, psoas) for hip fractures. *Cochrane Database of Systematic Reviews* (1):CD001159.

Parker, M.J., Handoll, H.H. & Griffiths, R. (2004). Anaesthesia for hip fracture surgery in adults. *Cochrane Database of Systematic Reviews* Oct 18;(4):CD000521.

Pecci, M. & Kreher, J.B. Clavicle fractures. (2008). Clavicle fractures. *American Family Physician* Jan; Vol. 77(No. 1): 65-70.

Pintaric, T.S., Potocnik, I., Hadzic, A., Stupnik, T., Pintaric, M. & Jankovic, V.N. (2011). Comparison of continuous thoracic epidural with paravertebral block on perioperative analgesia and hemodynamic stability in patients having open lung surgery. *Regional Anesthesia and Pain Medicine* May-Jun; Vol. 36(No. 3): 256-260.

Postacchini, F., Gumina, S., De Santis, P. & Albo, F. (2002). Epidemiology of clavicle fractures. *Journal of Shoulder and Elbow Surgery* Oct; Vol. 11(No. 5): 452-456.

Purcell-Jones, G., Pither, C.E. & Justins, D.M. (1989). Paravertebral somatic nerve block: a clinical, radiographic and computed tomographic study in chronic pain patients. *Anesthesia and Analgesia* Jan; Vol. 68(No. 1): 32-39.

Richards, H., Langston, A., Kulkarni, R. & Downes, E.M. (2004). Does patient controlled analgesia delay the diagnosis of compartment syndrome following intramedullary nailing of the tibia? *Injury* Mar; Vol. 35(No. 3): 296-298.

Richardson, J., Jones, J. & Atkinson, R.. (1998). The effect of thoracic paravertebral blockade on intercostal somatosensory evoked potentials. *Anesthesia and Analgesia* Aug; Vol. 87(No. 2): 373-376.

Richardson, J., Lonnqvist, P.A. & Naja, Z. (2011). Bilateral thoracic paravertebral block: potential and practice. *British Journal of Anaesthesia* Feb; Vol. 106(No.2): 164-171.

Robinson, C.M. Fractures of the clavicle in the adult. (1998). Epidemiology and classification. *Journal of Bone and Joint Surgery British* May; Vol. 80(No. 3): 476-484.

Rogers, F.B., Cipolle, M.D., Velmahos, G .& Rozycki, G. Practice management guidelines for the management of venous thromboembolism in trauma patients, Accessed July 12, 2011, Available from: http://www.east.org/tpg/dvt.pdf.]

Saito, T., Den, S., Cheema, P.S., Tanuma, K., Carney, E., Carlsson, C. & Richardson, J. (2001). A single injection, multi-segmental paravertebral block- extension of somatosensory and sympathetic block in volunteers. *Acta Anaesthesiologica Scandinavica* Jan; Vol. 45(No. 1): 30-33.

Schiferer, A., Gore, C., Gorove, L., Lang, T., Steinlechner, B., Zimpfer, M. & Kober, A. (2007). A randomized controlled trial of femoral nerve blockade administered preclinically for pain relief in femoral trauma. *Anesthesia and Analgesia* Dec; Vol. 105(No. 6): 1852-1854.

Schuerer, D.J.E., Whinney, R.R., Freeman, B.D., Nash, J., Prasad, S., Krem, M.M., Mazuski, H.E. & Buchman, T.G. (2005). Evaluation of the applicability, efficacy, and safety of a thromboembolic event prophylaxis guideline designed for quality improvement of the traumatically injured patient. *Journal of Trauma* Apr; Vol. 58(No. 4): 731-739.

Shorr, R.M., Rodriguez, A., Indeck, M.C., Crittenden, M.D., Hartunian, S. & Cowley, R.A. (1989). Blunt chest trauma in the elderly. *Journal of Trauma* Feb; Vol. 29(No. 2): 234-237.]

Sia, S., Pelusio, F., Barbagli, R. & Rivituso, C. (2004). Analgesia before performing a spinal block in the sitting position in patients with femoral shaft fracture: a comparison between femoral nerve block and intravenous fentanyl. *Anesthesia and Analgesia* Oct; Vol. 99(No. 4): 1221-1224.

Simon, B.J., Cushman, J., Barraco, R., Lane, V. & Luchette, F.A., Miglietta, M., Roccaforte, D.J., Spector, R., EAST Practice Management Guidelines Work Group. (2005). Pain management guidelines for blunt thoracic trauma. *Journal of Trauma* Nov; Vol. 59(No. 5): 1256-1267.

Thonse, R, Ashford, RU, Williams, TI, Harrington, P. (2004). Differences in attitudes to analgesia in post-operative limb surgery put patients at risk of compartment syndrome. Injury 2004; Vol. 35 (No.3): 290-295.

Thurston, T.J. (1982). Distribution of nerves in long bones as shown by silver impregnation. *Journal of Anatomy* Jun; Vol. 134(Pt 4): 719-728.]

Trunkey, D.D., Lewis, F.R. (1980). Chest trauma. *Surgical Clinics of North America* Dec; Vol. 60(No.6): 1541-1549.

Ulmer, T. The clinical diagnosis of compartment syndrome of the lower leg: are clinical findings predictive of the disorder? Journal of Orthopaedic Trauma 2002; Vol. 16 (No. 8): 572-577.

Wang, K., Dowrick, A., Choi, J., Rahim, R. & Edwards, E. (2010). Post-operative numbness and patient satisfaction following plate fixation of clavicular fractures. *Injury* Oct; Vol. 41(No. 10): 1002-1005.

Wathen, J.E., Gao, D., Merritt, G., Georgopoulos, G. & Battan, F.K. (2007). A randomized controlled trial comparing a fascia iliaca compartment nerve block to a traditional systemic analgesic for femur fractures in a pediatric emergency department. *Annals of Emergency Medicine* Aug; Vol. 50(No. 2): 162-171.

Wisner, D.H. (1990). A stepwise logistic regression analysis of factors affecting morbidity and mortality after thoracic trauma: effect of epidural analgesia. *Journal of Trauma* Jul; Vol. 7(No. 7): 799-804.

World Health Organization. (2004). *Global Burden of Disease (GBD)*, Accessed July 11, 2011, Available from: www.who.int/healthinfo/global_burden_of_disease/en/.

Yun M.J., Kim, Y.H., Han, M.K., Kim, J.H., Hwang, J.W. & Do, S.H. (2009). Analgesia before a spinal block for femoral neck fracture: fascia iliaca compartment block. *Acta Anesthesiologica Scandinavica* Nov; Vol. 53(No. 10): 1282-1287.

11

Propofol and Postoperative Pain: Systematic Review and Meta-Analysis

Antigona Hasani, Hysni Jashari, Valbon Gashi and Albion Dervishi
University Clinical Center of Kosova,
Department of Anesthesiology and Department of Pediatric Surgery, Prishtina,
Republic of Kosova

1. Introduction

If an intravenous or inhalator anesthetic, would include in itself all the components of general anesthesia, like hypnoses, analgesia, amnesia etc. it would represent a really ideal anesthetic.

Propofol is the drug of choice for induction and/or maintenance of anesthesia and sedation in the operating room and intensive care unit. It is a short-acting intravenous anaesthetic that features high blood-tissue solubility and allows a rapid induction and rapid emergence. Propofol has γ-aminobutyric acid agonist activity and produces dose dependent central nervous system depression resulting in sedation and hypnosis.

Analgesic properties of propofol are discussed in many studies, in recent years. However, evidence suggesting that the drug possesses analgesic activity still remains questionable (Fassoulaki, 2011).

The objective of this study is to systematically determine the effects of propofol in postoperative pain.

We have included double-blind, randomized, and controlled trials in humans, where postoperative analgesic effect of propofol was compared with another anesthetic or non-drug intervention.

The study was carried out according to the methods recommended by the Cochrane Collaboration (Higgins et al., 2009) and written in accordance with the PRISMA statement for reporting systematic reviews (Liberati et al., 2009, Moher et al., 2009).

Reports of randomized controlled trials were systemically sought using the Cochrane Library, PubMed, Embase, www.clinicaltrials.gov, and hand searching from the reference lists of identified papers.

Data were analyzed from 25 randomized controlled trials totaling 2033 adults and children. We developed standard data collection sheets to record details of trial design, interventions, and outcome measures for every trial. We extracted information about propofol and control group. Information about number of patients enrolled, type of surgical intervention and side effects, were also noted. Data on postoperative pain relief using pain scores time to first analgesic request and consumption of supplementary analgesics was taken from each report.

Qualitative analysis of postoperative effectiveness was evaluated by significant difference ($P < 0.05$ as reported in the original investigation) in pain relief using pain scores, time to first analgesic request, and consumption of supplementary analgesics between the treatment groups, and by assessment of the clinical importance of observed differences.

Quantitative analyses of combined data were intended by calculation of the number of patients reporting any pain or no pain (pain response rate) between treatment groups.

Each trial was assessed for different measures of internal sensitivity. First, trials were checked for magnitude of pain intensity. Because it is difficult to detect an improvement with low or no pain, it was noted that pain scores were less than 30 mm on a visual analog scale (VAS) or less than moderate pain on a verbal rating scale or similar score. Second, it was noted that a power calculation of the statistical tests was performed. Trials with sample sizes less than 10 patients per treatment group were not considered in the study.

Meta-analyses were carried out by direct comparisons of intervention versus control and indirect comparisons between the networks of interventions shown to be significant individually.

2. Propofol

Propofol (2,6-diisopropyl phenol) is chemically inert phenolic compound with anesthetic properties. It has high lipid solubility, but is almost insoluble in water. The original preparation contained the solubilizing agent Ctenophore EL (polyethoxylated Castrol oil). Reformulation of the drug in an egg-oil-glycerol emulsion has eliminated hypersensitivity reactions that occurred with the original formulation (Sebel, 1989). The dose of propofol required to induce anesthesia measured by loss of eyelash reflex in 95% of healthy unpremedicated patients was 1.5-2.5 mg/kg. The range of induction times was 22-125 seconds. The rapid loss of consciousness was realized due to the immediate uptake of the lipid – soluble drug by the central nervous system (CNS).Within several minutes of intravenous administration, the plasma concentration of propofol decreases due to the distribution of the drug throughout the body and its uptake by peripheral tissues. As the plasma concentration falls, propofol diffuses from the CNS into the systemic circulation; when bolus doses of the anesthetic are used to induce anesthesia, there is a rapid recovery of full consciousness and awareness. These advantageous properties have contributed to the popularity of propofol as an induction agent for short procedures and day – case surgery (Short, 1999).

Propofol is also indicated for the maintenance of anesthesia computer-assisted continuous infusion and target-controlled infusion of propofol using a monitor of the hypnotic effects of propofol on the brain electroencephalographic Bispectral Index [BIS] monitor; it is possible to create a closed-loop delivery system for improving the titration of propofol during general anesthesia (Kwan, 1989, Singh, 1999).

Infusions of subanesthetic doses of propofol have been used to sedate patients for surgery under regional anesthesia, in diagnostic centers for sedation during gastroenterology and pulmonary medicine procedures, as well as in critical care areas for sedation of ventilator-dependent patients as an alternative to benzodiazepines and/or opioid analgesics (Mazurek, 2004).

Propofol is extensively bound to plasma proteins; approximately 97-98% is bound to albumin. After intravenous injection the plasma concentration of propofol decline. The initial fall is extremely rapid (half life 1-3 min), reflecting the distribution of the lipid - soluble drug from plasma to tissue.

Approximately 70% of a dose is excreted in the urine within 24 hours after administration, and 90% is excreted within 5 days. Clearance of propofol ranges from 1.6 to 3.4 liters per minute in licultiy 70 kg patients. As the age of the patient increases, total body clearance of propofol may decrease. Clearance rates ranging from 1.4 to 2.2 liters per minute in patients 18 to 35 years of age have been reported, in contrast to clearance rates of 1 to 1.8 liters per minute in patients 65 to 80 years of age. The propofol mean total body clearance rate was 2.09 +/- 0.65 1/min (mean SD), the volume of distribution at steady state was 159 +/- 57 I, and the elimination half-life was 116 +/- 34 min. Elderly patients (patients older than 60 yr) had significantly decreased clearance rates (1.58 +/- 0.42 vs. 2.19 +/- 0.64 1/min), whereas women (vs. men) had greater clearance rates (33 +/- 8 vs. 26 +/- 7 1 kg⁻¹ min⁻¹) and volumes of distribution (2.50 +/- 0.81 vs. 2.05 +/- 0.65 1/kg). Patients undergoing major intraabdominal surgery had longer elimination half-life values (136 +/- 40 vs. 108 +/- 29 min). Patients required an average blood propofol concentration of 4.05 +/- 1.01 µg/ml for major surgery and 2.97 +/- 1.07 g/ml for nonmajor surgery. Blood propofol concentrations at which 50% of patients were awake and oriented after surgery were 1.07 and 0.95 µg/ml, respectively. The metabolic clearance of propofol exceeds hepatic blood flow, which has leaded to suggestion that propofol is also metabolized in extrahepatic sites. Approximately 70% of a dose is excreted in the urine within 24 hours after administration, and 90% is excreted within 5 days. Psychomotor performance returned to baseline at blood propofol concentrations of 0.38-0.43 g/ml (Shafer et al., 1988, White, 1989, Deegan, 1992; Zuppa et al., 2003).

Propofol causes a significant reduction in systemic blood pressure (more than 50% of preoperative level). This increase in blood pressure is a result of decrease in systemic vascular resistance. In addition to arterial vasodilatation, propofol produces venodilation (due both to a reduction in sympathetic activity and to a direct effect on the vascular smooth muscle), which contributes to its hypotensive effect. The fall in cardiac output is manifested with decrease in heart rate. (Machała & Szebla, 2008; Frolich, 2011).

Respiratory depression and apnea are more pronounced with propofol than thiopental. Propofol decreases tidal volume and increases respiratory rate. The ventilatory response to carbon dioxide and hypoxia is also significantly decreased, but propofol does not inhibit hypoxic pulmonary vasoconstriction. Propofol can produce bronchodilation in patients with chronic obstructive pulmonary disease and in patients with acute laryngospasm during emergence from anesthesia (Zeller et al., 2005).

Propofol decreases CMRO2 and CBF, as well as ICP.33 However, when larger doses are administered, the marked depressant effect on systemic arterial pressure can significantly decrease CPP. Cerebrovascular autoregulation in response to changes in systemic arterial pressure and reactivity of the cerebral blood flow to changes in carbon dioxide tension are not affected by propofol. Evidence for a possible neuroprotective effect has been reported in vitro preparations, and the use of propofol to produce EEG burst suppression has been proposed as a method for providing neuroprotection during aneurysm surgery. Its neuroprotective effect may at least partially be related to the antioxidant potential of propofol's phenol ring structure, which may act as a free-radical scavenger, decreasing free-radical induced lipid peroxidation. Recent studies reported that this antioxidant activity may offer many advantages in preventing the hypoperfusion/reperfusion phenomenon that can occur during surgery (Dagal & Lam, 2009; Girard et al., 2009; Ozturk et al., 2009; Menku et al., 2010).

Propofol produces cortical EEG changes that are similar to thiopental. However, sedative doses of propofol increase â-wave activity analogous to the benzodiazepines. Induction of anesthesia with propofol is occasionally accompanied by excitatory motor activity (so-called nonepileptic myoclonia). In a study involving patients without a history of seizure disorders, excitatory movements following propofol were not associated with EEG seizure activity.

Propofol appears to possess profound anticonvulsant properties. Propofol has been reported to decrease spike activity in patients with cortical electrodes implanted for resection of epileptogenic foci and has been used successfully to terminate status epilepticus. The duration of motor and EEG seizure activity following electroconvulsive therapy is significantly shorter with propofol than with other IV anesthetics. Propofol produces a decrease in the early components of somatosensory and motor evoked potentials but does not influence the early components of the auditory evoked potentials (Modica et al., 1990).

There is no evidence to suggest that propofol has any significant effects on renal or hepatic function.

Propofol is known to possess direct antiemetic effects. Its use for induction and maintenance of anesthesia has been shown to be associated with a lower incidence of postoperative nausea and vomiting (PONV) when compared to any other anesthetic drug or technique. The precise mechanism of propofol antiemetic effect of propofol has not been elucidated, several mechanisms have been proposed, including a direct depressant effect on the chemoreceptor trigger zone (CTZ), the vagal nuclei, and other centers implicated in PONV (Becker, 2010). A systematic review of PONV following maintenance of anesthesia with propofol or an inhalational anesthetic agent found that patients receiving propofol had a significantly lower frequency of PONV, regardless of induction agent, choice of inhalational agent, use of nitrous oxide, patient age, or use of an opioid (Soppitt et al., 2000). Another systematic review found that propofol may be effective in reducing PONV in the short term, but only when given as a continuous infusion for maintenance of anesthesia and when the PONV event rate is greater than 20% (Eberhart et al., 2006). There is evidence of a relationship between plasma propofol concentration and antiemetic efficacy. Gan et al., 1999, found that a median plasma propofol concentration of 343 ng/mL was associated with a reduction in PV in surgical patients. After a typical induction dose, plasma propofol levels remain above this antiemetic serum concentration threshold for approximately 30 minutes. Therefore, the common practice of selecting propofol for inducing anesthesia because of its antiemetic effects provides little benefit to a patient in terms of reducing the likelihood that the patient will develop PONV during the stay in the postanesthesia care unit and after discharge from the ambulatory surgery center.

Anticonvulsant effect of propofol is always described (Simpson et al., 1988). Theoretically, propofol should be strongly anticonvulsant, as it exhibits both GABAergic effects and persistent sodium current and calcium current blockade. However, a literature search of propofol associated tonic-clonic seizures retrieved more than 500 case reports, of which 81 were analyzed in more detail. The denominator is missing from these case reports, and hence the true incidence is unknown. Among the 172,592 anesthetics analyzed there were 53 generalized convulsions, of which 16 were thought to be primarily due to anesthesia. Fifteen of these cases were attributed to local anesthetic drug error, anti-epileptic drug withdrawal or cerebral anoxia/hypercarbia. This left a single case where the seizure was thought to be due to the anesthetic, propofol, an incidence of 1 per 172,592 anesthetics (Fredman et al, 1994).

Propofol has a remarkable safety profile (Sarani B, Gracias, 2008). Dose dependent hypotension is the commonest complication; particularly in volume depleted patients. Hypertriglyceridemia and pancreatitis are uncommon complications. Allergic complications, which may include bronchospasm, have been reported. High dose propofol infusions have been associated with the "propofol syndrome"; this is a potentially fatal complication characterized by severe metabolic acidosis and circulatory collapse (Murdoch &, Cohen, 1999). This is a rare complication first reported in pediatric patients and believed to be due to decreased transmembrane electrical potential and alteration of electron transport across the inner mitochondrial membrane. And, of course pain during injection of propofol which could prevent in several ways (Jalota et al., 2011).

Finally, the favorable pharmacokinetic properties, like short half-life and high clearance rate, minimal side effects and other nonhypnotic positive effects make it safe and usefull in clinical practice.

3. Analgesic effects of propofol

General anesthetics and propofol modulate the function of the gama (γ)-aminobutyric acid (GABA)$_A$ receptors, the inhibitory neurotransmitter receptors in the central nervous system. GABA is the major inhibitory neurotransmitter in the central nervous system, with fast synaptic inhibition mediated by postsynaptic GABA$_A$ receptors. GABA$_A$ receptors are members of the superfamily of ligand-gated ion channels and are thought to consist of five subunits (α, β, and γ). The GABA-induced chloride current can be potentiated by some general anesthetics. The actions of propofol appear to be mediated by β3-containing GABA$_A$ receptors. Specific residue is located within the second transmembrane region of the β3 subunit of the GABA$_A$ receptor and has a influence in determining the action of propofol (Krasowski et. Al., 1998; Siegwart et al. 2002).

The hypnotic effect of propofol and probably analgesic effect is related to GABA accumulation and occupation of the GABA receptor. Occupation of receptors produced hyperpolarisation of the postsynaptic cell membrane and neuronal inhibition. Propofol at low concentration enhance the amplitude of response of GABA and prolong the duration of GABA mediated synaptic inhibition. At supraclinical concentrations propofol directly activate the receptors anion channel.

The analgesic effect of propofol may result as it acts at GABA$_A$ receptors (Dong & Xu, 2002). On the other hand, propofol induced potentiation of glycin receptors at the spinal level and might contribute to its antinociceptive actions and general anesthesia (Xu et al., 2004).

Spinal (NMDA) receptors were reported to be involved in the antinociceptive action of propofol. Prolonged firing of C-fiber nociceptors causes release of glutamate which acts on N-methyl-D-aspartate (NMDA) receptors in the spinal cord. Activation of NMDA receptors causes the spinal cord neuron to become more responsive to all of its inputs, resulting in central sensitization. NMDA-receptor antagonists can suppress central sensitization. NMDA-receptor activation not only increases the cell's response to pain stimuli, it also decreases neuronal sensitivity to opioid receptor agonists. In addition to preventing central sensitization, co-administration of NMDA-receptor antagonists with an opioid may prevent tolerance to opioid analgesia. Was reported that intrathecal administration of an NMDA receptor agonist inhibited the antinociceptive effect of propofol; in contrast, an NMDA receptor antagonist enhanced the antinociceptive action of propofol (Cheng et al., 2008). These studies demonstrated that propofol has a synergistic action with several nociceptive transmission cascades including amino acid and opioid systems in the spinal cord.

The above mentioned methods determined the probable way of analgesic action of propofol.

4. Methods

We followed the PRIZMA statement that recommends standards to improve the quality of reporting of meta-analyses.

Systematic search

The study was carried out according to the methods recommended by the Cochrane Collaboration and written in accordance with the PRISMA statement for reporting systematic reviews (Higgins et al., 2009 & Liberati et al., 2009).

This systematic review included studies published up to December 2010. We conducted a systemic search of the electronic databasas: PubMed, Cochrane Library, and Embase, www.clinicaltrials.gov, and hand searching from the reference lists of identified papers. We used the search terms "propofol" and ("postoperative analgesia" OR "analgesic effect"). Abstracts and unpublished studies were not considered. The search was limited to clinical trials and randomised controlled trials. Reference lists from identified studies and journals which appeared to be associated with the most retrieved citations were then hand-searched. The trials in languages other than English were not excluded. We prepared a flow diagram to summarize the study selection process according to PRISMA (Jaded et al., 1996) (Figure 1.).

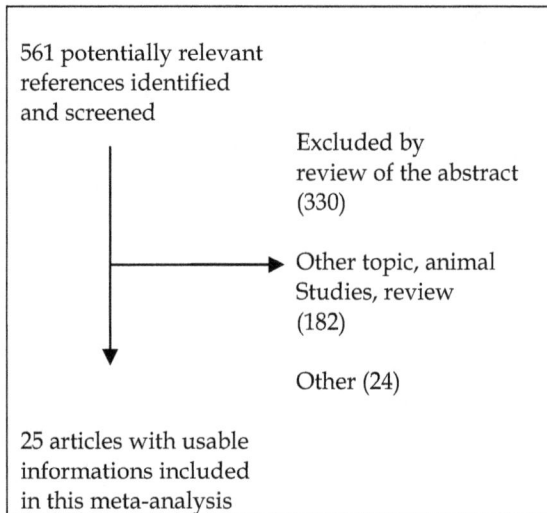

Fig. 1. Flow diagram of excluded and included studies according to PRIZMA statement

To minimize data duplication as a result of multiple reporting we compared papers from the same author. In addition, we searched www.clinicaltrials.gov for studies. Two authors (HJ and AD) screened and retrieved reports and excluded irrelevant studies. Relevant data were extracted by one author (VG) and checked by another (AH).

From each study we extracted details on patients' characteristics (adults and children, ASA status, age), type of surgery or no surgery and use of anesthetics in control group (Table 1.). Pain score, pain score method and use of postoperative analgesics, were also noted (Table 2). Side effects were noted in Table 3.

Study selection

To be considered for the review, the study was evaluated with regard to randomization method, allocation concealment, details of blinding measures, and withdrawals and dropouts using the modified 7-point 4-item Oxford scale (Figure 2) (Dong et al., 2002). This meant that adequate randomization was an absolute requirement for selection. However,

///////////-//////////, was ///// // ///////////// because adequate blinding was not felt to be possible in most studies. Each study was evaluated independently by authors and agreement was reached by consensus.

Selected studies included 25 randomised controlled trials that compared the use propofol during anesthesia and any drug or non-drug intervention, or a combination, with an active or inactive control, and reported the response rate and severity of pain after propofol anesthesia.

VALIDITY SCORE (0-7)	
Randomisation	Double blinding
0 None	0 None
1 Mentioned	1 Mentioned
2 Described and adequate	2 Described and adequate
Concealment of allocation	Flow of patients
0 None	0 None
1 Yes	1 Described but incomplete
	2 Described and adequate

Fig. 2. Modified Oxford Scale

Selected studies included 25 randomised controlled trials that compared the use propofol during anesthesia and any drug or non-drug intervention, or a combination, with an active or inactive control, and reported the response rate and severity of pain after propofol anesthesia.

The studies included in this review enrolled 1970, male and female patients, 1 to 80 year old, ASA I-III, who underwent surgical or non-surgical treatment resulting in the need for acute pain control. Relevant pain outcomes included number of patients who express pain, pain intensity, time to first analgesic request and supplemental analgesic demand were noted. All included studies had numerical data presented in the text or a table; if data were not presented as such, we extracted the information from the graphs if the scale allowed a sufficiently precise estimation.

We excluded trials including less than 10 patients and those reporting on chronic pain. Data from animal studies, abstracts, letters or reviews were not considered.

Information on number of patients, anesthetics and type of surgery was obtained from each report.

The data extracted from each of the included trials included: eligibility and exclusion criteria, study design, duration and degree of follow-up, randomization, allocation concealment, blinding, number and characteristics of participants, type of surgery, pain score, time to first analgesic request, and consumption of supplementary analgesics between the propofol and other treatment groups, and by assessment of the side effects (Table 1, 2 & 3).

Meta analyses

Qualitative analysis of postoperative effectiveness was evaluated by significant difference ($P < 0.05$ as reported in the original investigation) in pain relief using pain scores, time to first analgesic request, and consumption of supplementary analgesics between the treatment groups, and by assessment of the clinical importance of observed differences.

Reference	VS	Treatment	Control	No. of Patients	Type of Intervention
Briggs al. 1982	3	Propofol	Thiopentone	40	Gynecologic procedures
Doze el 1988	4	Propofol	thiopental/isoflurane	120	Abdominal surgery
Borgeal al. 1990	4	Propofol	thiopental/halothane	40	ENT surgery
Anker-Møller et al. 19	4	Propofol	thiopental/saline	19	laser stimulation
V Hemelrick et al. 19	4	Propofol	desflurane	92	gynecological laparoscopy
Hendolin et al. 1994	5	Propofol	thiopental/isoflurane	41	uvuloplasty
Jellish et al. 1995	5	Propofol	thiopental/isoflurane	102	middle ear surgery
Petersen Felix et al. 199	2	Propofol	alfentanyl	12	electric/laser/acoustical stimulation
Eriksson et al. 1996	5	desflurane	propofol	90	gynecological laparoscopy
Zacny et al. 1966	3	propofol	fentanyl	12	ice-cold water
Davis et al. 1997	5	reifentanil	alfentanil/isofl/prop	129	strabismus surgery
Boccara el al. 1998	5	propofol	isoflurane	40	cosmetic abdominoplasty
Ozkose et al. 2001	6	Propofol,/fentanyl	sevoflurane/isofl & alfentanyl	60	laminectomy and discectomy operations
Hand et al. 2001	3	propofol	intralipids	48	tourniquet pain
Mukherjee et al. 2003	6	propofol,fentanyl, isoflurane	pr, remifentanil	100	middle ear surgery
Hofer et al. 2003	7	propofol	sevoflurane	305	gynaecologic or orthopedic procedures
Coolong et al 2003	4	propofol	thiopental	84	laparascopic procedures
Frölich et al. 2005	4	propofol	placebo	80	thermal pain
Cheng et al. 2008	7	propofol	isoflurane	80	open uterine surgery
Fassoulaki et al. 2008	7	sevofl/desfl	propofol	105	gynecological operations
Hasani et al. 2009	5	propofol	halothane	83	abdominal surgery
Bandschapp et al. 2010	7	propofol	intralipid/saline	14	electrical stimulation
Tan et al. 2010	6	propofol	sevoflurane	80	gynecological laparoscopic
Pieters et al. 2010	7	propofol	sevoflurane	42	adenotonsillectomy
Shin et al. 2010	7	propofol & remifentanyl	sevoflurane and remifentanyl	214	brest cancer surgery

VS-Validity Score (Modified Oxford Scale)
NS - no significant difference between treatment groups or no significant difference in favor of the treatment; $P< 0.05$ - significant difference between treatment groups in favor of the treatment; NE - not evaluated.

Table 1. Details of study included.

References	Pain Score Method	Pain Score	Time to First Analgesic Request	Supplemental Analgesic Demand
Briggs et al. 1982	tibial pressure algesimetry	P<0.001	NE	NE
Doze et al. 1988	NE	NE	p>0.05	p>0.05
Borgeat et al. 1990	VAS	P<0.05	p>0.05	p>0.05
Anker-Møller et al. 1991	laser power meter	NS	NE	NE
Van Hemelrijck etal. 1991	VAS	NS	NS	NS
Hendolin et al. 1994	VAS	P<0.05	NS	NS
Jellish et al. 1995	VAS	NS	NS	NS
Petersen-Felix et al. 1996	VAS	NS	NE	NE
Eriksson et al. 1996	VAS	NS	NS	NS
Zacny et al. 1966	VAS	P<0.05	NE	NE
Davis et al. 1997	OPDS	NS	NS	NS
Boccara et al. 1998	VAS	P<0.05 for Iso	P<0.05 for Iso	P<0.05 for Iso
Ozkose et al. 2001	VAS	P<0.05	P<0.05	P<0.05
Hand et al. 2001	NRS	NE	P<0.05	P<0.05
Mukherjee et al. 2003	VAS	P<0.05	P<0.05	P<0.05
Hofer et al. 2003	VAS	NS	NS	NS
Coolong et al 2003	VNRS	NS	NS	NS
Frölich et al. 2005	VAS	P<0.05 more pain with propofol	NE	NE
Cheng et al. 2008	NAS	p<0.01	p<0.01	p<0.01
Fassoulaki et al. 2008	VAS	NS	NS	NS
Hasani et al. 2009	FPS	NS	NE	NE
Bandschapp et al. 2010	NRS	P<0.05	NE	NE
Tan et al. 2010	VAS	P=0.01	NS	NS
Pieters et al. 2010	CHEOPS	P<0.05	P<0.05	P<0.05
Shin et al. 2010	VAS	P> 0.001	P> 0.001	P> 0.001

NS - no significant difference between treatment groups or no significant difference in favor of the treatment; $P<0.05$ - significant difference between treatment groups in favor of the treatment; NE - not evaluated.

Table 2. Details of study included.

	Nauzea			Vomiting			Other side effects		
Study	Propofol n/N	Control n/N	P	Propofol n/N	Control n/N	P	Propofol n/N	Control n/N	P
Doze 1988	1/ 60	8 /60	P<0.05	3/ 60	16/60	P<0.05	10 në 60	34/60	P<0.05
Borgeat 1990	0/20	2/20	NS	0/20	2 në 20	NE	16/20	20/20	P<0.05
Vhemelrijck 1991			P<0.05			P<0.05	9/46	46/46	P<0.05
Hendolin 1994	0/20	2/21	NS	0/20	1/21		2 /21	2 /21	NS
Jellish 1995	3/34	20/68	P<0.05	5/34	15/68	NS			
Eriksson 1996			NS			NS			NS
Davis 1997				6/20	32/57	P<0.05	0/20	23/57	P<0.05
Boccara 1998	5/ 20	12/ 20	P<0.05						NS
Ozkose 2001				1 /20	22/40	P<0.05			
Mukherjee 2003			NS			NS			NS
Hofer 2003	50/155	75/146	P<0.001	34/155	50/146	P<0.01			
Coolong 2003			NS			NS			NS
Cheng 2008			NS			NS			NS
Hasani 2009			NS			NS			NS
Tan 2010			NS			NS			NS
Pieters 2010	1/19	7/19	P<0.05	1/19	7/19	P<0.05			NS
Shin 2010	29/96	40/90	P<0.005	29/ 96	40/90	P<0.005	50/96	42/90	NS

NS - no significant difference between treatment groups or no significant difference in favor of the treatment;
$P<0.05$ - significant difference between treatment groups in favor of the treatment; NE - not evaluated.

Table 3. Details of study included (side effects).

Quantitative analyses of combined data were intended by calculation of the number of patients reporting any pain or no pain (pain response rate) between treatment groups. For studies with multiple intervention groups, we partitioned the count of events and patients in the control group into two or more control groups within any meta-analysis to avoid a unit of analysis error. For the studies participating in the indirect comparisons, we partitioned the comparator group according to how many times it was used for indirect comparisons (across meta-analyses). The summary relative risks and 95% confidence intervals were estimated using a random effects Mantel-Haenszel method in RevMan 5.0 (Cochrane Collaboration). Statistical heterogeneity was assessed by the I^2 value.

The weight given to each study in this analysis (*i.e.*, how much influence each study had on the overall results) was determined by the precision of its estimate by taking into account study size and SDs of the pain in the individual trials. For the current use, a mean for each treatment group was calculated in every trial from all available recordings performed after anesthesia with propofol. Verbal rating pain scores and similar scores were converted to VAS pain scores (*e.g.*, a four-point verbal rating score including no, light, moderate, and severe pain was converted to 0, 25, 50, and 75 mm VAS, respectively).

5. Results

The systematic search in the databases identified 561 relevant articles. After screening, 25 studies potentially met the inclusion criteria. The full-text publications of these studies were examined in more detail. Four study was excluded, because it was reviews or editorial articles. In 90 studies the subject of investigation were animals and also were excluded. (Fig. 1).

The data of 25 randomized controlled studies were included in the present meta-analysis (Table 1,2 &3). A total of 1970 patients (909 with propofol), male and female were included. The patients were 1-85 year old. The 294 patients were children, aged 1-18 year (Borgeat et al.,1990, Pieters et al., 2010, Davis et al., 1997 & Hasani et al., 2009). The participans undergoing brest, ginecologic, orthopedic, ENT, abdominal, urogenital, spine, cosmetic or eye surgery. In 7 studies the participants were volunteer and have no surgery (total 163 volunteers) (Briggs et al., 1982, Anker-Møller et al., 1991, Zacny et al., 1996, Petersen-Felix et al., 1996, Hand et al., 2001, Frolich et al., 2005 & Bandschapp et al. ,2010).

The participants were randomly   assigned to receive propofol and in control group: thiopental (Briggs et al.,1982 & Coolong et al.,2003); thiopental and saline (Anker-Møller et al., 1991); thiopental with halothane (Borgeat et al.,1990); or, thiopenthal with isoflurane (Doze et al., 1988 , Hendolin et al.,1994 & Jellish et al.,1995). In control grup the inhalation anesthetics used were halothane (Hasani et al., 2009), isoflurane (Boccara et al., 1998& Cheng et al.,2008), sevoflurane (Ozkose et al.,2001, Hofer et al., 2003, Tan et al., 2010, Pieters et al., 2010 & Shin et al., 2010) and desflurane (Van Hemelrijck et al.,1991&Fassoulaki et al., 2010). Also, the control groups contained opioids: fentanyl, remifentanil (Davis et al., 1997, Mukherjee et al., 2003 & Shin et al., 2010) and alfentanil (Petersen-Felix et al., 1996& Davis et al., 1997).

Intensity of pain scores was considered adequate (>30 mm VAS) in all trials. VAS (visual analogue score) pain score was not present in 9 studies. The pain scores used in studies was NRS-numeric rating scale (Hand et al., 2001&Bandschapp et al. ,2010), NAS-Numerical analogue score (Cheng et al., 2008), CHEOPS-Children's Hospital of Eastern Ontario Scale (Pieters et al., 2010), tibial pressure algesimetry (Briggs et al., 1982), VNSR-verbal numeric rating scale (Coolong et al., 2003), laser power meter (Anker-Møller et al., 1991), FPS- faces pain scale (Hasani et al., 2009) and OPDS-Objective Pain Discomfort Scale (Davis et al., 1997).

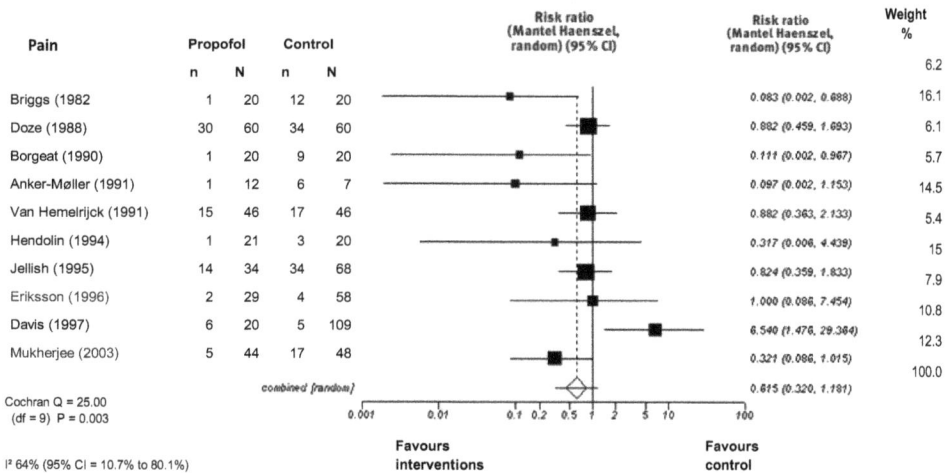

Pain	Propofol		Control		Risk ratio (Mantel Haenszel, random) (95% CI)	Risk ratio (Mantel Haenszel, random) (95% CI)	Weight %
	n	N	n	N			6.2
Briggs (1982	1	20	12	20		0.083 (0.002, 0.688)	16.1
Doze (1988)	30	60	34	60		0.882 (0.459, 1.693)	6.1
Borgeat (1990)	1	20	9	20		0.111 (0.002, 0.967)	5.7
Anker-Møller (1991)	1	12	6	7		0.097 (0.002, 1.153)	14.5
Van Hemelrijck (1991)	15	46	17	46		0.882 (0.363, 2.133)	5.4
Hendolin (1994)	1	21	3	20		0.317 (0.008, 4.439)	15
Jellish (1995)	14	34	34	68		0.824 (0.359, 1.833)	7.9
Eriksson (1996)	2	29	4	58		1.000 (0.088, 7.454)	10.8
Davis (1997)	6	20	5	109		6.540 (1.476, 29.384)	12.3
Mukherjee (2003)	5	44	17	48		0.321 (0.086, 1.015)	100.0
combined (random)						0.615 (0.320, 1.181)	

Cochran Q = 25.00
(df = 9) P = 0.003

I² 64% (95% CI = 10.7% to 80.1%)

Favours interventions   Favours control

Fig. 3. Risk of postoperative pain after propofol anesthesia.

In selected 25 randomized controlled trials the postoperative pain was evaluated in patients treated with propofol. In 15 of them the degree of pain was given as the mean and, in our research to find risk ratio (Mantel Haenszel, random) we included 10 researches in which pain was expressed as present or absent.

Pain was rarely present in the groups treated with propofol 0.615 (95% CI 0.320-1.181) (Fig. 3).

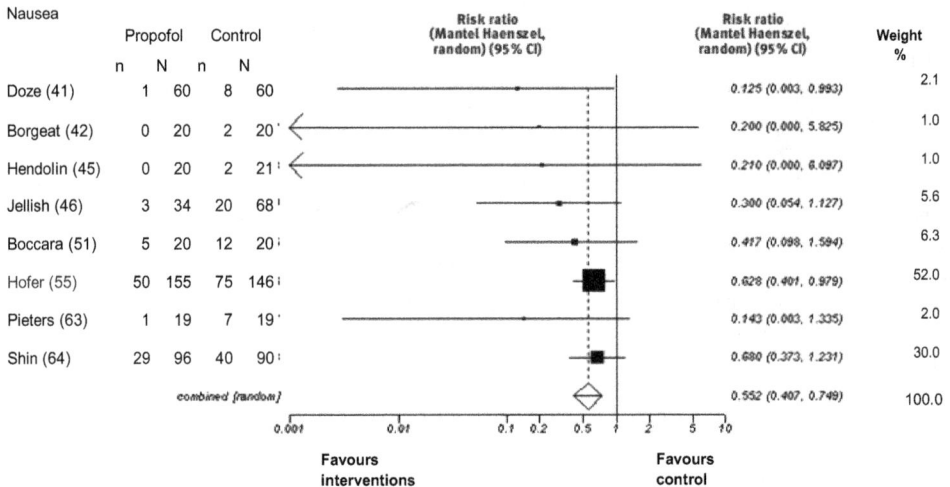

Fig. 4. Risk of postoperative nauzea after propofol anesthesia.

To study the presence of nausea we analyzed eight researches that have investigated this symptom in postoperative period. Nausea was the rare risk ratio 0.552 in intervention group (95% CI 0.407-0.749) (Fig. 4).

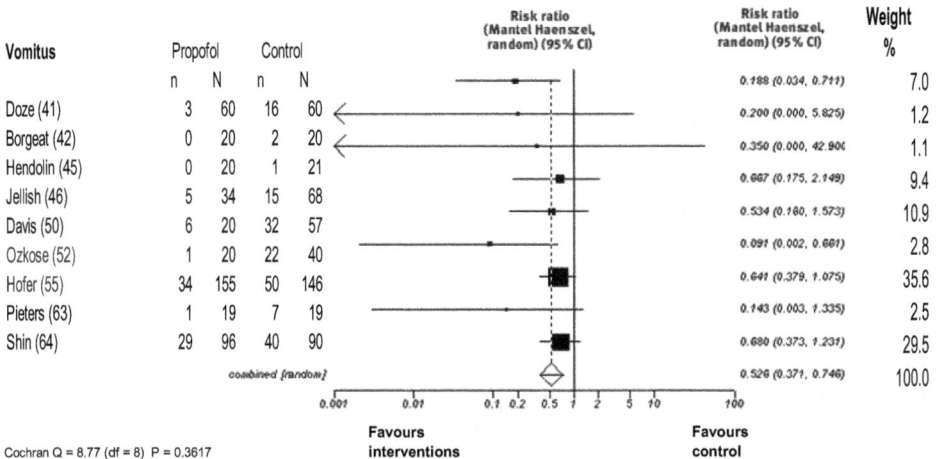

Fig. 5. Risk of postoperative vomiting after propofol anesthesia.

The presence of vomiting was analyzed in 9 researches. The risk ratio for vomiting was RR= 0.526 (95% CI 0.371-0.746) in intervention group with propofol (Fig. 5).

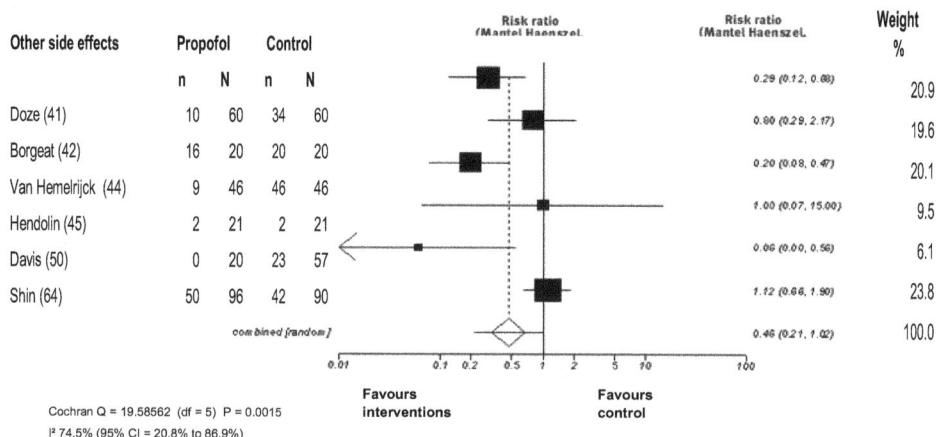

Other side effects	Propofol		Control		Risk ratio (Mantel Haenszel)	Risk ratio (Mantel Haenszel)	Weight %
	n	N	n	N		0.29 (0.12, 0.68)	20.9
Doze (41)	10	60	34	60		0.80 (0.29, 2.17)	19.6
Borgeat (42)	16	20	20	20		0.20 (0.08, 0.47)	20.1
Van Hemelrijck (44)	9	46	46	46		1.00 (0.07, 15.00)	9.5
Hendolin (45)	2	21	2	21		0.06 (0.00, 0.56)	6.1
Davis (50)	0	20	23	57		1.12 (0.66, 1.90)	23.8
Shin (64)	50	96	42	90			
			combined (random)			0.46 (0.21, 1.02)	100.0

Cochran Q = 19.58562 (df = 5) P = 0.0015
I² 74.5% (95% CI = 20.8% to 86.9%)

Favours interventions   Favours control

Fig. 6. Risk of the other side effects after propofol anesthesia during the postoperative period.

The other side effects which occurred in patients anesthetized with propofol were analyzed in 9 researches. In the term "the other side effects" was included: pain during propofol injection in induction period, bradycardia, hypotension, and spontaneous movements also described in perioperative period. Apnea, hypersalivation, laryngospasm and bronchospasm are also included in possible complications in postoperative period. The other side effects were also rare in the propofol anesthesia treated patients with the risk ratio 0.46 in intervention group (95% CI 0.21 to 1.02) (Fig. 6).

6. Discussion

Is propofol analgesic? ; still remain unclear. Experts held very different opinions on the value and clinical utility of an analgesic effect of propofol. The answers for this question were evaluated with pro *versus* con debates.

PRO: Propofol has analgesic effect

Discussions about analgesic effect of propofol restarted with the study published in *Anesthesia & Analgesia* in January 2008 by Cheng et al. The trial was based in hypothesis that women scheduled for hysterectomy or myomectomy and anesthetized with volatile anesthesia, isoflurane induces a hyperalgesic state, and that patients anesthetized with propofol was neutral in its modulation of pain sensitivity. They found that patients anesthetized with isoflurane reported more postoperative pain than those anesthetized with propofol. The other finding was the difference in postoperative opioid use with more requirements in those anesthetized with isoflurane.

Two years later, in 2010 issue of *Anesthesia & Analgesia*, Tan et al. report on a trial that tests the hypothesis that patients undergoing day surgery anesthetized with propofol have less pain and a better quality of recovery compared with patients anesthetized with sevoflurane. In this prospective, double-blind, randomized trial, the authors used a study design in which one group had an induction with inhalation of sevoflurane followed by sevoflurane maintenance, whereas the other group had an IV induction with propofol followed by propofol maintenance. The subjects were treated during surgery with alfentanil, paracetamol, and diclofenac for pain and dexamethasone and ondansetron for nausea. Pain was treated after surgery using morphine until visual analog scale score was <4 and then oral oxycodone. The authors found that propofol provided a statistically significant ($P <$ 0.01) difference, decrease in postoperative pain. Hendolin et al., 1994, found that propofol significantly reduced pain in the second hour compared with patients receiving isoflurane, corroborating the results of the present study.

The other study published in *Anesthesiology* August 2010 by Bandschapp et al., investigated the pain perception or central sensitization effects of propofol and its solvent (10% Intralipid) in healthy volunteers. They experienced decreased pain, hyperalgesia and allodynia elicited by intra-cutaneous electrical stimulation when they received a target-control infusion of propofol (2μg/ml) compared with controls (the solvent 10% Intralipid and saline). However, the results provide no evidence for a modulatory role of the solvent of propofol (10% Intralipid) in the analgesic and antihyperalgesic properties of propofol.

Propofol reduced pain by 40% and nearly abolished hypersensitivity which disappears on discontinuation of the drug. The EC_{50} for the analgesic effect of propofol was 3.2 μg/ml.

There is animal literature that addresses the modulatory effects of anesthetics in different nociceptive models.

In the 1990s, Ewen et al., found that in rats an IV infusion of propofol resulted in an initial decline followed by a rise in nociceptive threshold as the plasma concentration and degree of sedation increased. They suggest that smaller concentrations of propofol than sedative doses are responsible for hyperalgesia. However, the similar experiments in a postoperative pain models in mice were unable to detect any hyperalgesic phase at lower than sedative doses of propofol or on emergence (Udesky et al., 2005). Other groups have found an analgesic response to propofol, particularly in inflammatory pain models (Daniels&Roberts, 1998). A study in rodents by Guindon et al., 2007, demonstrated that in a test of inflammatory pain, locally injected propofol decreased pain behavior in a dose-dependent manner. The authors hypothesized that this antinociceptive activity was mediated, in part, by cannabinoid receptors 1 and 2 (CB1 and CB2). Gilron et al., 1999, however, showed that propofol suppressed hindpaw formalin-evoked expression of fos-like immunoreactivity (FLI) in spinal neurons, suggesting an important analgesic effect.

Clearly, most of the animal and human data on nociceptive effects mediated by propofol may provide advantages.

CON: Propofol has not analgesic effect

On the other hand, many studies with propofol in both animals and humans have failed to demonstrate any evidence of analgesic-like activity.

In an animal study by Merrill et al., 2006, propofol produced anesthesia but failed to produce the experimental findings typically associated with nociception, suggesting that propofol lacks analgesic properties. Accurately, propofol sufficient to produce immobility did not prevent increased activation (c-fos expression) of spinal neurons by intraplantar formalin injection, a finding consistent with propofol lacking analgesic properties. Mice with a mutation of the gamma-aminobutyric acid type A receptor were resistant to propofol anesthesia, supporting the importance of this receptor for propofol's action. Another rodent study (Ng & Antognini, 2006) found that isoflurane and propofol both had similar effects on neuronal "windup" in the spinal cord, a factor associated with persistent pain. The study from Goto et al., 1994, reported that propofol, unlike pentobarbital, had no effect on second-phase nocifensive behavioral responses elicited by formalin injection in the hind paws of rats. Wilder-Smith et al. , 1995, also determined that propofol infusions did not affect thermal pain thresholds.

The human studies of interest, (Boccara et al., 1998) compared postoperative pain and analgesic requirements in patients receiving propofol or isoflurane for maintenance of anesthesia and reported that patients receiving propofol actually had increased pain and opioid requirements for the first 6 hours after surgery compared with patients receiving isoflurane. These findings were exactly the opposite of the findings of Cheng et al.

We conduct a more recent clinical study, published in *Anesthesia & Analgesia* in November 2008, by Fassoulaki et al., in patients undergoing abdominal hysterectomy or myomectomy under sevoflurane, desflurane or propofol anesthesia. Anesthesia was induced with propofol, morphine and cisatracrium; and maintained with sevoflurane or desflurane or propofol. Postoperative analgesia was maintained with morphine. They were unable to demonstrate any difference in postoperative pain scores or in the requirement for opioid analgesic medication among patients maintained with propofol, sevoflurane, or desflurane.

Presented data explained the inconsistency between the studies regarding the post-operative analgesic effect of propofol.

Our findings support the analgesic effect of propofol.

Postoperative nausea and vomiting (PONV) are unpleasant, often underestimated side effects of anesthesia and surgery, not devoid of medical complications. Prevention with antiemetics is only partially effective. Propofol has been shown recently to possess antiemetic properties in several situations.

The limitation of our analysis is mainly related to the methodological heterogeneity of several studies. The dose of propofol varied between the studies and my influenced the postoperative analgesic effect. The methods of postoperative pain assessment my bias the results of our meta-analyses. On the other hand, the number of analyzed clinical trials may also bias our results.

7. Conclusions

Our meta-analysis indicates that propofol provides a prolonged and improved postoperative analgesia with few adverse effects compared with an other inhalation and intravenous anaesthetics. However, propofol have improved antiemetic effect. The other side effects are minimal, with exception of pain during injection of propofol.

Propofol changed the practice of anesthesia, nevertheless postoperative analgesia with ordinary analgesics must be sustained.

Finally, we accomplished that propofol is not an analgesic, but many studies have certainly demonstrated analgesic properties of propofol.

8. References

Anker-Møller, E; Spangsberg, N; Arendt-Nielsen, L; Schultz, P; Kristensen, MS & Bjerring, P. (1991). Subhypnotic doses of thiopentone and propofol cause analgesia to experimentally induced acute pain. *Br J Anaesth* 66:185-8.

Bandschapp, O, Filitz, J, Ihmsen, H, Koppert, W & Ruppen W. (2010). Analgesic and antihyperalgesic properties of propofol in a human pain model. *Anesthesiology* 113:421–428.

Becker, DE. (2010) Nausea, vomiting, and hiccups: a review of mechanisms and treatment. Anesth Prog 57:150-6

Boccara, G, Mann, C, Pouzeratte, Y, Bellavoir, A, Rouvier, A & Colson, P. (1998). Improved postoperative analgesia with isoflurane than with propofol anaesthesia. *Can J Anaesth* 45:839–42.

Borgeat ,A, Popovic, V, Meier, D& Schwander, D. (1990). Comparison of propofol and thiopentone/halothane for short duration ENT surgical procedures in children. *Anesth Analg* 71:511–5.

Briggs, LP, Dundee, JW, Bahar, M & Clarke, RS.(1982). Comparison of the effect of diisopropyl phenol (ICI 35, 868) and thiopentone on response to somatic pain. *Br J Anaesth* 54:307–1.

Cheng, SS, Yeh, J& Flood, P. (2008). Anesthesia matters: patients anesthetized with propofol have less postoperative pain than those anesthetized with isoflurane. *Anesth Analg* 106:264-9.

Coolong, KJ, McGough, E, Vacchiano, C& Pellegrini, JE. (2003). Comparison of the effects of propofol versus thiopental induction on postoperative outcomes following surgical procedures longer than 2 hours. *AANA J* 71:215-22.

Dagal, A& Lam, AM. (2009). Cerebral autoregulation and anesthesia. *Curr Opin Anaesthesiol* 22:542-52.

Daniels, S& Roberts, RJ. (1998). Post-synaptic inhibitory mechanisms of anaesthesia; glycine receptors. *Toxicol Lett* 100–101:71–6.

Davis, PJ, Lerman, J, Suresh, S, McGowan, FX, Coté, CJ, Landsman, I & Henson LG. (1997). A randomized multicenter study of remifentanil compared with alfentanil, isoflurane, or propofol in anesthetized pediatric patients undergoing elective strabismus surgery. *Anesth Analg.* 84:982-9.

Deegan, RJ. (1992). Propofol: a review of the pharmacology and applications of an intravenous anesthetic agent. *Am J Med Sci* 304:45-9.

Dong, XP& Xu, TL. (2002). The actions of propofol on gamma-aminobutyric acid-A and glycine receptors in acutely dissociated spinal dorsal horn neurons of the rat. *Anesth Analg* 95:907-14.

Doze, VA, Shafer, A& White, PF. (1988). Propofol-nitrous versus thiopental-isoflurane-nitrous oxide for general anesthesia. *Anesthesiology* 69:63–71

Eberhart, LH; Frank, S; Lange, H; Morin, AM; Scherag, A; Wulf, H & Kranke, P. (2006). Systematic review on the recurrence of postoperative nausea and vomiting after a first episode in the recovery room - implications for the treatment of PONV and related clinical trials. *BMC Anesthesiol* 13;6:14

Ewen, A, Archer, DP, Samanani, N& Roth, SH. (1995). Hyperalgesia during sedation: effects of barbiturates and propofol in the rat. Can J Anaesth 42:532–40.

Fassoulaki, A. (2011). Is propofol an analgesic. *Eur J Anaesthesiol* 28:481-2.

Fassoulaki, A, Melemeni, A, Paraskeva, A, Siafaka, I& Sarantopoulos, C. (2008). Postoperative pain and analgesic requirements after anesthesia with sevoflurane, desflurane or propofol. *Anesth Analg* 107:1715–9.

Fredman, B; Husain, MM & White, PF. (1994). Anaesthesia for electroconvulsive therapy: use of propofol revisited. *Eur J Anaesthesiol* 11:423-5.

Frölich, MA; Arabshahi, A; Katholi, C; Prasain, J & Barnes S. (2011). Hemodynamic characteristics of midazolam, propofol, and dexmedetomidine in healthy volunteers. *J Clin Anesth* 23:218-23.

Gan, TJ; El-Molem, H; Ray, J & Glass, PS. (1999). Patient-controlled antiemesis: a randomized, double-blind comparison of two doses of propofol versus placebo. *Anesthesiology* 90:1564-70.

Gilron, I, Quirion, R& Coderre, TJ.(1999). Pre- versus postinjury effects of intravenous GABAergic anesthetics on formalin-induced Fos immunoreactivity in the rat spinal cord. *Anesth Analg* 88:414–20

Girard, F; Moumdjian, R; Boudreault, D; Chouinard, P; Bouthilier, A & Ruel, M. (2009). The effect of sedation on intracranial pressure in patients with an intracranial space-occupying lesion: remifentanil versus propofol. *Anesth Analg* 109:194-8.

Goto, T, Marota, JJ & Crosby, G. (1994). Pentobarbitone, but not propofol, produces pre-emptive analgesia in the rat formalin model. *Br J Anaesth* 72:662–7.

Guindon,J, LoVerme, J, Piomelli,D & Beaulieu,P. (2007). The antinociceptive effects of local injections of propofol in rats are mediated in part by cannabinoid CB1 and CB2 receptors. *Anesth Analg* 104:1563–9.

Hendolin, H, Kansanen, M, Kosk, E& Nuutinen, J. (1994).Propofol-nitrous oxide versus thiopentone-isoflurane-nitrous oxide anaesthesia for uvulopalatopharyngoplasty in patients with sleep apnea. *Acta Anaesthesiol Scand* 38:694–8.

Higgins, JPT & Green, S; eds. (2009). Cochrane handbook for the systematic reviews of interventions. Version 5.0.2. Cochrane Collaboration.

Jaded, AR, Moore, RA, Carroll, D, Jenkinson, C, Reynolds, DJ, Gavaghan, DJ & McQuay HJ.(1996). Assessing the quality of reports of randomized clinical trials: is blinding necessary? *Control Clin Trials* 17:1-12.

Jalota, L; Kalira, V; George, E; Shi, YY; Hornuss, C; Radke, O; Pace, NL & Apfel, CC. (2011). Prevention of pain on injection of propofol: systematic review and meta-analysis. Perioperative Clinical Research Core. *BMJ* 15;342:d1110.

Jewett, BA, Gibbs, LM, Tarasiuk, A& Kendig JJ. (1992). Propofol and barbiturate depression of spinal nociceptive neurotransmission.[see comment].*Anesthesiology* 77:1148–54

Krasowski, M. D., Koltchine, V. V., Rick, C. E., Ye, Q., Finn, S. E.& Harrison, N. L. (1998) Propofol and other intravenous anesthetics have sites of action on the γ-aminobutyric acid type A receptor distinct from that for isoflurane. *Mol. Pharmacol.* 53, 530-538.

Kwan, JW. (1989). High-technology i.v. infusion devices. Am *J Hosp Pharm* 46:320-35.

Liberati, A; Altman, DG; Tetzlaff, J; Mulrow, C; Gotzsche, PC; Ioannidis JP, et al. (2009). The PRISMA statement for reporting systematic reviews and meta-analyses of studies that evaluate healthcare interventions: explanation and elaboration. *BMJ* 339: b2700.

Machała, W & Szebla, R. (2008) . Effects of propofol induction on haemodynamics. *Anestezjol Intens Ter* 40:223-6.

Matsuki, A. (1991). A review of recent advances in total intravenous anesthesia. *Masui* 40:684-91.

Menku, A; Ogden, M & Saraymen, R.(2010). The protective effects of propofol and citicoline combination in experimental head injury in rats. *Turk Neurosurg* 20:57-62.

Merrill,AW, Barter,LS, Rudolph, U, Eger, EI II, Antognini, JF, Carstens,MI&Carstens,E. (2006). Propofol's effects on nociceptive behavior and spinal c-fos expression after intraplantar formalin injection in mice with a mutation in the gamma-aminobutyric acid-type (A) receptor beta3 subunit. *Anesth Analg* 103:478–83.

Modica, PA, Tempelhoff, R & White, PF. (1990). Pro- and anticonvulsant effects of anesthetics (Part I) *Anesth Analg* 70:303-15.

Modica, PA, Tempelhoff, R & White, PF (1990). Pro- and anticonvulsant effects of anesthetics (Part II) *Anesth Analg*. 70:433-44.

Moher, D; Liberati, A; Tetzlaff, J & Altman DG. (2009). PRISMA Group. Preferred reporting items for systematic reviews and meta-analyses: the PRISMA statement. *J Clin Epidemiol* 62:1006-12.

Murdoch, SD & Cohen, AT. (1999). Propofol-infusion syndrome in children. *Lancet* 12;353:2074-5.

Ng, KP& Antognini, JF.(2006). Isoflurane and propofol have similar effects on spinal neuronal windup at concentrations that block movement. Anesth Analg 103:1453–8.

Ozturk, E;l Demirbilek, S; Kadir But, A; Saricicek, V; Gulec, M; Akyol, O & Ozcan Ersoy, M. (2005). Antioxidant properties of propofol and erythropoietin after closed head injury in rats. Prog *Neuropsychopharmacol Biol Psychiatry* 29:922-7.

Sarani, B & Gracias, V. (2008). Safety and efficacy of propofol. *J Trauma* 64:242.

Siegwart, R., Jurd, R., Rudolph, U. (2002) Molecular determinants for the action of general anesthetics at recombinant α2β3γ2 γ-aminobutyric acidA receptors. *J. Neurochem* 80, 140-148.

Simpson, KH; Halsall, PJ; Carr, CM & Stewart, KG. (1988). Propofol reduces seizure duration in patients having anaesthesia for electroconvulsive therapy. *Br J Anaesth* 61:343-4.

Singh, H. (1999). Bispectral index (BIS) monitoring during propofol-induced sedation and anaesthesia. *Eur J Anaesthesiol* 16:31-6.

Sebel, PS& Lowdon& JD. (1989) Propofol: a new intravenous anesthetic. Anesthesiology. 71:260-77.

Shafer, A; Doze, VA; Shafer, SL & White PF. (1988). Pharmacokinetics and pharmacodynamics of propofol infusions during general anesthesia. *Anesthesiology* 69:348-56.

Short, CE & Bufalari A. (1999). Propofol anesthesia.Vet *Clin North Am Small Anim Pract* 29:747-78.

Soppitt, AJ; Glass, PS; Howell, S; Weatherwax, K & Gan, TJ. (2000). The use of propofol for its antiemetic effect: a survey of clinical practice in the United States. *J Clin Anesth* 12:265-9.

Sun YY, Li KC, Chen J.(2005). Evidence for peripherally antinociceptive action of propofol in rats: behavioral and spinal neuronal responses to subcutaneous bee venom. *Brain Res* 1043:231–5

Tan, T, Bhinder, R, Carey, M & Briggs, L. (2010). Day-surgery patients anesthetized with propofol have less postoperative pain than those anesthetized with sevoflurane. *Anesth Analg* 111:83–5.

Trame`r, M; Moore, A & McQuay, H. (1997). Propofol anaesthesia and postoperative nausea and vomiting: quantitative systematic review of randomized controlled studies. *Br J Anaesth* 78:247-255.

Udesky, JO, Spence, NZ, Achiel,R, Lee, C& Flood, P. (2005). The role of nicotinic inhibition in ketamine-induced behavior. Anesth Analg 101:407–11.

Xu AJ, Duan SM & Zeng, YM. (2004). Effects of intrathecal NMDA and AMPA receptors agonists or antagonists on antinociception of propofol. *Acta Pharmacol Sin*, 25:9-14.

White, PF. (1989). Clinical uses of intravenous anesthetic and analgesic infusions. *Anesth Analg* 68:161-71.

White, PF. (2008). Propofol: its role in changing the practice of anesthesia. *Anesthesiology* 109:1132–1136.

Wilder-Smith, OH, Kolletzk, M & Wilder-Smith, CH.(1995). Sedation with intravenous infusions of propofol or thiopentone: effects on pain perception. *Anaesthesia*;50:218–22

Zeller, A; Arras, M; Lazaris, A; Jurd, R & Rudolph U. (2005). Distinct molecular targets for the central respiratory and cardiac actions of the general anesthetics etomidate and propofol. *FASEB J* 19:1677-9.

Zuppa, AF; Helfaer, MA & Adamson, PC. (2003). Propofol pharmacokinetics. *Pediatr Crit Care Med* 4:124-5.

Anker-Møller, E; Spangsberg, N; Arendt-Nielsen, L; Schultz, P; Kristensen, MS & Bjerring, P. (1991). Subhypnotic doses of thiopentone and propofol cause analgesia to experimentally induced acute pain. *Br J Anaesth* 66:185-8.

Bandschapp, O, Filitz, J, Ihmsen, H, Koppert, W & Ruppen W. (2010). Analgesic and antihyperalgesic properties of propofol in a human pain model. *Anesthesiology* 113:421–428.

Boccara, G, Mann, C, Pouzeratte, Y, Bellavoir, A, Rouvier, A & Colson, P. (1998). Improved postoperative analgesia with isoflurane than with propofol anaesthesia. *Can J Anaesth* 45:839–42.

Borgeat ,A, Popovic, V, Meier, D& Schwander, D. (1990). Comparison of propofol and thiopentone/halothane for short duration ENT surgical procedures in children. *Anesth Analg* 71:511–5.

Briggs, LP, Dundee, JW, Bahar, M & Clarke, RS.(1982). Comparison of the effect of diisopropyl phenol (ICI 35, 868) and thiopentone on response to somatic pain. *Br J Anaesth* 54:307–1.

Cheng, SS, Yeh, J& Flood, P. (2008). Anesthesia matters: patients anesthetized with propofol have less postoperative pain than those anesthetized with isoflurane. *Anesth Analg* 106:264-9.

Coolong, KJ, McGough, E, Vacchiano, C& Pellegrini, JE. (2003). Comparison of the effects of propofol versus thiopental induction on postoperative outcomes following surgical procedures longer than 2 hours. *AANA J* 71:215-22.

Davis, PJ, Lerman, J, Suresh, S, McGowan, FX, Coté, CJ, Landsman, I & Henson LG. (1997). A randomized multicenter study of remifentanil compared with alfentanil, isoflurane, or propofol in anesthetized pediatric patients undergoing elective strabismus surgery. *Anesth Analg.* 84:982-9.

Doze, VA, Shafer, A& White, PF. (1988). Propofol-nitrous versus thiopental-isoflurane-nitrous oxide for general anesthesia. *Anesthesiology* 69:63–71.

Eriksson, H & Korttila, K. (1996). Recovery profile after desflurane with or without ondansetron compared with propofol in patients undergoing outpatient gynecological laparoscopy. *Anesth Analg* 82:533–8.

Fassoulaki, A, Melemeni, A, Paraskeva, A, Siafaka, I& Sarantopoulos, C. (2008). Postoperative pain and analgesic requirements after anesthesia with sevoflurane, desflurane or propofol. *Anesth Analg* 107:1715–9.

Frölich, MA; Arabshahi, A; Katholi, C; Prasain, J & Barnes S. (2011). Hemodynamic characteristics of midazolam, propofol, and dexmedetomidine in healthy volunteers. *J Clin Anesth* 23:218-23.

Hand, R Jr, Riley, GP, Nick, ML, Shott, S & Faut-Callahan, M. (2001). The analgesic effects of subhypnotic doses of propofol in human volunteers with experimentally induced tourniquet pain. *AANA J* 69:466–70.

Hasani, A, Ozgen ,S & Baftiu, N. (2009). Emergence agitation in children after propofol versus halothane anesthesia. Med Sci Monit 2009; 15: CR302-CR306.

Hendolin, H, Kansanen, M, Kosk, E& Nuutinen, J. (1994).Propofol-nitrous oxide versus thiopentone-isoflurane-nitrous oxide anaesthesia for uvulopalatopharyngoplasty in patients with sleep apnea. *Acta Anaesthesiol Scand* 38:694–8.

Hofer, CK, Zollinger, A, Buchi,S, Klaghofer, R, Serafino, D, Buhlmann, S, Buddeberg, C, Pasch, T & Spahn, DR. (2003). Patient well-being after general anaesthesia: a prospective, randomized, controlled multi-centre trial comparing intravenous and inhalation anaesthesia. *Br J Anaesth* 91:631–7.

Jellish, WS, Leonetti, JP, Murdoch, JR & Fowles S. (1995). Propofol-based anesthesia as compared with standard anesthetic techniques for middle ear surgery. *J Clin Anesth* 7:292-6.

Mukherjee, K, Seavell, C, Rawlings, E & Weiss, A. (2003). A comparison of total intravenous with balanced anaesthesia for middle ear surgery: effects on postoperative nausea and vomiting, pain, and conditions of surgery. [see comment]. *Anaesthesia* 58:176–80.

Ozturk, E;l Demirbilek, S; Kadir But, A; Saricicek, V; Gulec, M; Akyol, O & Ozcan Ersoy, M. (2005). Antioxidant properties of propofol and erythropoietin after closed head injury in rats. Prog *Neuropsychopharmacol Biol Psychiatry* 29:922-7.

Petersen-Felix, S, Arendt-Nielsen, L, Bak, P, Fischer, M & Zbinden, AM. (1996). Psychophysical and electrophysiological responses to experimental pain may be influenced by sedation: comparison of the effects of a hypnotic (propofol) and an analgesic (alfentanil). *Br J Anaesth* 77:165-71.

Pieters, BJ, Penn, E, Nicklaus, P, Bruegger, D, Mehta, B &Weatherly, R. (2010). Emergence delirium and postoperative pain in children undergoing adenotonsillectomy: a comparison of propofol vs sevoflurane anesthesia. *Paediatr Anaesth* 20:944-50.

Shin, SW, Cho, AR, Lee, HJ, Kim, HJ, Byeon, GJ, Yoon, JW, Kim, KH & Kwon JY. (2010). Maintenance anaesthetics during remifentanil-based anaesthesia might affect postoperative pain control after breast cancer surgery. *Br J Anaesth* 105:661-7.

Tan, T, Bhinder, R, Carey, M & Briggs, L. (2010). Day-surgery patients anesthetized with propofol have less postoperative pain than those anesthetized with sevoflurane. *Anesth Analg* 111:83–5.

Van Hemelrijck, J, Smith, I & White, PF. (1991). Use of desflurane for outpatient anesthesia. A comparison with propofol and nitrous oxide. *Anesthesiology* 75:197-203.

Zacny, JP, Coalson, DW, Young, CJ, Klafta, JM, Lichtor, JL, Rupani, G, Thapar, P & Apfelbaum, JL. (1996). Propofol at conscious sedation doses produces mild analgesia to cold pressorinduced pain in healthy volunteers. *J Clin Anesth* 8:469-74.

12

The Effect of General Anesthesia and General Anesthesia Plus Epidural Levobupivacaine or Bupivacaine on Hemodynami Stress Response and Postoperative Pain

Semra Calimli, Ahmet Topal,
Atilla Erol, Aybars Tavlan and Seref Otelcioglu
Selcuk university Meram Medical Faculty,
Turkey

1. Introduction

Levobupivacaine, a new long-acting local anesthetic, is reported to achieve an effective and safe epidural anesthesia, similar to the anesthesia achieved by bupivacaine. Levobupivacaine with a pharmacological structure similar to that of bupivacaine was shown to have a wider confidence interval, and less neurotoxic and cardiotoxic effects.

A large number of trials have been conducted on determining the anesthetic methods that decrease the stress response of major surgery. These trials usually compared the effects of general, epidural and general + epidural anesthetic methods on the stress response occurring in major surgery with respect to mortality and morbidity. While some authors recommended general + epidural anesthesia, some only recommended the general anesthesia.

A combination of epidural and general anesthesia is reported to reduce the requirement for analgesic and anesthetic agents. Intraoperative hemodynamic stability can be better achieved and the metabolic, endocrine and immunologic responses better suppressed. Management of these responses is important in reducing postoperative morbidity and mortality. With the combination of epidural and general anesthesia, recovery is faster, a higher anesthetic quality can be achieved and patients can be mobilized earlier (1-4). There are no adequate trials on the novel agent, levobupivacaine.

This trial was designed to compare the epidural bupivacaine or levobupivacaine combined with general anesthesia and general anesthesia alone in patients who will undergo TAH-BSO, with respect to stress response to surgery, intraoperative hemodynamics, requirement for peroperative anesthetics and analgesic agents, the quality of the postoperative analgesia, recovery from anesthesia and postoperative side effects.

2. Methods

This trial included 54 ASA I-II group patients in the age range of 18-65 who were scheduled to undergo TAH-BSO and who gave written consent to participate in the trial. Those with severe cardiac, pulmonary, hepatic diseases, renal failure, hemorrhagic diathesis, fever, infection and those with known hypersensitivity to investigational drugs were excluded from the trial. Non-premedicated cases were randomly assigned to three groups: general anesthesia + epidural bupivacaine (Group I, n=18), general anesthesia + epidural levobupivacaine (Group II, n=18) and general anesthesia (Group III, n=18). All the patients were monitored for EKG, non-invasive blood pressure, peripheral oxygen saturation (SpO$_2$), end-tidal carbon dioxide pressure (EtCO$_2$) and body temperature.

In Groups I and II, the epidural space was entered by a 16-gauge Tuohy epidural needle before the surgery using the loss of resistance method through the L3-L4 space while the patient was in the sitting position and an 18-gauge epidural catheter was inserted (Perifix, Braun, Germany). As a test dose, 2 ml of 2% lidocaine (Aritmal Ampul® Osel) was administered; five minutes later, Group I and Group II were administered 5 ml of 0.25% bupivacaine (Marcaine flacon® Eczacıbaşı, Turkey) and 0.25% levobupivacaine (Chirocaine flacon® Abbott, USA) respectively via epidural catheter, followed by administration of 10 ml of 0.25% bupivacaine to Group I and 10 ml of 0.25% levobupivacaine to Group II via epidural catheter five minutes later. The sensory block upper level, time to achieve sensory block at T6 dermatome and the Bromage Scale values were assessed.

Anesthetic induction was achieved in all patients (when reached the sensorial block level dermatome of T6 in Group I and Group II) by 2 mg kg^{-1} propofol (Propofol ampul® Fresenius Kabi) and 1 µg kg^{-1} remifentanil (Ultiva® Glaxo Wellcome) administered in 60 seconds. 0.6 mg kg^{-1} rocuronium (Esmeron® Organon) was used for achieving neuromuscular block. For all three groups, the maintenance of anesthesia was achieved using 1% sevoflurane (Sevorane® Abbott, USA) in 50% O$_2$-air mixture and 0.1 µg kg^{-1} min^{-1} remifentanil infusion (Perfusor Compact-Braun). Regarding the patients who would require an anesthesia duration of more than two hours, Group I was scheduled to receive an additional 5 ml of 0.25% bupivacaine and Group II was scheduled to receive an additional 5 ml of 0.25% levobupivacaine from the epidural catheter.

When the heart beat rate (HBR) and the mean blood pressure (MBP) was reduced by 20% of the control value, the concentration of the inhalation agent was reduced by 50%. 250 ml of ringer lactate solution was rapidly administered. In case of absence of improvement, the dose of remifentanil was decreased by 50%. If the low level persisted, atropine or ephedrine was administered as required. When the HBR and MBP increased by more than 20% of the control value, the concentration of the inhalation agent was increased by 50%. In the case of persistence of the high level, the dose of remifentanil was increased by 50%. For maintenance of the neuromuscular blockage, 0.15 mg kg^{-1} rocuronium iv was administered, where necessary.

The hemodynamic parameters, systolic blood pressure (SBP), diastolic blood pressure (DBP), MBP, HBR, and SpO$_2$ were recorded 2 and 5 minutes after the intubation, 2, 5, 10, 15, 30, 45, 60, 90 and 120 minutes after the skin incision and after the extubation. For measuring the glucose, cortisol, insulin and CRP levels, preoperative venous access was achieved followed by blood sampling in the first and 24th hours of operation. The glucose, glucose oxidase, cortisol and insulin values were measured by chemiluminescent immunoassay, CRP, and the immunoturbidimetric methods.

The postoperative recovery was evaluated by the spontaneous breathing time, extubation time, eye opening time and the time to reach an Aldrete recovery score of ≥9. Data were recorded on the amount of sevoflurane used (ml) (Datex Ohmeda, S5. Sweden), the total dose of remifentanil (mg), whether muscle relaxant was added and whether atropine or ephedrine were required. Pain intensity was evaluated by the visual analogue scale (VAS) and the motor block was assessed by the Bromage scale; the hemodynamic data and the side effects (hypotension, respiratory depression, motor block, nausea-vomiting, itching, tremor) were recorded at 0 and 30 minutes, and 2, 6, 12 and 24 hours after the operation.

To relieve the postoperative pain, Group III was administered iv morphine and PCA at a concentration of 1 mg ml^{-1} concentration with a loading dose of 1 mg and a lock-out period of 6 minutes. In Group I, 0.125% bupivacaine + 0.025 mg ml^{-1} morphine, in Group II, 0.125% levobupivacaine + 0.025 mg ml^{-1} morphine and 5 ml of h^{-1} basal infusion were prepared for PCA with a 1 ml loading and a lock-out period of 20 minutes and PCA administration was initiated in the recovery room. The total amount of anesthetics used and the administered and requested amounts were recorded.

Statistical analysis were performed using the SPSS 12.0 software. The data were summarized as mean ± standard deviation and percentage. Comparisons between the three groups were assessed by one way variance analysis (Anova) in cases where the parametric conditions could be met and by Kruskal Wallis variance analysis in non-parametric conditions. In the three-group comparisons, post-hoc Tukey-HSD test and Bonferroni correction Mann-Whitney U test were used for significantly differing parameters. The comparison between the two groups was made with a t test. The chi-square test was used for comparing categorical data. Variance analysis was used to analysis the parametric data and Wilcoxon Signed Ranks test Bonferroni correction was used to analyze the non-parametric data for the analysis of the repeated measurements. The level of significance was set at $p<0.05$.

3. Results

The groups showed similarity in the mean values for age, weight, height, the ASA score and the duration of surgery ($p>0.05$) (Table 1).

	GROUP I	GROUP II	GROUP III	P
Age (year)	46.55 ± 4.97	47.53 ± 6.87	48.44 ± 8.75	0.246
Weight (kg)	70.88 ± 8.58	75.50 ± 15.27	79.55 ± 8.05	0.075
Hight (cm)	160.55 ± 5.29	162.16 ± 5.95	160.27 ± 4.61	0.520
Surgery time (min)	74.88 ± 18.31	72.83 ± 20.47	80.94 ± 13.35	0.365
ASA I / II	11 / 7	13 / 5	10 / 8	0.574

Table 1. Patient characteristics (Mean ± SD)

Time to achieve sensory block at T6 dermatome was 18.72±4.41 and 21.27±4.48 in Group I and Group II, respectively; the sensory block upper levels were 5.66±0.68 and 5.88±0.32 dermatome, respectively ($p>0.05$). The pre-operative Bromage scores were 0 in Group I and II ($p>0.05$).

The total doses of the intra-operatively administered remifentanil and sevoflurane were similar between Group I and Group II, however, statistically higher in Group III ($p<0.000$) (Table 2). While there was no statistically significant difference between Group I and Group II in the postoperative recovery evaluated by spontaneous respiratory time, extubation time, eye opening time and the time to reach an Aldrete recovery score of ≥9, Group III had a significantly longer recovery time compared to Groups I and II ($p<0.000$) (Table 2).

	GROUP I	GROUP II	GROUP III	P
Remifentanil (mg)	0.78 ± 0.38	0.77 ± 0.27	1.24 ± 0.38 *	0.000
Sevoflurane (ml)	21.38 ± 7.63	21.94 ± 8.93	44.44 ± 14.84 *	0.000
Spontaneous breathing time (min)	4.58 ± 2.46	4.11 ± 1.17	7.58 ± 2.68 *	0.000
Extubation time (min)	5.19 ± 2.81	4.27 ± 1.14	8.36 ± 2.66 *	0.000
Eye opening time (min)	6.36 ± 3.27	5.16 ± 1.79	9.80 ± 3.79 *	0.000
Time to Aldrete Score ≥9 (min)	7.91 ± 3,19	7.75 ± 2.49	13.11 ± 3.67 *	0.000

* p< 0.05 Compared with Group I and Group II
(Mean ± SD)

Table 2. Mean doses of drugs used in the operation and recovery times.

There was no statistically significant difference between the groups with respect to requirement for atropine and ephedrine (p>0.05). One, two and nine patients received additional muscle relaxant administration in Group I, II and III respectively. There was a statistically significant difference between the groups with respect to the requirement of muscle relaxant (p=0.002), which was higher in Group III relative to Groups I and II.

Regarding the MBP values, Group III had the highest values at 5, 10, 15, 30, 45 and 60 minutes of incision and after extubation (p<0.05).

The intra-group MBP values showed significant reductions relative to the control values during induction, 2, 5 minutes after intubation and 2, 5, 10, 15, 30, 45, 60 and 90 minutes after the surgical incision in Group 1; during induction, five minutes after the intubation, and 2, 5, 10, 15, 30, 45 and 60 minutes after the surgical incision in Group II; and during induction, 2, 5 minutes after the intubation and 2, 30 and 45 minutes after the surgical incision in Group 3 (p<0.05). While there was no statistically significant difference between the post-extubation MBP values and the control MBP values in Groups I and II (p>0.05), Group III exhibited a significant increase relative to the control value in Group III (p<0.013).

The HBR values were lower in Group III compared to Groups I and II in the 2nd and 5th minutes of intubation (p<0.05).

The intra-group HBR values showed significant reductions relative to the control values during induction, and 2, 5, 10, 15, 30, 45 and 60 minutes after the surgical incision in Group I; during induction, and 10, 15, 30, 45 and 60 minutes after the surgical incision in Group II; and during induction, five minutes after intubation, and 2, 5, 10, 45 and 60 minutes after the surgical incision in Group III (p<0.05).

Since the duration of surgery was below 100 minutes in all patients, there was no requirement for additional epidural local anesthetic administration and the follow-ups at 120 minutes could not be conducted (Table 1).

The mean control values for the parameters used to assess the response to surgical stress including glucose, insulin, cortisol and the CRP values were statistically similar between the three groups (p>0.05).

While the postoperative glucose values in the first and 24th hours were not significantly different, they were higher in Group III relative to Groups I and II (p>0.05). Regarding the intra-group comparison, the glucose values exhibited a significant increase relative to the control values one hour after the operation in all groups, and 24 hours after the operation in Groups I and III (p<0.05) (Figure 1).

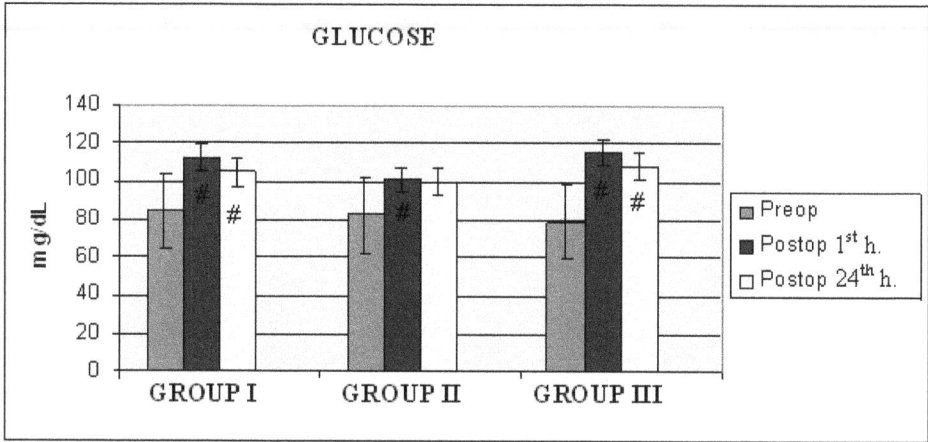

Compared with the control values (p<0.05)

Fig. 1. Changes in Glucose values when compared to Groups

There was no statistically significant difference between the groups in the 1st and 24th hour measurements of the insulin values (p>0.05). In Group I, the postoperative 1st and 24th hour values were different and the 24th hour values were higher (p<0.05). In Group III, the postoperative values in the first and 24th hours were higher than the control values (p<0.05) (Figure 2).

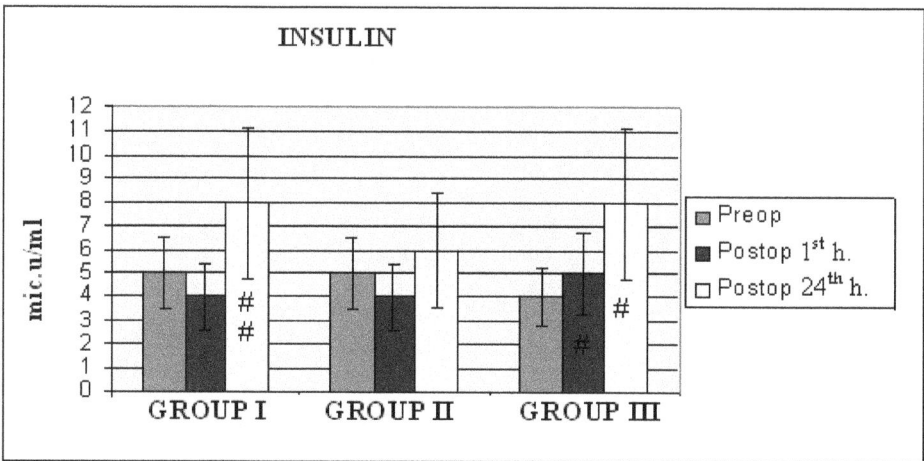

Compared with the control values (p<0.05)
Compared in Group I post op. 1th and 24th hours values (p<0.05).

Fig. 2. Changes in Insulin values when compared to Groups

The postoperative cortisol values at 1 hour differed between the groups and were highest in Group III (p<0.05). The intra-group comparison of the cortisol values revealed higher measurements one hour after the operation relative to the control values (p<0.05). The 24th hour postoperative cortisol values were higher than the control value only in Group III ($p<0.05$) (Figure 3).

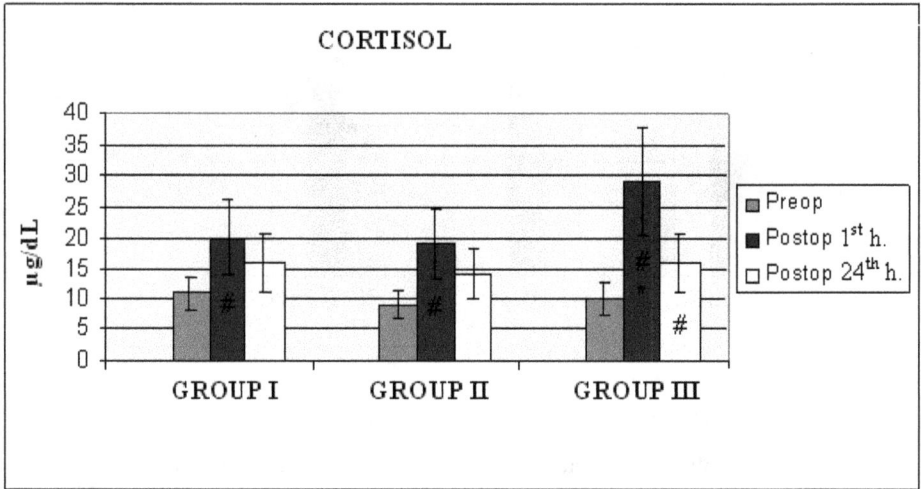

* Compared with the Groups ($p<0.05$)
# Compared with the control values ($p<0.05$).

Fig. 3. Changes in Cortisol values when compared to Groups

There was no difference between the groups in the CRP values. The intra-group comparison of the CRP values showed higher postoperative 24th hour values relative to the control values and the postoperative 1st hour values in all groups ($p<0.05$) (Figure 4).

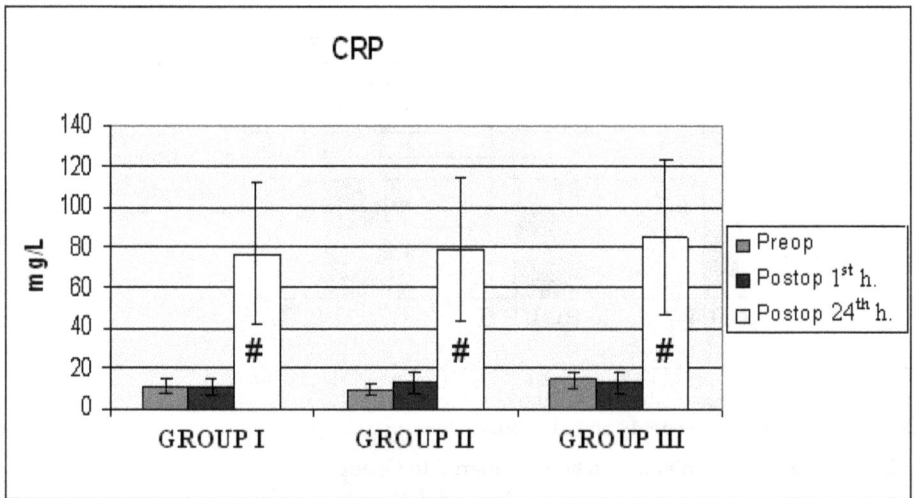

Compared with the control values ($p<0.05$)

Fig. 4. Changes in CRP values when compared to Groups

The comparison of the postoperative pain scores between the groups demonstrated the highest VAS value at minute 0 in Group III (p<0.000). Regarding the other measurement times, no significant difference was detected between the groups (p>0.05) (Table 3).

	GROUP I	GROUP II	GROUP III	P
Postop 0th min.	0.38 ± 1.14	1.33 ± 2.02	5.88 ± 1.99 *	0.000
Postop 30th min.	4.77 ± 1.95 #	4.50 ± 2.22 #	5.83 ± 1.75	0.172
Postop 2nd h	3.77 ± 2.21 #	3.22 ± 2.43	2.55 ± 1.72 #	0.388
Postop 6th h	2.11 ± 2.13	1.33 ± 1.74	1.33 ± 1.13 #	0.465
Postop 12th h	0.38 ± 0.69	0.50 ± 1.42	0.77 ± 1.16 #	0.325
Postop 24th h	0.25 ± 0.23	0.27 ± 0.75	0.33 ± 0.76 #	0.355
P	<0.05	<0.05	<0.05	

*Comparisons between-groups (p<0.05)
Comparison intra-groups (p<0.05).

Table 3. VAS values (Mean ± SD)

The comparison of the postoperative hemodynamic data revealed the highest MBP at minute 0 in Group III (p<0.002). None of the three groups exhibited postoperative hypotension or respiratory depression. Regarding the motor block, there was no significant difference between Groups I and II with respect to nausea-vomiting, itching, or tremor (p>0.05).

4. Discussion

In this trial investigating the extent of suppression of the stress response to surgery in patients undergoing general anesthesia + epidural anesthesia achieved with two different local anesthetics relative to the patients only receiving general anesthesia, the intraoperative hemodynamics, intraoperative anesthetic and analgesic agent requirement, the postoperative analgesia quality, the side effects and the recovery were also compared between the groups.

Bupivacaine is commonly used in epidural analgesia owing to its long-lasting effect and the sensory block it achieves that is more marked than the motor block. However, levobupivacaine was reported to be safer with respect to the central nervous system toxicity and cardiotoxicity in addition to exhibiting a local anesthetic effect similar to bupivacaine in the clinical trials. The tendency for sensory block is longer with levobupivacaine relative to bupivacaine. Following epidural administration of levobupivacaine, the duration of the motor block was observed to be shorter than that of the sensory block. Levobupivacaine was reported to be as effective as bupivacaine when combined with morphine or fentanyl in the treatment of postoperative pain. Some trials demonstrated that levobupivacaine exhibited small increases in the sensory block time relative to bupivacaine, in line with the results from this trial. This finding may be attributed to the relatively increased vasoconstrictor effect of levobupivacaine compared to bupivacaine (5-8).

In this trial, there was no difference between Group I and Group II in the time to achieve sensory block at T6. There was no difference between the two groups in the motor block levels measured until the time to achieve sensory block at T6 dermatome. The follow-ups conducted during the 24th postoperative hour revealed a smaller number of patients developing motor block in the group using levobupivacaine.

In the trial by Bader et al (9) where women undergoing cesarean section were administered 0.5% (150 mg) levobupivacaine or bupivacaine at the same dose via epidural anesthesia, the incidence of hypotension was detected to be lower in those receiving levobupivacaine (84.4% levobupivacaine, 100% bupivacaine).

Bardsley et al (10), upon administering 56.1 mg of levobupivacaine and 47.9 mg of bupivacaine via the iv route, and Kopacz and Allen (11), upon accidentally administering 17 ml of 0.75% of levobupivacaine intravenously to a patient, reported that levobupivacaine was safer for achieving direct depression of the myocardial contractility relative to bupivacaine.

In this trial, there was one patient in Group I and four patients in Group II who required intraoperative ephedrine for hypotension, although this was not statistically significant. In Group III, the arterial blood pressure values were higher at various measurement times and required higher anesthetic doses to achieve hemodynamic stability. None of the three groups exhibited EKG changes. The absence of EKG changes in Groups I and II may be attributed to the low concentration of the epidural local anesthetic used.

Luchetti M et al (12) compared epidural + general anesthesia and total intravenous anesthesia in patients undergoing laparoscopic cholecystectomy and reported that the epidural + general anesthesia group did not require intraoperative opioid use, did not exhibit an increase in side effects and had a faster recovery. In our trial, the amount of sevoflurane and remifentanil used was lower in the epidural + general anesthesia groups relative to the general anesthesia group and thus, recovery was faster in Groups I and II relative to Group III; this finding is in line with the literature.

In their trial where they compared general anesthesia combined with epidural anesthesia achieved by 2% lidocaine to general anesthesia alone, Lu CH et al (13) reported that the requirement for volatile anesthetics was lower in the epidural + general anesthesia group, in line with our results.

The stress response can be avoided and the mediator levels can be maintained at the preoperative values by epidural anesthesia administered before surgical stimulation (14). In addition, epidural analgesia achieved by local anesthetics or opioids should also be maintained in the postoperative period to be able to reduce the stress response at the maximum level (15). In this trial, Group I and Group II were administered local anesthetic solution from the epidural space approximately 20 minutes before the surgery. As the sensory block level reached the T6 dermatome, general anesthesia induction was performed and the surgery was initiated. Maintenance of analgesia was achieved by using postoperative epidural PCA. Postoperative iv morphine PCA was used in Group III. As such, suppression of the stress response was observed similarly to these trials (14, 15).

Latterman et al (16) demonstrated that the glucose response was more limited in the patients receiving epidural anesthesia relative to the group undergoing general anesthesia. In this trial, the plasma glucose value showed a limited increase relative to the control value at the 1st and 24th postoperative hours; this increase was slightly more in Group III. None of the groups exhibited an increase in the glucose level above 150 mg dL^{-1}.

The blood glucose level was detected to be lower with postoperative epidural fentanyl administration relative to iv fentanyl administration (17). Again after general anesthesia, the blood glucose level was observed to be better suppressed in association with general anesthesia + paravertebral anesthesia and analgesia versus postoperative iv morphine administration (18). In this trial, epidural morphine was combined with local anesthetic agents to achieve postoperative analgesia in Groups I and II. Iv morphine was used in Group III. Glucose level was better suppressed in Groups I and II relative to Group III.

The trials detected that the cortisol levels increased starting from the skin incision in cases undergoing general anesthesia + epidural analgesia; however, the blood cortisol levels were suppressed relative to the group receiving general anesthesia (19, 20). In another trial (21), epidural + general anesthesia and postoperative morphine administration were claimed to provide a better suppression of the blood cortisol level relative to the general anesthesia + postoperative iv morphine administration. In this trial, the postoperative 1st hour cortisol value was higher in Group III relative to Groups I and II. In all groups, the postoperative 1st hour cortisol value was higher than the control value; the postoperative cortisol value at 24 hours was significantly increased only in Group III. This shows that the cortisol response was better suppressed in the groups receiving epidural anesthesia and postoperative epidural analgesia relative to the group receiving general anesthesia and postoperative iv analgesia, even if partially.

Insulin, an anabolic and hypoglycemic hormone decreases following trauma as opposed to glucose and cortisol. This helps to maintain hyperglycemia and protect the metabolic status of the vital organs (22). In this trial, there was no difference between the groups in the insulin values measured preoperatively and in the first and 24th hours postoperatively. The increase in the insulin values in the 24th postoperative hour in Groups I and III may be related to the increase in glucose values.

Compared to general anesthesia, the increase in TNF-a and CRP levels was observed to be less with general + epidural anesthesia (1). In this trial, the 24th postoperative hour CRP values exhibited an increase compared to the control values in all groups. While there was no statistically significant difference between the groups, the values in Group III were higher relative to Groups I and II.

Chu CPW et al (2) compared general anesthesia followed by iv morphine, and combined spinal epidural anesthesia followed by epidural 1% bupivacaine and 2 µg ml-1 fentanyl, and detected lower VAS scores in the first, 12th and 48th postoperative hours in the group receiving epidural anesthesia and postoperative epidural analgesia (p<0.05).

In this trial, morphine was combined with low-dose local anesthetic in patients using epidural PCA. Iv morphine PCA was used in the general anesthesia group. In the treatment of postoperative pain, the VAS scores were higher during the first hours in Group III relative to Groups I and II (p<0.05). This may result from the postoperative maintenance of analgesia in groups receiving preoperative epidural anesthesia. In the group receiving intravenous morphine PCA, the VAS scores gradually decreased and exhibited no significant difference compared to the other groups.

Enquist et al (3) demonstrated that epidural anesthesia blocking the neural afferent conduction whether combined with general anesthesia or alone resulted in suppression of the stress response to surgery in their trial on the effects of epidural anesthesia at various doses on surgical stress. The blood pressure values were higher during the first postoperative hours in the group of patients receiving epidural + general anesthesia relative to the general anesthesia group with no difference detected between the groups after three hours. In this trial, the MBP values were similarly higher in Group III during the first two hours relative to Groups I and II.

Nabil W. Doss et al (4) compared the thoracic epidural anesthesia and general anesthesia techniques in their trial performed using 0.2% ropivacaine in patients undergoing mastectomy and detected higher rates of nausea and vomiting in the general anesthesia group. Regarding hemodynamics, hypertension was more common in the general anesthesia group. The Aldrete recovery scores measured 1, 2 and 3 hours after the operation exhibited significant differences between the groups only in the first hour and were better in the thoracic epidural anesthesia group. In our trial, nausea-vomiting was less and the time of recovery from anesthesia was shorter in Groups I and II relative to Group III.

Morphine-related postoperative complications were most commonly in the form of nausea-vomiting, similar to the other trials. There was no significant difference between Groups I and II, and Group III with respect to nausea and vomiting. However, the number of patients with nausea and vomiting was higher in Group III. None of the patients had hypotension that required postoperative rapid fluid replacement or vasopressor agent use. Similarly, none of the patients developed respiratory depression. While there was no difference between the groups in itching, there were more patients with this compliant in Group III. There was no significant difference between the groups in tremor and only one patient in Group II had tremor.

In avoiding stress response, individual differences, the type and duration of surgery, tissue injury in major surgeries, the type of analgesia and the drugs used are also important as well as the method of anesthesia used.

As a result, we concluded that bupivacaine and levobupivacaine used in epidural anesthesia had similar effects, epidural + general anesthesia provided a better intraoperative hemodynamic stability relative to general anesthesia and reduced the requirement for anesthetic agents, provided a faster recovery, resulted in less side effects and achieved a better analgesia, particularly during the first postoperative hours. We believe that the stress response can be better suppressed by epidural + general anesthesia.

5. References

[1] Foster RH, Markham A. Levobupivacaine: A review of its pharmacology and use a local anesthetics. Drugs 2000; 59:531-79.

[2] McCellan KJ, Spencer CM. Levobupivacaine. Drugs 1998; 56:355-62.

[3] McLeod GA, Burke D. Review Article: Levobupivacaine. Anaesthesia 2001; 56:331-41.

[4] O' Sullivan EP. Comparison of 0.75 % levobupivacaine with 0.75 % racemic bupivacaine for peribulbar anaesthesia (letter). Anaesthesia 1999; 54:610.

[5] Bader AM, Tsen LC, Camann WR, Nephew E, Datta S. Clinical effects and maternal and fetal plasma concentrations of 0.5 % epidural levobupivacaine versus bupivacaine for cesarean delivery. Anesthesiology 1999; 90:1596-601.

[6] Bardsley H, Gristwood R, Baker H, Watson N, Nimmo W. A comparison of the cardiovascular effects levobupivacaine and rac-bupivacaine following intravenous administration to healty volunteers. Br J Clin Pharmacol 1998; 46(3):245-9.

[7] Kopacz DJ, Allen HW. Accidental intravascular injection of 0.75 % levobupivacaine during lumbar epidural anaesthesia. Anaesth Analg 1999; 89:1027-9.

[8] Luchetti M, Palamba R, Sica G, Massa G, Tufano R. Effectiveness and safety of combined epidural and general anesthesia for laparoscopic cholecystectomy. Reg Anesth 1996; 21(5):465-9.

[9] Lu CH, Borel CO, Wu CT, Yeh CC, Jao SW, Chao PC, Wong CS. Combined general-epidural anesthesia decreases the desflurane requirement for equivalent A-line ARX index in colorectal surgery.Acta Anaesthesiol Scand 2005; 49(8):1063-7.

[10] Chernow B, Alexander HR, Smallridge RC, Thompson WR, Cook D, Beardsley D, Fink MP, Lake CR, Fletcher JR. Hormanal responses to graded surgical stress. Arch Intern Med 1987; 147:1273-8.

[11] Moller IW, Dinesen K, Sondergard S, Knigge U, Kehlet H. Effect of patient-controlled analgesia on plasma catecholamine, cortisol and glucose concertrations after cholecystectomy. Br J Anaesth 1988; 61:160-4.

[12] Lattermann R, Carli F, Wykes L, Schricker T. Epidural Blockade Modifies Perioperative Glucose Production without Affecting Protein Catabolism. Anesthesiology 2002; 97:374-81.

[13] Salomaki TE, Leppahuoto J, Laitinen JO, Vuolteenaho O, Nuutinen DS. Epidural versus intravenous fentanyl for reducing hormonal, metabolic and physiologic responses after thoracotomy . Anesthesiology 1993; 79:672-9.

[14] Engquist A, Fog-Moller F, Christiansen C, Thode J, Vester-Andersen T, Madsen SN. Influence of epidural analgesia on the catecholamine and cyclic AMP responses to surgery. Acta Anaesthesiol Scand 1980; 24:17-21.

[15] Naito Y, Tamai S, Shingo K, Shindo K, Matsui T, Segawa H, Nakai Y, Mori K. Responses of plasma adrenocorticotropic hormone, cortizol and cytokines during and after upper abdominal surgery. Anesthesiology 1992; 77(3):426-31.

[16] Hase K, Meguro K. Perioperative stres response in elderly patients for elective gastrectomy the comparison between isoflurane anesthesia and sevoflurane anesthesia both combined with epidural anaesthesia. Masui 2000; 49:121-9.

[17] Qu DM, Jin YF, Ye TH, Cui YS, Li SQ, Zhang ZY. The effects of general anesthesia combined with epidural anesthesia on the stres response in thoracic surgery. Zhonghua Yi Xue Za Zhi 2003; 83(5):408-11.

[18] Christensen NJ, Hilsted J, Hegedus L, Madsbad S. Effects of surgical stress and insulin on cardiovascular function and norepinephrine kinetics. Am J Physiol. 1984; 247(1):29-34.

[19] Christopherson R, Beattie C, Frank SM, Norris EJ, Meinert CL, Gottlieb SO, Yates H, Rock P, Parker SD, Perler BA, et al. Perioperative morbidity in patients randomized to epidural or general anesthesia for lower extremity vascular surgery. Perioperative ischemia randomized anesthesia trial study group. Anesthesiology 1993; 79(3):422-34.

[20] CPW Chu, JCCM Yap, PP Chen, HH Hung. Postoperative outcome in Chinese patients having primary total knee artroplasty under general anaesthesia / intravenous patient-controlled analgesia compared to spinal-epidural anaesthesia / analgesia. Hong Kong Med J 2006; 12:442-7.

[21] Engquist A, Brant MR, Fernandez A. The blocking effect of epidural analgesia on the adrenocortical and hyperglisemic responses to surgery. Acta Anaesthesiol Scand 1977; 231:330-5.

[22] Doss NW, Ipe J, Crimi T, Rajpal S, Cohen S, Fogler RJ, Michael R, Gintautas J. Continuous thoracic epidural anesthesia with 0.2 % ropivacaine versus general anesthesia for perioperative management of modified radical mastectomy. Anesth Analg. 2001; 92(6):1552-7.

13

Efficacy of Continuous Femoral Nerve Block with Stimulating Catheters Versus Nonstimulating Catheters - A Systematic-Narrative Review

Mario Dauri, Ludovica Celidonio, Sarit Nahmias,
Eleonora Fabbi, Filadelfo Coniglione and Maria Beatrice Silvi
Departement of Anesthesia and Intensive Care Unit, Tor Vergata University, Rome,
Italy

1. Introduction

A femoral nerve block is simple to perform, has a high rate success, carries a low risk of complications, and it is widely used technique for surgical anesthesia and post-operative pain management of the lower extremity. It provides analgesia to the anterior thigh, including the flexor muscles of the hip and extensor muscles of the knee and therefore, it is well suited for surgeries that involve the hip, the knee or the anterior thigh zone. The femoral nerve block is often associated with sciatic nerve block in order to achieve a lower extremity analgesia.

The anterior approach to the femoral nerve block initially described as a 3-in-1 block by Winnie et al (Winnie et al., 1973), suggested that the femoral, lateral femoral cutaneous, and obturator nerves could be blocked from a single paravascular injection at a point inferior to the inguinal crease. Studies have since showed that the femoral can be reliably blocked by a single injection, the lateral femoral cutaneous nerves is blocked in 95%, but the obturator nerve is almost always spared (Parkinson et al., 1989). Therefore, a 3-in-1 block with the paravascular approach seems difficult to obtain, and, as a consequence, when all three nerves need to be anesthetized a posterior lumbar plexus block or a multitruncular block should be performed. The anterior approach to the femoral nerve is similar for "single shot" or continuous nerve blocks. A femoral nerve block can be obtained with single shot of local anesthetic or by using a continuous catheter technique. The localization of the femoral nerve can be obtained by the use of nerve stimulator or with ultrasound guidance. When using single shot technique, the local anesthetic agent is injected through the needle after location of the nerve with the nerve stimulator. When using continuous catheter techniques, the nerve can be stimulated via the needle through which the catheter is placed, or via both the needle and the catheter itself.

This narrative review summarizes the evidence derived from randomized controlled trials (RCTs) and retrospective analysis, in order to determine the efficacy of continuous femoral nerve block comparing the use of stimulating catheters with non-stimulating catheters for lower-extremity surgery. Furthermore, we explore the adjunctive use of ultrasonography for femoral nerve block.

1.1 Anatomy (Gray & Henry, 1918)

The Femoral Nerve, the largest branch of the lumbar plexus, arises from the dorsal divisions of the second, third, and fourth lumbar nerves. It descends through the fibers of the Psoas major, emerging from the muscle at the lower part of its lateral border, and passes down between it and the Iliacus, behind the iliac fascia; it then runs beneath the inguinal ligament, into the thigh, and splits into an anterior and a posterior division. At this level it is located lateral and posterior to the femoral artery.

The anterior division of the femoral nerve gives off (Table 1):

- Anterior cutaneous branches. The anterior cutaneous branches comprise the intermediate and medial cutaneous nerves
  - o The intermediate cutaneous nerve pierces the fascia lata (and generally the Sartorius) and divides into two branches which supply the skin as low as the front of the knee. Here they communicate with the medial cutaneous nerve and the infrapatellar branch of the saphenous, to form the patellar plexus.
  - o The medial cutaneous nerve passes obliquely across the upper part of the sheath of the femoral artery, and divides into two branches, an anterior and a posterior. Before dividing it gives off a few filaments, which supply the integument of the medial side of the thigh, accompanying the long saphenous vein. The anterior branch divides into two branches: one supplies the integument as low down as the medial side of the knee; the other crosses to the lateral side of the patella. The posterior branch descends along the medial border of the Sartorius muscle to the knee, where it pierces the fascia lata, communicates with the saphenous nerve, and gives off several cutaneous branches. It then passes down to supply the integument of the medial side of the leg.
- Muscular branches – The nerve to the Pectineus and the nerve to the Sartorius

The posterior division of the femoral nerve gives off (Table 1):

- The saphenous nerve - the largest cutaneous branch of the femoral nerve. It approaches the femoral artery where this vessel passes beneath the Sartorius, and lies in front of it, behind the aponeurotic covering of the adductor canal, as far as the opening in the lower part of the Adductor magnus. It descends vertically along the medial side of the knee behind the Sartorius, pierces the fascia lata, between the tendons of the Sartorius and Gracilis, and becomes subcutaneous. The nerve then passes along the tibial side of the leg, accompanied by the great saphenous vein, descends behind the medial border of the tibia, and, at the lower third of the leg, divides into two branches: one continues its course along the margin of the tibia, and ends at the ankle; the other passes in front of the ankle, and is distributed to the skin on the medial side of the foot, as far as the ball of the great toe. The saphenous nerve, about the middle of the thigh, gives off a branch which joins the subsartorial plexus. At the medial side of the knee it gives off a large infrapatellar branch, which pierces the Sartorius and fascia lata, and is distributed to the skin in front of the patella. Below the knee, the branches of the saphenous nerve are distributed to the skin of the front and medial side of the leg, communicating with the cutaneous branches of the femoral, or with filaments from the obturator nerve.
- Muscular branches supply the four parts of the Quadriceps femoris. The branch to the Rectus femoris enters the upper part of the muscle, and supplies a filament to the hip-joint. The branch to the Vastus lateralis enters the lower part of the muscle and gives off an articular filament to the knee-joint. The branch to the Vastus medialis enters the

muscle about its middle, and gives off a filament to the knee-joint. The branches to the
Vastus intermedius, two or three in number, enter the muscle about the middle of the
thigh and give off filament to the Articularis genu and the knee-joint.

* Articular branches
    o articular branch to the hip-joint is derived from the nerve to the Rectus
    femoris.
    o articular branches to the knee-joint are three in number. One is derived
    from the nerve to the Vastus lateralis, the second derived from the nerve
    to the Vastus medialis and the third branch is derived from the nerve to
    the Vastus intermedius.

Femoral Branches	

Anterior division provides sensory innervation to the skin of the anterior and medial thigh and motor innervation to the Sartorius and Pectineus muscles.	• Anterior cutaneous branches
	   o intermediate cutaneous nerves
	   o medial cutaneous nerves
	• Muscular branches
	   o nerve to the Pectineus
	   o nerve to the Sartorius

Posterior division provides sensory innervation to the medial part of the lower leg and motor innervation to the quadriceps muscle	• Saphenous nerve
	• Muscular branches (individual heads of the quadriceps muscle)
	• Articular branches
	   o to the hip-joint
	   o branches to the knee-joint

Table 1. Anatomy of femoral nerve

1.2 Indications
The femoral nerve block is mainly indicated for the pain control associated with unilateral
anterior knee surgery (total knee arthroplasty, ACL). It is also ideal for surgery that
involves the hip (femoral fracture repair) or anterior thigh. The block is often combined
with a sciatic nerve block or with obturator nerve block if surgery is distal or posterior to
the knee join.

1.3 Contraindications
* Infection or haematoma In the puncture site
* Local anesthetic allergy
* Lesion of the nerves to be stimulated distal to the puncture site
* Neurological deficit of the leg to be anaesthetised
* Refusal of the procedure by the patient

2. History of continuous nerve blocks

The first attempt to practice a continuous peripheral nerve blockade was done by Ansbro in
1946, who described a continuous block of the brachial plexus at a supraclavicular level
(Ansbro, 1946). A continuous axillary block was performed in 1977 by Selander in patients
who underwent hand surgery. (Selander, 1977).

The first use of an epidural catheter at the level of the lumbar plexus was reported by Brands and Callanan. Their conclusion was that continuous lumbar plexus blockade reduced administration of opioids and resulted in effective pain relief. (Brands E& Callanan VI, 1987 as cited in Navas et al., 2005). A continuous sciatic nerve block to relieve pain from ischaemic gangrene of the foot was described in 1984 by Smith et al. (Smith et al, 1984 as cited by Navas et al., 2005).

In order to provide reliable post-operative analgesia and prevent readmission due to failed catheter placement, it was necessary to develop methods to ensure accurate catheter positioning and to prevent catheter dislodgment.

Improvements in techniques and instruments have led to a painless, longer-lasting postoperative analgesia, with reduction of Opioids consumption, better functional recovery, increased patient satisfaction and reduced side-effects. New techniques and devices are increasingly appearing, and catheters are constantly being developed and improved (Navas et al., 2005)

3. Continuous femoral catheter placement technique (Fig 1- 2)

The patient should be in the supine position with legs spread slightly apart. After aseptic skin disinfection and sterile draping of the inguinal region, a local anesthetic is injected superficially. The stimulating needle insertion site is immediately below the inguinal crease, 1 to 2 cm lateral to the femoral artery pulsation. A 50-mm 18-gauge insulated stimulating needle is then connected to the peripheral nerve stimulator (PNS) with an initial current output of 1 mA (2 Hz, 0.1 ms). The stimulating needle has to be inserted with a 45° angle and advanced in a cephalad direction until quadriceps femoris muscle contractions were elicited (as evidenced by cephalad patellar movements). The needle position has to be adjusted until quadriceps femoris contractions are still elicited at a current of 0.5 mA or less. At this point, a 20-gauge catheter is introduced through the needle. The catheter is then advanced for 10 to 15 cm beyond the needle tip, needle is withdrawn and the catheter has to be secured in place. The local anesthetic of choice, has to be injected slowly through the catheter.

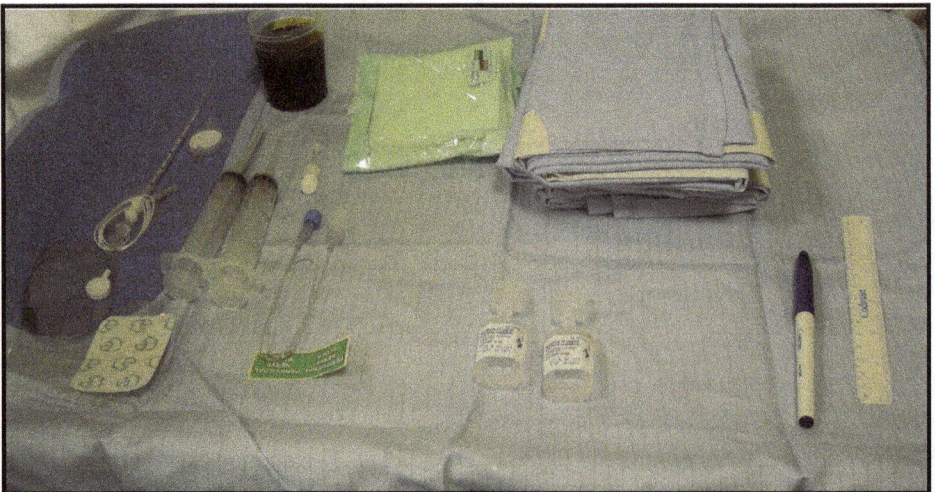

Fig. 1. Equipement

When stimulating catheter is being used, the catheter has to be connected to the PNS without changing the current output. The catheter is advanced 5 to 15 cm past the needle tip, and its position is adjusted until quadriceps femoris contractions are still elicited at a current output between 0.4 to 0.5 mA. At this point, the needle is withdrawn and quadriceps contractions are elicited via the catheter again to confirm the final perineural position of the catheter. (Dauri et al., 2007)

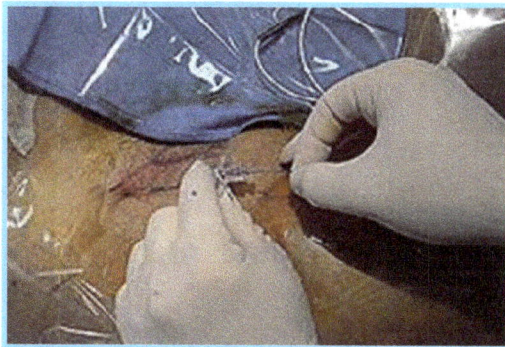

Fig. 2. Catheter placement

3.1 Local anesthetics
A number of local anesthetics may be used for femoral nerve blocks. In general, the volume of local anesthetic used to achieve a surgery anesthesia for a femoral nerve block will range from 15-20 ml. For 3-in-1 nerve block, the volume ranges from 25-30 ml. When postoperative analgesia is required, 0.5% of long acting anesthetic agents ropivacaine or levobupivacaine is often used. For postoperative analgesia, 1-2 mg/ml ropivacaine or 0.625-1.25 mg/ml levobupivacaine are used. The drugs are best administered by PCA pump with a basal rate infusion of 5-8 ml/h and bolus option.

3.2 Complications
- Vascular puncture
- Local infection
- Seizures (from systemic injection and local anesthetic toxicity)
- Neural ischemia and/or neural toxicity
- Local anesthetic toxicity:
  - CNS: tinnitus, confusion, metallic taste in the mouth
  - Cardiac: tachycardia, hypertension, arrhythmia
- Dislocation of the catheter
- Catheter breakage, formation of knots or loops
- Local anesthetic leakage (Gurnaney et al., 2011)

4. Continuous femoral block versus other techniques

Many studies were conducted in order to explore the benefits arising from continuous femoral nerve block compared with other analgesic techniques. Some of the studies conclusions are reported below:

- Continuous peripheral nerve blocks improve postoperative analgesia, patient satisfaction, and rehabilitation compared with IV narcotic therapy for lower extremity procedures (Capdevila et al., 1999; Singelyn et al., 1998; Ganapathy et al., 1999)
- Continuous femoral nerve blocks have been demonstrated to improve the outcome of total knee arthroplasty (capdevila et al., 1999; Chelly et al, 2001)
- Continuous femoral nerve block technique provides similar or better analgesia with fewer undesirable effects than intravenous PCA and the epidural technique during the first 48 h of postoperative management after total knee arthroplasty and after total hip arthroplasty (Singelyn et al., 1998; Singelyn et al., 1999).
- Outcome with continuous femoral nerve block has shown to be better than "single shot" femoral block and continuous epidural anesthesia. For analgesia after proximal lower limb orthopedic surgery, continuous three-in-one nerve blockade is as effective as epidural analgesia, with fewer side effects (urinary retention, nausea, and risk of spinal subarachnoid hemorrhage in anticoagulated patients) (Capdevila et al., 1999; Singelyn et al 1998)

5. Correlation between catheter position and the rate of effective sensory and motor blockades

Continuous femoral nerve block is commonly obtained with a peripheral nerve stimulator connected to a stimulating needle to localize the femoral nerve. The localization of the nerve is then followed by insertion of the catheter through the needle. Studies using blind advancement of femoral catheters indicate that catheter position in relation to the nerve is unpredictable. (Ganapathy et al., 1999; Capdevila et al., 2002) Therefore, even if the initial injection of local anesthetic through the needle produces adequate intraoperative anesthesia/analgesia, subsequent infusion through the catheter may not provide adequate postoperative analgesia. Furthermore, it is difficult to determine the correct catheter's position in order to obtain an effective postoperative analgesia; on the other side the proximity of the catheter to the femoral nerve could guarantee a better analgesia.
Few studies were conducted on the matter:
- Marhofer et al. used MRI scans in order to verify the distribution of local anesthetic. They showed that there is no evidence of cephalad spread of 30 ml of local anaesthetic when a 3-in-1 blockade is performed (Marhofer et al., 2000) .
- Ganapathy et al. used CT scans to verify the catheter position. They observed that only 40% of catheters are located in an 'ideal' position, defined as catheter-tip position at 2 cm of the cephalad extremity of the sacroiliac joint or between the sacral promontory and the lateral portion of the vertebral bodies of L4 and L5. (Ganapathy et al., 1999)
- Capdevila et al. used anteroposterior pelvic radiograph to determine the location of the distal tip of the catheter. They showed catheter location in a continuous 3-in-1 block to be unpredictable. Their conclusion was that during a continuous three-in-one block, the threaded catheter rarely reached the lumbar plexus and that the quality of sensory and motor blockade and initial pain relief depend on the location of the catheter tip under the fascia iliaca. (Capdevila et al., 2002) .

The reported results may highlight the theoretical advantages of using a stimulating catheter to ensure proper perineural catheter placement. The catheter's position could be fixed at a point where the desired motor response is observed at a stimulation intensity that guarantees its proximity to the femoral nerve.

6. Aim of the review

This narrative review summarizes the evidence derived from randomized controlled trials (RCTs) and retrospective analysis, in order to determine the benefits and harm comparing continuous femoral nerve block with stimulating catheters versus non-stimulating catheters for lower-extremity surgery; moreover we will explore the association with adjunctive ultrasonography (US) and stimulating perineural catheters for femoral nerve block.

7. Methods of searching literature

We searched PubMed, EMBASE, and the Cochrane Database using the following search terms: "ACL or anterior cruciate ligament" OR "knee arthroplasty" OR "knee surgery" AND "femoral nerve block" OR " peripheral nerve block" OR "regional anesthesia" AND "stimulating catheters" OR "non-stimulating catheters" AND "ultrasonography". Study were included in the review if they were randomized clinical trial (RCTs) and non randomized clinical trial comparing femoral nerve block with stimulating catheters versus non-stimulating catheters for elective knee surgery or RCTs comparing the insertion of stimulating catheters with or without ultrasonographic guidance; limits: English language, human adults. In addition to the systematic search of the bibliographic databases, the reference lists of all retrieved articles were screened for additional relevant trials.

8. Study description and results (Table 2)

An initial search yielded 8 potentially relevant clinical trial that were further examined. Two of these was subsequently excluded because it did not meet the inclusions criteria. A total of 733 patients were investigated: 311 patients with stimulating and 422 with nonstimulating catheters .

Salinas et Al. in 2004 (Salinas et al., 2004) published a prospective comparison of continuous femoral nerve block with nonstimulating catheter placement versus stimulating catheter-guided perineural placement, randomizing twenty volunteers; a stimulating catheter was placed on one side and an identical non-stimulating catheter on the contralateral side. Success of femoral block was defined as loss of sensation to cold and pinprick stimuli. Quality of successful block was determined by tolerance to transcutaneous electrical stimulation and force dynamometry of quadriceps strength. Despite the trial shown that block success was 100% via the stimulating catheters versus 85% via the nonstimulating catheters, they concluded that there was no statistically significant difference in block success between the two techniques.

Morin et Al. (Morin et al., 2005) in the following year published the results from the comparison between femoral nerve catheters inserted under continuous stimulation and catheters that were placed using the conventional technique of blind advancement in 81 patients undergoing major knee surgery. The aim of his randomized double blind trial was to determine whether accurate catheter positioning under continuous stimulation accelerates the onset of sensory and motor block, improves the quality of postoperative analgesia, and enhances functional recovery. He concluded that with continuous femoral nerve blocks, blind catheter advancement is as effective as the stimulating catheter technique with respect to onset time of sensory and motor block as well as for postoperative pain reduction and functional outcome.

A retrospective non randomized study of 419 patients was published in 2005 (Jack et al., 2005) comparing stimulating versus nonstimulating femoral catheter; it demonstrated no differences in term of visual analogue scale score and total morphine consumption with 3 days follow up. The conclusion was that the practical advantages of the stimulating catheter, as reported by previous investigators, were not obvious in this clinical situation.

In 2006 (Hayek et al., 2006) a randomized study was performed to evaluate whether a stimulating catheter allowed the use of lesser amounts of local anesthetics than a nonstimulating catheter concluding that the use of stimulating catheters in continuous femoral nerve blocks for TKA does not offer significant benefits over traditional nonstimulating catheters.

The experience from our department   (Dauri et al., 2007) is about the evaluation of the efficacy of stimulating catheter to perform continuous femoral nerve block for anterior cruciate ligament reconstruction; data collection from 70 patient regarded pain scores, adverse effects, and need for supplemental anesthesia and analgesia other than a continuous postoperative infusion of ropivacaine 2 mg/mL through the continuous femoral nerve catheter set at 7 mL/h. Data collected shown that although the use of a stimulating catheter was associated with faster onset time for the femoral nerve block and lower additional analgesics postoperatively, the conclusions was that the clinical superiority (analgesia; lateral femoral cutaneous, and obturator nerve block) of stimulating catheters was not evident in this clinical setting.

	Study design	Results	Conclusions
Salinas et al., 2004	• Prospective , randomized double blind study in volounteers • SC= 20, NSC=20 Outcomes: • Block success • Overall tolerance to transcutaneous electrical stimulation • Overall depth of motor block	• Block success : • SC 100% , NSC 85%(p0.07) • Overall tolerance to transcutaneous electrical stimulation (p 0.009) and • overall depth of motor block(p 0.03) was significantly higher in the stimulating catheter-guided femoral nerve blocks	There was no statistically significant difference in block success between the two techniques. Stimulating catheter-guided placement provided an increased overall quality of continuous femoral perineural blockade.
Morin et al., 2005	• Randomized,controlled observer blinded trial in patients after major knee surgery • SC=38, NSC=43 Outcomes: • onset of sensory and motor block, • quality of postoperative analgesia • functional recovery	• onset time of sensory and motor block similar in both groups • no differences in the postoperative IV opioid consumption, and visual analog scale pain scores at rest and movement • No differences in maximal bending and stretching of the knee joint during the 5 days after surgery.	With continuous femoral nerve blocks, blind catheter advancement is as effective as the stimulating catheter technique with respect to onset time of sensory and motor block, for postoperative pain reduction and functional outcome.

	Study design	Results	Conclusions
Hayek et al., 2006	• randomized prospective study of patients undergoing TKA • SC=19, NSC=22 Outcomes: • amounts of local anesthetics • postoperative pain scores, • opioid use • side effects • acute functional orthopedic outcomes	• no statistically significant differences in the amount of ropivacaine administered (MD – 0.6, CI – 2.3 to 0.6. P=0.26) • No significant differences between groups for the amount of fentanyl dispensed by the IV patient-controlled anesthesia • No differences in numeric pain rating scale scores • No differences in acute functional orthopedic outcomes, side effects, or amounts of oral opioids consumed.	The use of stimulating catheters in continuous femoral nerve blocks for TKA does not offer significant benefits over traditional nonstimulating catheters.
Dauri et al., 2007	• prospective randomized controlled trial in patients undergoing anterior cruciate ligament reconstruction • SC=35, NSC=35 Outcomes: • pain score • adverse effects • need for supplemental anesthesia and analgesia other than a continuous postoperative infusion of ropivacaine 2 mg/mL set at 7 mL/h.	• Onset time was faster in the SC group (SC: 6.4± 2.5, NSC: 8.3±2.9 min, P 0.006). • No differences in Visual analog scale. • The number of patient-controlled regional analgesia boluses (SC: 14.6 ± 12.6, NSC:23.2±13.6 mg ropivacaine 2 mg/mL, P_.008) as well as intravenous rescue ketorolac (SC: 34.3±35.7, NSC: 54±39.7 mg, P 0 .033) administered were higher in the NSC group.	Although the use of a stimulating catheter was associated with faster onset time for the femoral nerve block and lower additional analgesics postoperatively, the clinical superiority (analgesia; lateral femoral cutaneous, and obturator nerve block) of stimulating catheters was not evident in this clinical setting.
Barrington et al., 2008	• randomized, controlled, double-blind trial in patient undergoing TKA • SC=40, NSC=42 Outcomes: • Sensory blockade at 10 min, 20 min after injection of, lidocaine via femoral catheter and at postoperative days 1 (POD 1) and 2 (POD 2) • Morphine requirements • pain scores • markers of early recovery	• No differences on sensory blockade in the femoral nerve distribution • At 24 h, the 95% confidence interval for difference in morphine consumption between groups was -8 to 5 mg. • No difference between groups in visual analog scale scores at rest on POD 1 and POD 2, during active and passive physiotherapy • No differences in markers of early recovery after surgery.	In this study, blind catheter advancement was as reliable as a SC technique for establishing and maintaining CFNB for postoperative analgesia as a part of multimodal analgesia technique after TKA.

Table 2. Study included in analysis (SC= stimulating catheter, NSC= non stimulating catheter, TKA= Total knee arthroplasty, CFNB= continuous femoral nerve block)

Recently, a randomized clinical trial (Barrington et al., 2008) compared a stimulating catheter with a nonstimulating catheter technique for institution of continuous femoral nerve block and its effects on quality of analgesia after total knee arthroplasty performed under general anesthesia in 82 patients. Patients were randomized to have continuous femoral nerve block instituted using either a non-stimulating or a stimulating catheter technique. There were no differences in term of included morphine requirements, pain scores, and markers of early recovery. There was an increase in procedural time required for insertion of a SC compared with a NSC (10 and 6 min, respectively); however, this is of debatable clinical significance.

They concluded that blind catheter advancement was as reliable as a stimulating catheter technique for establishing and maintaining continuous femoral nerve block for postoperative analgesia as a part of multimodal analgesia technique after total knee arthroplasty.

In summary, although advantageous from a theoretical standpoint and in experimental designs (Salinas et al., 2004), randomized controlled trials in the clinical environment have yielded limited evidence to justify use of stimulating catheters for continuous femoral nerve block after knee surgery. The increased cost and need for additional catheter adjustments compared with nonstimulating catheter also make it hard to justify their use in this clinical setting.

9. Discussion: Focus on

Postoperative pain after major knee surgery is a major concern. It is severe in 60% of patients and moderate in another 30% (Singelyn et al., 1998; 2000). Pain has a major impact on patient satisfaction and postoperative well-being. In addition, pain impairs early intensive physical therapy and rehabilitation, probably the most influential factor for good postoperative knee rehabilitation (Singelyn & Gouverneur, 2000; Capdevila et al., 1999).

Continuous peripheral nerve blocks offer the potential benefits of extended postoperative analgesia, few side effects, improved patient satisfaction, and accelerated functional recovery after major knee surgery (Liu & Salinas, 2003); for this reason continuous femoral nerve block is often used to provide postoperative analgesia in this clinical setting (Singelyn et al.,1998; Capdevila et al., 1999)

9.1 Catheter tip
When performing a continuous femoral nerve block, efforts are made to place the catheter close to the nerve to achieve effective perioperative analgesia. Traditionally, catheter placement is performed through a stimulating needle, followed by injection of the local anesthetic and then blind advancement of the peripheral catheter beyond the needle tip. Secondary analgesic block failure rate (failure of a catheter to produce postoperative analgesia after having provided sufficient intraoperative analgesia with the bolus administration) with this technique ranges from 10% (Grant et al., 2001; Chelly & Casati, 2003) up to 40% (Salinas, 2003). This may be explained by the fact that the catheter can curl away from the needle during uncontrolled advancement (Salinas 2003). Correct catheter placement is confirmed by testing for a clinical effect of satisfactory analgesia or by sensory modality testing within the desired sensory distribution after injection of the local anesthetic. However, in case of insufficient block, the catheter cannot be further redirected.

The rational for using stimulating catheters, introduced in 1999 (Boezaart et al., 1999) is based on the assumption that catheter tips are directed close to nerves; in fact it provide the possibility to verify the position the catheter takes during advancement through the cannula. A study performed by Pham Dang et al (Pham Dang et al., 2003) concluded that the ability to electrostimulate nerves using an in situ catheter increases success rate in catheter placement for continuous peripheral nerve blocks. However, they were surprised to find that the amperage required to elicit motor responses is higher with the stimulating catheter than with the introducer needle. In a study performed by Morin et al (Morin et al., 2005), the authors did not find a relationship between the current that had to be applied via the stimulating catheter to evoke a motor response and any of the variables determined to judge the success of the catheter positioning. Viewing this works, doubts may arise regarding the reliability of stimulating catheter to elucidate motor contruction and to determine correct catheter positioning. Furthermore, A stimulation current 0.5mA or less is considered safe in order to avoid nerve injury and to deliver adequate stimulus to provoke a motor response. A stady performed by Bigeleisen et al (Bigeleisen et al., 2009) suggest that stimulation currents of more than 0.2 and no more than 0.5 mA could not rule out an intraneural position of the needle or catheter tip. Therefore, even with the use of low stimulation (0.2-0.5 mA) the tip of the stimulating catheters are not ascertained to be in the vicinity of the nerve of might be inside the nerve.

Placement of the catheter tip should ideally be as close as possible to the nerve to attain the minimal blocking concentration that will block the fibers responsible for transmission of painful stimuli. From a practical point, use of larger volumes may permit more successful blocks when nerves are less than ideally localized. This concept is expressed also by Pham Dang et al. (Pham Dang et al., 2009) affirming that interpretation of their data suggests that the failure of previous studies to show a superiority of stimulating catheters has perhaps been masked by methodological problems in previous investigations on the subject. In fact in their study, stimulating catheters seem to provide early analgesia within the femoral nerve distribution using low-dose initial bolus and subsequent low-volume infusion. Small doses of local anesthetics suffice if a catheter is correctly placed next the femoral nerve and that pain from unblocked obturator and sciatic nerves should be treated specifically (Pham Dang 2009).

Moreover, use of larger volumes of local anesthetics may potentially increase the risk of systemic toxicity and potentially increase motor block (Borgeat et al., 2001; Bergman et al., 2000).

More importantly, minimal motor weakness is desired for continuous femoral analgesia after total knee arthroplasty, because excessive quadriceps motor block may impair active knee extension required for rehabilitation protocols and potentially delay achievement of predetermined functional physical therapy goals. To better ascertain the difference between a well placed and a poorly placed catheter, one should use smaller amounts of local anesthetics. Hayek et al. (Hayek et al., 2006), analyzed data regarding the total amount of local anesthetic used in patient treated with stimulating catheter versus nonstimulating group founding no statistically significant differences in the amount of ropivacaine administered .

The question arises whether nerve proximity is really needed for the femoral nerve to be blocked effectively in routine clinical use. Several reasons argue against this necessity, particularly when larger volumes (40 ml) of local anaesthetic are used. Firstly, anatomical review suggests that, once the iliac fascia is penetrated, there are no relevant diffusion barriers for local anaesthetics. Secondly, catheters threaded 16–20 cm from the inguinal level radiographically deviated in 77% of cases but were as effective in motor blockade of the femoral nerve, and only marginally less effective in sensory blockade of the femoral nerve, compared with radiographically well placed catheters (Capdevila et al., 2002). Thirdly, iliac fascia blocks performed without any nerve stimulation are as effective as femoral nerve blocks, in both children (Dalens et al.,1989) and adults (Capdevila et al., 1998), suggesting no clinically meaningful reason for placing catheter tips in close proximity to the femoral nerve. For these reasons, Birbaum affirmed that well designed studies should to be done to prove the superiority of stimulating catheters, but not for the femoral nerve (Birnbaum & Volk., 2006).

However , without direct visualization, catheter positions corresponding to the various stimulating tip-to-nerve distances could only be inferred on the basis of the neurostimulation recently developed by Johnson et al. (Jonson et al., 2007).

Another common problem to underling is the lack of control of the pain transmitted by the unblocked obturator nerve in all studies (Morin et al., 2005; Barrington et al., 2008) and the unblocked sciatic nerve in 2 studies (Morin et al., 2005; Hayek et al., 2006). These unblocked nerves constitute major confounding factors during assessment of the femoral block based on pain scores, given that the knee is innervated principally by the femoral, obturator, and sciatic nerves. In contrast to these studies, ours used a low dose of ropivacaine (0.2%) for initiation and maintenance of femoral nerve block and eliminated pain from obturator and sciatic nerves by blocking them.(Pham Dang et al., 2009).

It is conceivable that clinicians with less experience might find that the ability to verify accuracy of catheter placement with the stimulating catheter system improves their clinical outcomes. However the introduction of the stimulating catheter requires more expertise than introduction of the non-stimulating catheter. Placing the catheter to give good contractions often involves extra manipulation, reintroduction of the needle, or both. Thus, it would not (necessarily) expect the stimulating catheter to give better results in inexperienced hands.

9.2 Effect on neurostimulation of injectates used for perineural space expansion

A randomized clinical trial (Pham Dang et al., 2009) clinically assessed the electrophysiologic effect of dextrose 5% in water and of normal saline used for expansion of the perineural space before placing a stimulating catheter. They questioned if higher current was required with normal saline but not with dextrose 5% in water, as has been observed experimentally. This was a prospective randomized double-blind study of ASA I to II patients scheduled for total knee replacement. Patients were randomly assigned to receive unidentified injectate dextrose 5% in water (n = 25) or normal saline (n = 25). The primary outcome was the minimal intensity of stimulation (MIS) recorded before and after 2 and 5 mL of study injectates were flushed through the needle before placing a stimulating catheter for continuous femoral and sciatic nerve blocks. Secondary outcomes included, among other parameters, minimal intensity of stimulation recorded during placement of stimulating catheters.

Analysis of the primary outcome using a between-group comparison showed that minimal intensity of stimulation recorded during electrostimulation via the needle was significantly higher after normal saline than after dextrose 5% in water in all blocks and at each volume of injectate. This presumably reflects the electrophysiologic properties of normal saline versus dextrose 5% in water given the absence of difference between groups with all other parameters assessed in this study. To conclude, the use of normal saline for expanding the perineural space led to increased intensity for nerve electrostimulation, which may lead to potential errors when electrolocating the nerve. Dextrose 5% in water seemed to be a superior medium for perineural space expansion, which is in agreement with the animal and clinical studies of Tsui et al.(Tsui et al., 2005).

9.3 An alternative: Ultrasonographic guidance

Continuous femoral nerve blocks, have recently evolved towards being the gold standard for acute pain therapy after major reconstructive knee surgery, including total knee arthroplasty and certain techniques for anterior cruciate ligament reconstruction. As shown previously, accurate placement of femoral nerve catheters in close proximity to the femoral nerve, allows for a therapy with low infusion rates and minimal boluses, thus increasing its effectiveness and allowing for prolonged analgesia (48-72hours) with small portable disposable pumps in the outpatient setting. Neuro-stimulation and stimulating catheters, were the basis for perfecting continuous femoral blocks. While usually a simple technique, with minimal risks, occasionally, even in experienced hands, stimulating catheters present several shortcomings: lack of placement time consistency, increased costs, lack of direct visualization of local anesthetic spread, variability in stimulating catheter design and quality, uncertainty about nerve stimulation endpoints (Hayek, 2006; Jack et al., 2005; Morin et al., 2005; Salinas et al., 2004; Birnbaum et al., 2007).

An alternative for assisting with correct catheter placement is ultrasonographic guidance (Fig. 3- 4- 5).

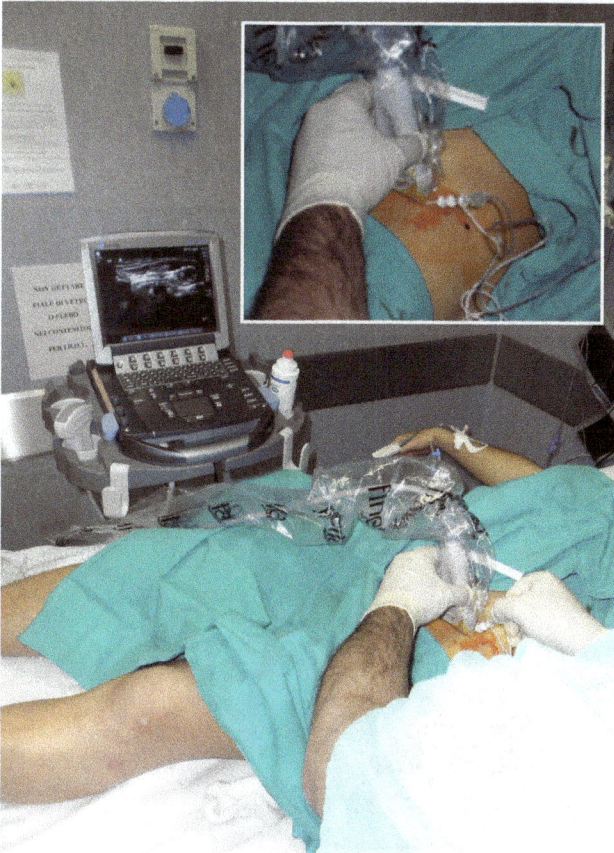

Fig. 3. Ultrasound-guided femoral nerve block: in plane approach

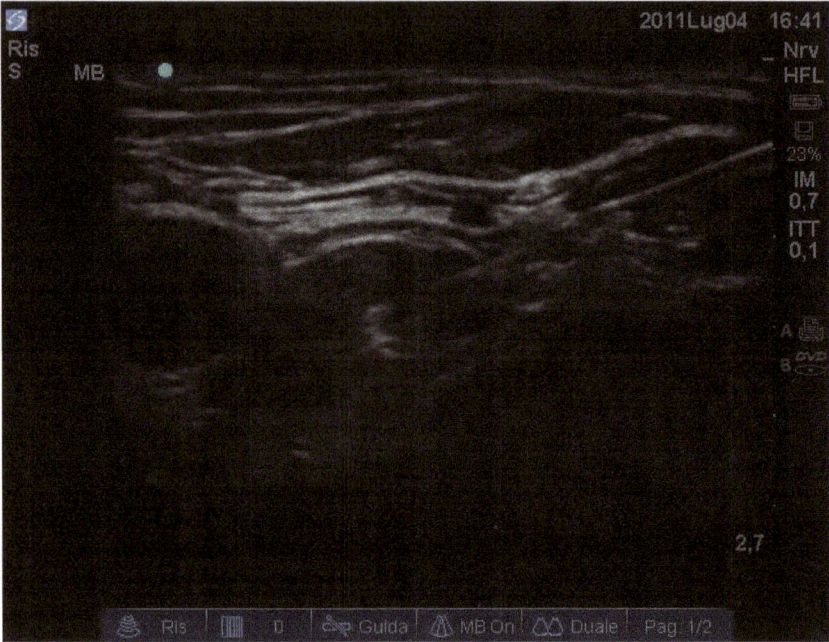

Fig. 4. Ultrasound guided femoral nerve block: needle insertion

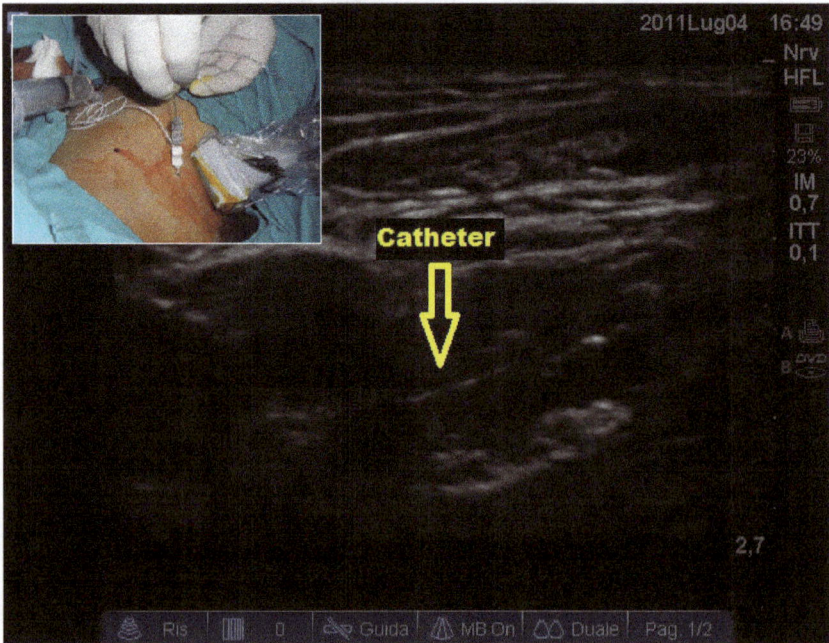

Fig. 5. Ultrasound guided femoral nerve block: catheter insertion

Ultrasound-guided regional anesthesia is an evolving field and its use has gained enormous popularity in the last 10 years. In one investigation, the onset of sensory blockade with ultrasound guidance was significantly shorter and the quality of sensory block significantly better compared with the nerve stimulator needle-assisted application of local anesthetic (Marhofer et al., 1997). Addition of ultrasound guidance to nerve stimulation could offer the benefits of rapid localization and visualization of local anesthetic spread, at the cost of several disadvantages: need for multiple assistants, increased time and cost; moreover the tip position can suggest proximity even though sufficient nerve stimulation is not achieved, injection of local anaesthetic usually produces a clinically effective block.

Other authors have reported both increased block density and lower anesthetic dose requirements with US-guided techniques when compared with conventional techniques using nerve stimulators (Marhofer, 1997-1998).

Mariano et al. (Mariano et al., 2009) performed a study were patients receiving a femoral perineural catheter for knee surgery were randomly assigned to either ultrasound guidance with a nonstimulating catheter or electrostimulation guidance with a stimulating catheter. The primary outcome was the catheter placement procedure time (minutes) starting when the ultrasound transducer (ultrasound group) or catheter insertion needle (electrostimulator group) first touched the patient and ending when the catheter insertion needle was removed after catheter insertion. He concluded that for femoral perineural catheter placement, an ultrasound-guided technique decreases the procedure time compared with nerve electro-stimulation alone while maintaining a similar success rate. Furthermore, patients in the ultrasound group reported less procedure-related pain during perineural catheter placement and had fewer inadvertent vascular punctures (20% less).

It is possible that using a combination of both approaches may offer additional benefits over either technique alone for brachial plexus perineural catheters (Mariano et al., 2009;Fredricksonet al., 2008). For continuous femoral nerve block the needle is inserted at the level of the inguinal crease along the long axis of the ultrasound probe. The needle shaft and needle tip are clearly visible with this approach during advancement of the needle toward the femoral nerve. Once the needle pierces the fascia iliaca lateral to the nerve, the needle tip is advanced 2 to 3 mm toward the nerve. This is contrary to the common method of placing the needle tip in close proximity to the nerve. At this point, 5 mL of dextrose 5% solution is injected to expand the perineural space, and electrical stimulation conforms a quadriceps or patellar twitch. The position of the needle in conjunction with the injected dextrose provides a path for catheter advancement toward the nerve and the catheter tip to lie in close approximation to the nerve. Had the needle tip initially been placed next to the femoral nerve, the catheter would have advanced medially past the nerve.

Another method to possibly improve catheter advancement is slight withdrawal of the catheter guide wire by 1 to 2 cm from the tip. This will provide more flexibility to the catheter tip but stiffness to the remainder of the catheter during advancement. This may further decrease the likelihood of catheter advancement away from the tract formed by the injected dextrose solution, thereby improving the ease of catheter insertion (Niazi et al., 2009). To date, however, the need for electro-stimulation in addition to ultrasound guidance remains controversial, especially for lower extremity perineural catheter placement (Chan et al., 2007; Walker & Roberts, 2007; Beach et al., 2006; Gürkan et al., 2008; Dingemans et al., 2007).

Moreover combining ultrasound with electro-stimulation does negate any cost advantages attributed to ultrasound guidance alone (Sandhu et al., 2004).

10. Conclusions

Randomized controlled trials in the clinical environment have yielded limited evidence to justify use of stimulating catheters for continuous femoral nerve block after knee surgery. It can be affirmed that failure of previous studies to show a superiority of stimulating catheters has perhaps been masked by methodological problems, above all regarding the dose and volume of local anesthetics used. However ultrasound guidance offer a safe and cost/effective technique for femoral catheter placement.

11. Future directions

It is important to design future trials in a consistent manner to make studies comparable and to enable a standard quantitative meta-analysis. Future study designs need to account for differences between the primary anesthetic block (bolus or a relatively large mass of concentrated local anesthetic via either the needle or catheter, typically with a long-acting agent) and the secondary analgesic block (infusion of a dilute local anesthetic). Injection of long-acting local anesthetic as the primary block renders interpretation of the secondary analgesic infusion difficult if not impossible for the first 12 to 24 hrs as the residual analgesic effects of the primary block may still be effective.

12. References

Ansbro P. A method of continuous brachial plexus block. *American Journal of Surgery* 1946; 121: 716 – 722

Barrington MJ, Olive DJ, McCutcheon CA, Scarff C, Said S, Kluger R, et al. Stimulating catheters for continuous femoral blockade after total knee arthroplasty: a randomized, controlled, double blind trial. *Anesth Analg.* 2008;106:1316Y1321.

Beach ML, Sites BD, Gallagher JD. Use of a nerve stimulator does not improve the efficacy of ultrasound-guided supraclavicular nerve blocks. *J Clin Anesth* 2006; 18:580–584.

Bergman BD, Hebl JR, Kent J, Horlocker TT. Neurologic complications of 405 consecutive continuous axillary catheters. *Anesth Analg* 2000;96:247-252.

Bigeleisen P.E, Moayeri N, Groen G.J. Extraneural versus Intraneural Stimulation Thresholds during Ultrasound-guided Supraclavicular Block. *Anesthesiology 2009; 110:1235–43*

Birnbaum J et al. "Electrical nerve stimualtion for plexus and nerve blocks" *Anaesthesist.* 2007 Nov; 56(11): 1156-62 .

Birnbaum J., Volk T. Use of a stimulating catheter for femoral nerve block. *British Journal of Anaesthesia* 96 (1): 139–42 (2006)

Boezaart AP, de Beer JF, duToit C, van Rooyen KA. New technique of continuous interscalene nerve block. *Can J Anaesth* 1999;46:275–81.

Borgeat A, Ekatodramis G, Kalberer F, Benz C. Acute and nonacute complications associated with interscalene block: A prospective study. *Anesthesiology* 2001;95:875-880.

Capdevila X, Barthelet Y, Biboulet P, et al. Effects of perioperative analgesic technique on the surgical outcome and duration of rehabilitation after major knee surgery. *Anesthesiology* 1999; 91:8–15.

Capdevila X, Biboulet P, Bouregba M, Barthelet Y, Rubenovitch J, d'Athis F. Comparison of the three-in-one and fascia iliaca compartment blocks in adults: clinical and radiographic analysis. *Anesth Analg* 1998; 86: 1039–44.

Capdevila X, Biboulet P, Morau D et al. Continuous three-inone block for postoperative pain after lower limb orthopedic surgery: where do the catheters go? *Anesth Analg* 2002; 94: 1001–6

Chan VW, Perlas A, McCartney CJ, Brull R, Xu D, Abbas S. Ultrasound guidance improves success rate of axillary brachial plexus block. *Can J Anaesth* 2007; 54:176–182..9,26–29.

Chelly JE, Casati A. Are nonstimulating catheters really inappropriate for continuous nerve block techniques? *Reg Anesth Pain Med* 2003;28:483–5.

Chelly JE, Greger J, Gebhard R et al. Continuous femoral blocks improve recovery and outcome of patients undergoing total knee arthroplasty. *J Arthroplasty* 2001; 16: 436 – 45.

Dalens B, Vanneuville G, Tanguy A. Comparison of the fascia iliaca compartment block with the 3-in-1 block in children. *Anesth Analg* 1989; 69: 705–13

Dauri M, Sidiropoulou T, Fabbi E, Giannelli M, Faria S, Mariani P, Sabato AF. Efficacy of continuous femoral nerve block with stimulating catheters versus nonstimulating catheters for anterior cruciate ligament reconstruction. *Reg Anesth Pain Med.* 2007 Jul-Aug;32(4):282-7.

Dingemans E, Williams SR, Arcand G, et al. Neurostimulation in ultrasound-guided infraclavicular block: a prospective randomized trial. *Anesth Analg* 2007; 104:1275–1280.

Fredrickson MJ, Ball CM, Dalgleish AJ. Successful continuous interscalene analgesia for ambulatory shoulder surgery in a private practice setting. *Reg Anesth Pain Med* 2008; 33:122–128.

Ganapathy S, Wasserman RA, Watson JT, et al. Modified continuous femoral three-in-one block for postoperative pain after total knee arthroplasty. *Anesth Analg* 1999;89:1197–202

Grant SA, Nielsen KC, Greengrass RA, et al. Continuous peripheral nerve block for ambulatory surgery. *Reg Anesth Pain Med* 2001;26:209–14.

Gray, Henry. Anatomy of the Human Body. Philadelphia: *Lea & Febiger,* 1918; Bartleby.com, 200.

Gürkan Y, Acar S, Solak M, Toker K. Comparison of nerve stimulation vs. ultrasound-guided lateral sagittal infraclavicular block. *Acta Anaesthesiol Scand* 2008; 52:851–855.

Gurnaney H, Kraemer FW, Ganesh A. Dermabond decreases pericatheter local anesthetic leakage after continuous perineural infusions. *Anesth Analg.* 2011 Jul;113(1):206.

Hayek SM, Ritchey RM, Sessler D, Helfand R, Samuel S, Xu M, Beven M, Bourdakos D, Barsoum W, Brooks P. Continuous femoral nerve analgesia after unilateral total knee arthroplasty: stimulating versus nonstimulating catheters. *Anesth Analg.* 2006 Dec;103(6):1565-70.

Jack NT, Liem EB, Vonhögen LH. Use of a stimulating catheter for total knee replacement surgery: preliminary results. *Br J Anaesth.*2005 Aug;95(2):250-4. Epub 2005 May 27.

Johnson CR, Barr RC, Klein SM. A computer model of electrical stimulation of peripheral nerves in regional anesthesia. *Anesthesiology.* 2007;106:323Y330.

Liu SS, Salinas FV. Continuous plexus and peripheral nerve blocks for postoperative analgesia. *Anesth Analg* 2003;96:263–72.

Marhofer P, Nael C, Sitwohl C et al. Magnetic resonance imaging of the distribution of local anesthetic during the three-in-one block. *Anesth Analg* 2000; 90: 119 – 24.

Marhofer P, Schrogendorfer K, Koinig H, et al. Ultrasonographic guidance improves sensory block and onset time of three-in-one blocks. *Anesth Analg* 1997;85:854-7.

Mariano ER, Afra R, Loland VJ, et al. Continuous interscalene brachial plexus block via an ultrasound-guided posterior approach: a randomized, triple-masked, placebo-controlled study. *Anesth Analg* 2009; 108:1688–1694.

Mariano ER, Loland VJ, Sandhu NS, Bellars RH, Bishop ML, Afra R, Ball ST, Meyer RS, Maldonado RC, Ilfeld BM. Ultrasound guidance versus electrical stimulation for femoral perineural catheter insertion. *J Ultrasound Med.* 2009 Nov;28(11):1453-60.

Morin AM, Eberhart LH, Behnke HK, Wagner S, Koch T, Wolf U, Nau W, Kill C, Geldner G, Wulf H. Does femoral nerve catheter placement with stimulating catheters improve effective placement? A randomized, controlled, and observer-blinded trial. *Anesth Analg.* 2005 May;100(5):1503-10.

Navas A.M, Gutieirrez T.V, Moreno M.E. Continuous peripheral nerve blockade in lower extremity surgery. *Acta Anaesthesiol Scand* 2005; 49: 1048 – 1055

Niazi AU, Prasad A, Ramlogan R, Chan VW. Methods to ease placement of stimulating catheters during in-plane ultrasound-guided femoral nerve block. *Reg Anesth Pain Med.* 2009 Jul-Aug;34(4):380-1.

Parkinson SK, Mueller JB, Little WL, Bailey SL. Extent of blockade with various approaches to the lumbar plexus. *Anesth Analg* 1989;68:243-248.

Pham-Dang C., Kick o, Collet T, et al. Continuous peripheral nerve blocks with stimulating catheters. *Reg Anesth Pain Med 2003;28:83-88.*

Pham Dang C, Difalco C, Guilley J, Venet G, Hauet P, Lejus C. Various possible positions of conventional catheters around the femoral nerve revealed by neurostimulation. *Reg Anesth Pain Med.* 2009 Jul-Aug;34(4):285-9.

Pham Dang C, Lelong A, Guilley J, Nguyen JM, Volteau C, Venet G, Perrier C, Lejus C, Blanloeil Y. Effect on neurostimulation of injectates used for perineural space expansion before placement of a stimulating catheter: normal saline versus dextrose 5% in water.*Reg Anesth Pain Med.* 2009 Sep-Oct;34(5):398-403.

Salinas FV, Neal JM, Sueda LA, Kopacz DJ, Liu SS. Prospective comparison of continuous femoral nerve block with nonstimulating catheter placement versus stimulating catheter-guided perineural placement in volunteers. *Reg Anesth Pain Med.* 2004 May-Jun;29(3):212-20

Salinas FV. Location, location, location: continuous peripheral nerve blocks and stimulating catheters. *Reg Anesth Pain Med* 2003;28:79–82.

Sandhu NS, Sidhu DS, Capan LM. The cost comparison of infraclavicular brachial plexus block by nerve stimulator and ultrasound guidance. *Anesth Analg* 2004; 98:267–268.

Selander D. Catheter technique in axillary block. *Acta Anaesth Scand* 1977;21:324–329.

Singelyn F, Deyaert M, Pendeville E et al. Effects of intravenous patient-controlled analgesia with morphine, continuous epidural analgesia and continuous three-in-one block on postoperative pain and knee rehabilitation after unilateraltotal knee arthroplasty. *Anesth Analg* 1998; 87: 88 – 92.

Singelyn F, Gouverneur JM. Postoperative analgesia after total hip arthroplasty: i.v. PCA with morphine, patientcontrolled epidural analgesia, or continuous '3-in-1' block?: a prospective evaluation by our acute pain service in more han 1,300 patients. *J Clin Anesth* 1999; 11: 550 – 4.

Singelyn FJ, Gouverneur JM. Extended "three-in-one" block after total knee arthroplasty: continuous versus patient-controlled techniques. *Anesth Analg* 2000;91:176–80.).

Tsui BC, Kropelin B, Ganapathy S, Finucane B. Dextrose 5% in water: fluid medium maintaining electrical stimulation of peripheral nerve during stimulating catheter placement. *Acta Anaesthesiol Scand.* 2005;49:1562Y1565.

Walker A, Roberts S. Stimulating catheters: a thing of the past? *Anesth Analg* 2007; 104:1001-1002.

Winnie AP, Ramamurthy S, Durrani Z. The inguinal paravascular technique of lumbar plexus anesthesia: The "3 in 1" block. *Anesth Analg* 1973;52:989-996.

Part 3

Opioids

14

Opioid Analgesics

Maree T. Smith[1,2] and Wei H. Goh[1]
*[1]Centre for Integrated Preclinical Drug Development,
The University of Queensland, St Lucia Campus, Brisbane, Queensland
[2]School of Pharmacy, The University of Queensland,
St Lucia Campus, Brisbane, Queensland
Australia*

1. Introduction

Intensive research on the neurobiology of pain over the past two decades has revealed many receptors, ion channels and enzymes with potential as novel targets for development of a new generation of analgesic agents. However, despite large investment in preclinical and clinical development of small molecules and biologics as potential novel pain therapeutics, very few have reached the clinic. Hence, drugs used in the clinical setting for the pharmacological management of pain continue to be those that were first recommended in 1986 by the World Health Organisation (WHO) for the management of chronic cancer pain (WHO, 1986). Twenty-five years on, the WHO 3-step Analgesic Ladder (Figure 1) is still used widely to guide the pharmacological management of pain and opioid analgesics are the mainstay for alleviation of moderate to severe nociceptive pain.

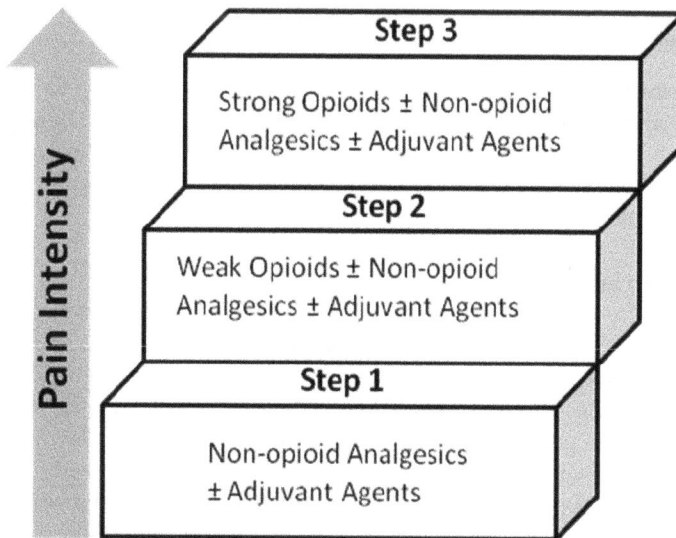

Fig. 1. World Health Organisation 3-Step Analgesic Ladder (WHO, 1986)

2. WHO Analgesic Ladder

The WHO Analgesic Ladder provides a succinct encapsulation of the guidelines for the management of chronic pain according to intensity (WHO, 1986). Specifically, for mild pain, non-opioid analgesics on Step 1 of the Analgesic Ladder including acetaminophen, aspirin and nonsteroidal anti-inflammatory drugs such as ibuprofen, are recommended. When the pain has a neuropathic component, addition of an adjuvant agent such as a tricyclic antidepressant, anticonvulsant or anti-arrhythmic agent, is recommended. Weak opioid analgesics such as codeine, tramadol and dextropropoxyphene are added to non-opioid analgesics when mild pain progresses to moderate pain (Step 2); adjuvants are again co-administered when the pain has a neuropathic component. Strong opioid analgesics are recommended for the management of moderate to severe nociceptive pain (Step 3) with morphine the strong opioid analgesic of choice due to its ready availability world-wide at low cost. Strong opioid analgesics are often co-administered with non-opioids, and adjuvants are added when pain has a neuropathic component (WHO, 1986).

According to the WHO guidelines, each patient should receive a period of individualized dose titration on a 'round the clock' rather than an 'as required' basis as this facilitates dosage optimization for the selected analgesic and/or adjuvant (WHO, 1986). Although many opioid analgesics have relatively short elimination half-lives (Table 1), most are available as sustained-release formulations that are administered once or twice-daily to optimize patient compliance as well as pain relief. For patients who experience break-through pain during ambulation or activities of daily living, additional bolus doses of immediate-release formulations are given on an "as required" basis. For most patients, the oral dosing route is preferred except where impaired gastrointestinal transit makes this impractical as in the immediate post-operative period or during labor.

3. Opioid analgesics

Opioid analgesics commonly used for the control of clinical pain include morphine, codeine, oxycodone, hydromorphone, buprenorphine, tramadol, fentanyl, remifentanil, pethidine and methadone. The potencies of these opioid analgesics differ markedly. Equi-analgesic doses and usual starting doses for the oral route derived from the acute pain setting are shown in Tables 2 and 3 respectively.

3.1 Opioid-related adverse effects

Apart from their desired analgesic action, clinically prescribed opioids also produce many undesired effects including respiratory depression, sedation, nausea, vomiting, constipation, pruritus, tolerance and dependence, to name but a few (Zollner & Stein, 2007). Although studies using μ-opioid (MOP) receptor knockout mice suggest that the analgesic and adverse effects of opioid analgesics are all produced by activation of the MOP receptor, clinical experience shows that there are marked between-opioid differences with respect to analgesic and tolerability profiles within the same patient (Smith, 2008). However, the precise mechanistic basis underpinning these observations is not well understood.

Opioid Analgesic	Elimination Half-life (h)	Duration of Action (h)
Codeine	3	4-6
Meperidine	3.5	4-6
Fentanyl	3.7	0.5-1 (IV); 72 (TD); 2-4 (TM)
Hydromorphone	2-3	4-5
Methadone	24#	4-6
Morphine	2.5	3-4
Oxycodone	3	8-12 (CR), 3-4 (IR)
Tramadol	5-7	4-6 (IR), 24 (ER)
Buprenorphine	3	6

#large inter-individual variability in range 12-150 h
IV = intravenous; TD = transdermal; TM = transmucosal
IR = immediate release; ER = extended release; CR = controlled release

Table 1. Typical Mean Elimination Half-lives and Durations of Action for Commonly Prescribed Opioid Analgesics (adapted from Mather & Smith 1998; Trescot et al., 2008; Argoff & Silvershein, 2009)

Opioid Analgesic	Dose × Conversion Factor
Codeine	x 0.16
Meperidine (IV)	× 0.4
Methadone	× 1.5
Oxycodone	× 1.5
Buprenorphine	× 50
Morphine (IV)	× 3
Morphine (oral)	× 1

IV = intravenous

Table 2. Opioid Analgesic Dose Conversion Table to Oral Morphine (adapted from Nissen et al., 2011)

Opioid Analgesic	Oral Administration	
	Dose	Inter-dosing Interval (h)
Codeine	15-60 mg	3-6
Fentanyl	100-200 µg (IV)	6a
Hydromorphone	2-4 mg	3-4
Methadone	5-10 mg	24
Morphine	15-30 mg (IR)	4 (IR)
Oxycodone	10 mg (CR), 5-10 mg (IR)	12 (CR), 4-6 (IR)
Tramadol	50-100 mg (IR), 100 mg (ER)	4-6 (IR), 24 (ER)

CR = controlled-release; ER = extended-release; IR = immediate-release; IV = intravenous;
aNot more than 4 doses per day.

Table 3. Common Starting Doses for Selected Opioid Analgesics (adapted from Mather & Smith; Argoff & Silvershein, 2009)

3.1.1 Respiratory depression
Opioid-related deaths continue to be reported in the acute pain setting underpinned by opioid-induced ventilatory impairment that often develops due to a combination of factors including opioid-induced central respiratory depression, sedation and/or upper airway obstruction (Macintyre et al., 2011). It is recommended that all patients be monitored for opioid-induced ventilatory impairment using sedation scores as a '6th vital sign' so that it can be detected early and appropriate intervention initiated (Macintyre et al., 2011).

3.2 Strategies for minimizing opioid-related adverse effects
It is essential to assess patients to ensure that adverse effects are genuinely opioid-related rather than being due to another medical problem. Strategies recommended (Swegle & Logemann, 2006) for minimizing opioid-related adverse effects are as follows:
1. Titrating opioid doses slowly
2. Dose reduction to assess if satisfactory analgesia can be obtained with tolerable side-effects
3. Symptom management including pro-active preventative treatment of nausea and constipation
4. Addition of, or increasing non-opioid or adjuvant analgesic doses for an opioid sparing effect
5. Opioid rotation
6. Changing the route of administration
7. Frequent re-assessment

3.3 Strategies for managing intolerable opioid-related adverse effects
For patients experiencing poor pain relief together with intolerable opioid-related side-effects such as severe vomiting, severe dysphagia or bowel obstruction, changing from the oral to the parenteral (e.g. intravenous, subcutaneous, intramuscular), rectal, buccal, sublingual, transdermal or spinal (epidural, intrathecal) route of administration, may reduce adverse effects to a tolerable level and restore satisfactory analgesia (Walsh, 2005). Another strategy for restoring satisfactory analgesia with tolerable side-effects in such patients is 'opioid rotation' that involves switching from one strong opioid analgesic to another (Smith, 2008; Knotkova et al., 2009; Vissers et al., 2010). Additional clinical strategies for restoring analgesia in patients experiencing inadequate pain relief and intolerable opioid-related side-effects include use of neurolytic blocks as an adjunct or alternative to pharmacotherapy (Eisenberg et al., 2005) or progression to use of anaesthetic intervention if 'opioid rotation' fails (Riley et al., 2007).

3.4 Tolerance to the analgesic effects of opioids
In the absence of disease progression, tolerance to the analgesic effects of an opioid manifests in patients with clinical pain as the need for progressively higher opioid doses in order to maintain the same level of pain relief (South & Smith, 2001). In rodent studies, analgesic tolerance is demonstrated by a rightward shift in the analgesia dose-response curve for a particular opioid administered after a period of chronic dosing relative to the dose-response curve determined for the same opioid in opioid-naïve animals (South & Smith, 2001).

3.5 Tolerance to opioid-related side-effects
As already noted, opioid-related adverse effects that may occur after the initation of opioid analgesic treatment in opioid-naïve patients include respiratory depression, somnolence,

nausea, vomiting, miosis, pruritus, constipation, and euphoria/dysphoria. With chronic dosing, tolerance often develops to sedation, nausea and respiratory depression whereas tolerance to constipation and miosis is minimal (Chang et al., 2007).

3.6 Opioid analgesics and renal impairment

Several opioid analgesics including morphine, hydromorphone and meperidine are metabolized in the liver to pharmacologically active metabolites that may accumulate in patients with renal impairment. Hence, for patients with renal impairment, opioid analgesics including oxycodone and fentanyl that are devoid of active metabolites, are preferred (King et al., 2011).

4. Weak opioid analgesics

4.1 Codeine

Codeine (7,8-didehydro-4,5-epoxy-3-methoxy-17-methylmorphinan-6-ol) is an opioid alkaloid found in opium, the dried exudate of the unripe seed capsule of the opium poppy, *Papaver somniferum*, at 0.7 to 2.5% (Boerner, 1975). Due to its high consumption rates globally, codeine is generally synthesized by O-methylation of morphine, an abundant opium constituent at 10-15% (Lenz et al., 1986).

Codeine is a weak opioid analgesic that binds to the μ-opioid (MOP) receptor with low affinity (Ki = 0.7 μM) (Volpe et al., 2011). Its analgesic properties are generally thought to be derived from the fact that it is a prodrug for morphine as up to 10% of oral doses are O-demethylated to morphine by cytochrome P450 2D6 (CYP2D6), an enzyme subject to genetic polymorphism (Kadiev et al., 2008, Somogyi et al., 2007, Zollner & Stein, 2007). Supporting this notion, plasma morphine concentrations are virtually undetectable and codeine lacks efficacy in individuals with the poor metabolizer (PM) CYP2D6 phenotype (Poulsen et al., 1996). By contrast, codeine is extensively metabolized to morphine in those with the ultra-metabolizer (UM) phenotype who also have an increased risk of respiratory depression after regular doses of codeine (Kirchheiner et al., 2007).

Doses of codeine generally do not exceed 60 mg (Trescot et al., 2008). Codeine is available in a range of prescription and over-the-counter medicines, often in combination with paracetamol, aspirin or ibuprofen for pain relief (Moore et al., 1997; Moore et al., 2011). It is also the active ingredient in many cough suppressant mixtures and anti-diarrhoeal products (Schiller, 1995; Wee, 2008). Codeine is susceptible to metabolic drug-drug interactions with other commonly prescribed medications that are also metabolized by CYP2D6 including both CYP2D6 inhibitors (e.g. cimetidine) and CYP2D6 inducers (e.g. rifampicin) (Caraco et al., 1997; Zhou, 2009).

4.2 Meperidine (pethidine)

Meperidine (pethidine; ethyl-1-methyl-4-phenylpiperidine-4-carboxylate), is a synthetic MOP receptor agonist that binds with low affinity (Ki = 450 nM) at the MOP receptor (Volpe et al., 2011). Meperidine is a weak opioid analgesic with potency at ~10% that of morphine for the relief of acute post-operative pain (Latta et al., 2002). Meperidine is metabolized by hepatic esterases to pethidinic acid, an inactive metabolite, and by N-demethylation to a neurotoxic metabolite, normeperidine (Gilman et al., 1980, Armstrong et al., 2009). After multiple doses, normeperidine may accumulate in plasma and cerebrospinal fluid causing tremors, twitches, myoclonus and seizures as it has a longer plasma half-life than meperidine itself (Plummer et al., 1995; Simopoulos et al., 2002). Meperidine is contra-indicated in patients with impaired renal function as they are at increased risk of normeperidine neurotoxicity due to its faster accumulation (Marinella, 1997; Reutens & Stewart-Wynne, 1989). Generally, meperidine use is discouraged in favour of more efficacious and less toxic opioid analgesics (Latta et al., 2002).

4.3 Tramadol

Tramadol ((1RS,2RS)-2-[(dimethylamino)methyl]- 1 -(3-methoxyphenyl)-cyclo-hexanol hydrochloride) is a synthetic analgesic that is a racaemic mixture of two enantiomers that bind to the MOP receptor with low (10 µM) affinity (Volpe et al., 2011). After systemic administration, tramadol is metabolized in the liver by the enzyme CYP2D6, to its O-demethylated M1 metabolite, a potent µ-opioid agonist that contributes to its analgesic actions (Subrahmanyam et al., 2001). The (-)-enantiomer of tramadol mainly inhibits noradrenaline reuptake in the central nervous system (CNS) to augment descending inhibition of pain transmission in the spinal cord whereas the (+)-enantiomer preferentially inhibits serotonin reuptake (Reimann & Hennies, 1994). Thus, the pharmacology of tramadol is complex with its analgesic action being due to the combined effects of its two enantiomers and the M1 metabolite. For this reason, the US Food and Drug Administration (FDA) has classified tramadol as a nontraditional, centrally acting analgesic (Grond & Sablotzki, 2004).

For the relief of post-operative pain relief, tramadol is regarded as a "weak" opioid analgesic with potency at ~10% that of morphine but it does not produce significant constipation or respiratory depression and it has low abuse potential (Grond & Sablotzki, 2004). When tramadol is given in doses larger than the recommended doses, or if it is co-administered with medications that lower the seizure threshold such as selective serotonin reuptake inhibitors, tricyclic antidepressants and antipsychotic drugs, seizures may be induced (Gardner et al., 2000).

5. Strong opioid analgesics

5.1 Morphine

Morphine (7,8-didehydro-4,5,-epoxy-17-methyl-(5α,6α)-morphinan-3,6-diol) is extracted from opium due to its relatively high abundance at ~10-15% by weight (Boerner, 1975). Morphine was first isolated from opium in 1805 by Freidrich Sertürner, a German pharmacist who named it "morphium" after Morpheus the Greek God of Dreams (Milne et al., 1996).

Morphine is the prototypic strong opioid analgesic that binds with high affinity (K_i = 1.2 nM) at the MOP receptor (Volpe et al., 2011). After oral administration in humans, morphine has low oral bioavailability at ~20% due to extensive first-pass metabolism in the liver to two major metabolites, viz morphine-6-glucuronide (M6G) and morphine-3-glucuronide (M3G) that account for ~10% and >50% of each dose, respectively (Milne et al., 1996). Morphine has a short elimination half-life at ~2 h consistent with its short duration of action at ~4 h (Mather & Smith, 1998).

M6G, like morphine, binds with high affinity at the MOP receptor and it is a more potent analgesic than morphine when given by central routes (Smith & South, 2001). By contrast, supraspinally administered M3G evokes dose-dependent neuro-excitatory effects and its actions generally oppose those of morphine in animal studies (Smith, 2000). The elimination half-lives of M3G and M6G are in the range 3-4 h (Mather & Smith, 1998).

After administration of single doses of morphine to patients with clinical pain, the plasma and CSF concentrations of M3G exceed those of morphine by several-fold (Hasselström & Säwe, 1993) and after chronic dosing, the plasma M3G concentrations exceed the corresponding morphine levels by as much as 10-20 fold (Smith et al., 1999). In patients with renal impairment, M6G and M3G may accumulate in the plasma and CSF, thereby increasing the risk of M6G-induced respiratory depression (Smith & South, 2001) and/or M3G-induced neuro-excitation (Smith, 2000).

Morphine is available in immediate-release and sustained-release oral tablet and capsule formulations as well as oral mixtures, rectal suppositories and sterile ampoules for parenteral administration by the intramuscular, intravenous, subcutaneous, epidural and intrathecal routes (Argoff & Silvershein, 2009). The duration of action for immediate-release oral morphine preparations is approximately 3-4 h whereas for oral sustained-released morphine tablets and capsules, the duration of action is 12-24 h (Mather & Smith, 1998). The convenience of once or twice daily dosing provided by sustained-release formulations improves patient compliance and pain relief outcomes (Argoff & Silvershein, 2009).

5.2 Oxycodone

Oxycodone ((5α-4,5-epoxy-14-hydroxy-3-methoxy-17-methylmorphinan-6-one) is a strong opioid analgesic that is a semi-synthetic derivative of the abundant opium alkaloid, thebaine (Lenz et al., 1986). After oral administration, the bioavailability of oxycodone is high at 60-87% (Leow et al., 1992; Lalovic et al., 2006). Oxycodone is extensively N-demethylated by the enzyme, CYP3A4, to the analgesically inactive metabolite, noroxycodone (Poyhia et al., 1992; Davis et al., 2003; Lalovic et al., 2004, 2006) with up to another 10% of each dose undergoing CYP2D6-catalyzed O-demethylation to the high affinity MOP receptor agonist oxymorphone (Lalovic et al., 2006). However, metabolically-derived oxymorphone does not contribute significantly to the analgesic actions of oxycodone for the relief of clinical pain because its circulating plasma concentrations are very low (~1 ng/mL) in both extensive metabolisers (EMs) and PMs (0.3 ng/mL) as it is rapidly further metabolized to its analgesically-inactive glucuronide conjugate (Lalovic et al., 2006; Zwisler et al., 2010). For patients with post-operative pain, there is no difference in analgesic outcomes between PMs and EMs (Zwisler et al., 2010), affirming earlier work by others showing that the analgesic effects of oxycodone are attributable to the parent opioid alone (Heiskanen et al., 1998; Lalovic et al., 1996).

Radioligand binding studies show that oxycodone has relatively low affinity (Ki = 26 nM) at the cloned MOP receptor (Volpe et al., 2011) and that it has a distinctly different binding profile from morphine in rat brain homogenate (Nielsen et al., 2007). This likely underpins the low extent of cross-tolerance between oxycodone and morphine in rodents (Nielsen et al., 2000) and the success of opioid rotation from morphine to oxycodone for the restoration of analgesia with tolerable opioid-related side-effects in humans (Narabayashi et al., 2008).

The potency of intravenous and oral oxycodone for the relief of both post-operative and chronic cancer pain is ~1.5 times that of morphine (Kalso et al., 1991; Heiskanen & Kalso, 1997; Bruera et al., 1998). However, when given by the epidural route for the relief of post-operative pain, the potency of oxycodone is much lower than that of morphine at ~11% (Backlund et al., 1997).

Oxycodone, like morphine, is available in immediate-release and sustained-release tablet formulations as well as in oral mixtures, rectal suppositories and ampoules for parenteral administration (Argoff & Silvershein, 2009).

5.3 Methadone

Methadone, 6-dimethylamino-4,4-diphenyl-heptan-3-one, is a synthetic, strong opioid analgesic that is a racaemic mixture of two enantiomers. The analgesic efficacy of methadone is multi-faceted as the R-enantiomer is a high affinity MOP receptor agonist (Ki = 3.4nM) whereas the S-enantiomer augments descending noradrenergic inhibition to block nociceptive signaling in the spinal cord, and both enantiomers have NMDA receptor antagonist activity (Davis and Walsh, 2001).

In humans, methadone has high but unpredictable oral bioavailability at ~80% (range 41-99%) with peak plasma concentrations observed at 2-4 h post-dosing (Trescot et al., 2008; Modesto-Lowe et al., 2010). There is a large degree of inter-individual variability in its long elimination half-life (12-150 h) (Trescot et al., 2008). These properties make it difficult to use for the relief of acute pain or for pain that is poorly controlled where rapid dose adjustments are needed (Davis & Walsh, 2001). Further adding to these difficulties, methadone is metabolized by CYP3A4-catalyzed N-demethylation to the analgesically inactive metabolite, normethadone, such that methadone is potentially subject to a large number of metabolic drug-drug interactions as many clinically used drugs are either CYP3A4 inhibitors or inducers (Fishman et al., 2002).

Apart from its use as a strong opioid analgesic for relief of moderate to severe pain, methadone is also widely used for opioid maintenance therapy in patients with heroin addiction (Fishman et al., 2002). Commercially available methadone formulations include oral tablets and mixtures, rectal suppositories and ampoules for parenteral administration (Manfredi et al., 2003). When converting patients from a strong opioid analgesic such as morphine to methadone, caution needs to be exercised. This is because morphine-methadone analgesic ratios vary significantly according to the previous morphine dosing regimen (Mancini et al., 2000).

For individuals receiving chronic methadone treatment for opioid dependence, cardiotoxicity characterized by prolonged QTc intervals are associated with methadone dose and concurrent stimulant use (Modesto-Lowe et al., 2010; Mayet et al., 2011). For individuals receiving methadone at doses exceeding 60 mg/day together with tricyclic antidepressants or other drugs that inhibit methadone metabolism, the QTc interval is lengthened thereby initiating Torsades de Pointes (Krantz et al., 2002, Ehret et al., 2007). QT prolongation with methadone is also influenced by other factors including hypokalaemia, hepatic failure and pre-existing heart disease (Ehret et al., 2007). Unfortunately, the general lack of awareness of the long and highly variable elimination half-life of methadone together with its many metabolic drug-drug interactions, has led to a dramatic increase in methadone-associated deaths (Trescot et al., 2008).

5.4 Hydromorphone

Hydromorphone, 4,5 alpha-epoxy-3-hydroxy-17-methyl morphinan-6-one, is a semi-synthetic opioid analgesic (Murray & Hagen, 2005) that binds with high affinity (Ki = 0.37 nM) at the MOP receptor (Volpe et al., 2011) and to a lesser extent at the δ-opioid (DOP) receptor but not at the κ-opioid (KOP) receptor (Murray & Hagen, 2005). Orally administered hydromorphone undergoes extensive first-pass metabolism in the liver to hydromorphone-3-glucuronide (H3G) that accounts for more than 50% of each dose. Although H3G, like M3G, is analgesically inactive, it produces dose-dependent neuro-excitatory effects after supraspinal administration in rodents with a potency ~2.5-fold higher than M3G (Wright et al., 2001). Chronic administration of hydromorphone in patients with renal impairment will result in H3G accumulation, raising the risk that neuro-excitatory side-effects will be produced (Smith, 2000; Mercadante & Arcuri, 2004).

The analgesic potency of parenteral hydromorphone is ~ 5-fold higher than that of morphine for the alleviation of moderate to severe acute pain (Bruera et al., 1996; Dunbar et al., 1996; Quigley, 2002; Horn & Nesbit, 2004) whereas for chronic cancer pain, the analgesic potency of hydromorphone is similar to that of morphine (Murray & Hagen, 2005).

Hydromorphone is available as immediate-release and controlled-release oral formulations (Guay, 2010) as well as ampoules for parenteral administration by either the epidural or intrathecal routes (Lee et al., 2011; Liu et al., 2011).

5.5 Buprenorphine

Buprenorphine, ((2S)-2-[(-)-(5R,6R,7R,14S)-9α-cyclopropylmethyl-4,5-epoxy-6,14-ethano-3-hydroxy-6-methoxymorphinan-7-yl]-3,3-dimethylbutan-2-ol), is also a semi-synthetic derivative of thebaine. Buprenorphine binds with high affinity (K_i = 0.2nM) at the MOP receptor (Volpe et al., 2011) and functionally it is a partial agonist (Pick et al., 1997). Buprenorphine also has antagonist actions at the κ-opioid (KOP) receptor and it interacts with the nociceptin (ORL-1) receptor (Pick et al., 1997). Buprenorphine produces dose-dependent analgesia with potency at ~25-50 times higher than morphine (Evans & Easthope, 2003). The slow onset and long duration of buprenorphine's pharmacodynamic actions are thought to be due to its slow binding to and dissociation from the MOP receptor (Evans & Easthope, 2003).

Consistent with its partial agonist activity at the MOP receptor, sublingual buprenorphine administered to healthy male volunteers in doses up to 70-fold higher than the recommended analgesic dose (0.3 mg) and 4-8 fold higher than doses (4-8 mg) used to treat opioid addiction, produced ceiling responses for subjective measures of drug liking in doses at 8 to 16 mg (Walsh et al., 1994). In the same subjects a ceiling effect for respiratory depression was observed at 16mg (Walsh et al., 1994). Because buprenorphine exhibited linear pharmacokinetics across the dose range tested, dose-limited sublingual absorption is not responsible for the ceiling effects (Walsh et al., 1994). The KOP antagonist activity of buprenorphine is thought to contribute to its good tolerability characterized by limited dysphoria or psychotomimetic effects (Johnson et al., 2005).

After oral administration, buprenorphine undergoes extensive first-pass metabolism in the liver catalyzed by the enzymes, CYP3A4 and CYP2C8 to produce the active N-dealkylated metabolite, norbuprenorphine (Picard et al., 2005). Consequently the oral bioavailability is low at ~14% and so buccal, sublingual, intranasal and transdermal formulations of buprenorphine have been developed that effectively by-pass first-pass metabolism and increase bioavailability to 30-60% (Evans & Easthope, 2003; Johnson et al., 2005; Davis, 2005). Due to its long half-life (~26 h) and ceiling pharmacodynamic effects, buprenorphine is used as an alternative to methadone for opioid maintenance therapy in opioid-dependent individuals (Robinson, 2002; Johnson et al., 2005). A combination product containing buprenorphine and naloxone in a 4:1 ratio respectively is available in some countries as a deterrent to illicit use of buprenorphine tablets for parenteral injection (Harris et al., 2004).

5.6 Fentanyl

Fentanyl, N-(1-(2-phenylethyl)-4-piperidinyl)-N-phenyl-propanamide, is a synthetic opioid analgesic (Horn & Nesbit, 2004) that binds with high affinity (Ki = 1.3 nM) at the MOP receptor (Volpe et al., 2011). Fentanyl is metabolized by CYP3A4 to its N-dealkylated metabolite, norfentanyl that is pharmacologically inactive (Horn & Nesbit, 2004).

After parenteral dosing, fentanyl is ~80-100 fold more potent than morphine with a rapid onset of action but only a short duration at < 60 min (Horn & Nesbit, 2004; Pasero, 2005; Stanley, 2005). For post-operative pain relief, fentanyl may be given by spinal routes whereas for breakthrough or procedural pain, the sublingual, transmucosal, intra-nasal, inhaled or parenteral routes are preferred (Lennernas et al., 2005; Hair et al., 2008; Peng & Sandler, 1999).

Fentanyl has high lipophilicity making it suitable for transdermal delivery. To this end, there are several transdermal patch formulations of fentanyl available for clinical use that effectively overcome fentanyl's short duration of action (Cachia & Ahmedzai, 2011). There is now a large body of evidence to support the use of fentanyl patches for the management of moderate to severe chronic cancer pain, with data suggesting improved pain relief and reduced opioid-related side-effects compared with sustained release oral morphine (Cachia & Ahmedzai, 2011).

5.7 Tapentadol

Tapentadol, [(-)-(1R,2R)-3-(3-dimethylamino-1-ethyl-2-methyl-propyl)-phenol], is a recently approved centrally acting analgesic with two complementary modes of action, viz moderate affinity activity at the MOP receptor (Ki = 0.1 µM) together with inhibitory effects on the NET transporter (Ki = 0.5 µM) to block the re-uptake of norepinephrine in the CNS and so augment descending inhibition to attenuate pain at the level of the spinal cord (Tzschentke et al., 2007; Hartrick, 2009; Wade & Spruill, 2009). After oral dosing, the oral bioavailability of tapentadol is relatively low at ~32% (Tzschentke et al., 2006) due to significant first-pass metabolism in the liver to the inactive glucuronide metabolite, tapentadol-O-glucuronide (Terlinden et al., 2010).

The immediate-release (IR) formulation of tapentadol was approved by the FDA in 2008 for the management of moderate-to-severe acute pain as the first new analgesic developed in over 25 years (Vadivelu et al., 2011). When compared with oxycodone in a head-to-head clinical trial for the relief of post-operative pain in patients following bunionectomy, tapentadol provided non-inferior analgesia to oxycodone with a superior gastrointestinal adverse effect profile characterized by significantly less nausea, vomiting, and constipation when compared with oxycodone (Hartrick, 2009; Vadivelu et al., 2011).

More recently, the FDA has approved an extended-release (ER) formulation of tapentadol for twice-daily oral administration for the management of moderate to severe chronic pain in adult patients (Vadivelu et al., 2011). In patients with end-stage joint disease administered IR tapentadol for two weeks followed by the ER formulation for a further 4-weeks, the superior gastrointestinal tolerability of tapentadol relative to oxycodone, was affirmed (Etropolski et al., 2011). Mechanistically, this may be due to an 'opioid-sparing' effect of the inhibitory actions of tapentadol at the NET transporter (Tzschentke et al., 2006).

5.8 Ultra-short acting opioid analgesics

For patients with cardiovascular instability, ultra-short acting structural analogues of fentanyl such as remifentanil, alfentanil and sufentanil are preferred for use as part of balanced analgesic regimens during anaesthesia (Horn & Nesbit, 2004).

5.8.1 Remifentanil

Remifentanil, 3-[4-methoxycarbonyl-4-[1-oxopropyl)phenylamino]-1-piperidine]propanoic acid, methyl ester) is a synthetic derivative of fentanyl with an ester function in its structure that makes it susceptible to hydrolysis by non-specific blood and tissue esterases (Egan et al., 1993). The very rapid metabolism of remifentanil to the inactive remifentanil acid metabolite by non-specific esterases underpins its activity as an ultra-short acting MOP agonist (Egan et al., 1993).

Parenteral remifentanil has a rapid onset of action (~1 min) and a rapid offset of action following discontinuation (~3–10 min) (Stroumpos et al., 2010) and it is indicated for the relief of pain associated with surgical procedures (Mesolella et al., 2004, Kucukemre et al., 2005).

Remifentanil's pharmacokinetics favour its use as an analgesic during labour (Leong et al., 2011), a notion supported by the findings of two recent clinical studies (Buehner et al., 2011; Ng et al., 2011). In the first study, 94% of 244 consecutive women in a small maternity unit who received remifentanil by patient-controlled analgesia (PCA) for relief of labour pain rated their analgesic outcomes as excellent, very good or good (Buehner et al., 2011). The safety profile of remifentanil was also good as the Apgar scores of neonates born to these women did not differ significantly from those for neonates born by normal vaginal delivery to women who received no analgesia (Buehner et al., 2011). In the second study, maternal satisfaction was higher in laboring women who received PCA remifentanil for analgesia compared with intramuscular pethidine (Ng et al., 2011) with no difference in the safety profile between these two opioid analgesics in the newborn infants (Ng et al., 2011).

6. Opioid rotation

For patients experiencing poor pain relief and intolerable opioid-related side-effects on one strong opioid analgesic, switching to a second strong opioid analgesic often results in restoration of satisfactory pain relief with tolerable opioid-related adverse effects (Knotkova et al., 2009; Vissers et al., 2010). The starting dose of the second opioid is selected to minimize potential risks whilst ideally restoring analgesic efficacy and must be informed by an estimate of its potency relative to the first opioid (Fine et al., 2009; Mercadante & Caraceni, 2011).

Both pharmacokinetic and pharmacodynamic factors may contribute to the clinical success of opioid rotation. For opioid analgesics such as morphine and hydromorphone that are avidly metabolized to the neuro-excitatory 'anti-analgesic' glucuronide metabolites, M3G and H3G respectively, opioid rotation facilitates clearance of these metabolites from the body enabling restoration of analgesia with the second opioid and resolution of neuro-excitatory side-effects (Smith, 2000). Additionally, opioid rotation exploits incomplete cross-tolerance between opioids possibly underpinned by subtle differences in their modulation of MOP receptor function (Smith, 2008; Slatkin, 2009).

7. Peripherally selective opioid antagonists for improving opioid-induced constipation

In patients receiving opioid analgesics for treatment of chronic pain, constipation is a very common side-effect that impairs quality of life and has a prevalence of >80% despite proactive laxative use (Clemens & Mikus, 2010; Diego et al., 2011). A recent approach to the treatment of opioid-induced constipation involves the recent development of quarternary ammonium opioid antagonists such as alvimopan and methylnaltrexone that have limited absorption across the gastrointestinal mucosa and do not cross the blood-brain-barrier, as well as products that incorporate low-dose oral naloxone that has very low oral bioavailability at 2% (Diego et al., 2011). These products selectively target opioid receptors in the gastrointestinal tract without affecting centrally-mediated analgesic mechanisms (Diego et al., 2011).

7.1 Alvimopan
Alvimopan, 2-([(2S)-2-([(3R,4R)-4-(3-hydroxyphenyl)-3,4-dimethylpiperidin-1-yl]methyl) -3-phenylpropanoyl]amino)acetic acid, is an orally active synthetic MOP receptor antagonist that is unable to cross the blood-brain-barrier due to the presence of a quaternary ammonium group in its chemical structure that is fully ionized at physiological pH (Foss et al., 2008; Diego et al., 2011). Thus after oral administration, its actions are confined to peripheral sites such as the gastrointestinal tract and it does not reverse centrally mediated analgesia (Foss et al., 2008; Karuppiah & Farrah, 2011). Alvimopan has been approved by the FDA for short-term use (maximum of 15 doses at twice-daily intervals) in hospitals to treat post-operative ileus that may be caused or exacerbated by opioid analgesics (Diego et al., 2011). Alvimopan accelerates the time to upper and lower gastrointestinal recovery following partial large or small bowel resection with primary anastomosis and decreases the time to hospital discharge by approximately one day (Diego et al., 2011; Karuppiah & Farrah, 2011).

The recommended dosing regimen for alvimopan is 12 mg at 0.5-5 h pre-surgery followed by 12 mg twice daily for a maximum of 15 doses (Karuppiah & Farrah, 2011). Alvimopan is generally well-tolerated when administered for seven days or less (Karuppiah & Farrah, 2011). However, with long-term use (e.g. 12 months) there is an increased risk of myocardial events (Bader et al., 2011; Karuppiah & Farrah, 2011).

7.2 Methylnaltrexone
Methylnaltrexone,   (5α)-17-(cyclopropylmethyl)-3,14-dihydroxy-17-methyl-4,5-epoxymorphinanium-17-ium-6-one, is a quaternary ammonium derivative of the opioid receptor antagonist, naltrexone (Bader et al., 2011; Diego et al., 2011). Due to the quaternary ammonium group in its chemical structure that is ionized at physiological pH, methylnaltrexone does not cross the blood-brain-barrier and so centrally mediated analgesia is not reversed (Bader et al., Diego et al., 2011).

Methylnaltrexone has 8-fold and 120-fold higher binding affinity at the MOP receptor relative to the KOP and DOP receptors respectively (Bader et al., 2011). Following administration by the subcutaneous route at 0.15-5 mg/kg in humans, mean peak plasma concentrations of methylnaltrexone are observed at 0.5 h post-dosing and the elimination half-life is in the range 8-9 h (Rotshteyn et al., 2011). The mean bioavailability is high at 82% with minimal metabolism and so it has low potential for drug-drug interactions (Rotshteyn et al., 2011).

Methylnaltrexone is approved by the FDA and the European Medicines Agency (EMA) to treat opioid induced constipation in patients with advanced disease where other laxative regimens have failed (Iskedjian et al., 2010; Bader et al., 2011). Methylnaltrexone causes laxation in at least 50% of patients in less than 24 h over the first two weeks of treatment without impairing analgesia or causing serious adverse events (Bader et al., 2011).

7.3 Oral naloxone

Naloxone, (1S,5R,13R,17S)-10,17-dihydroxy- 4-(prop-2-en-1-yl)-12-oxa-4-azapentacyclo [9.6.1.0^{1,13}.0^{5,17}.0^{7,18}]octadeca-7(18),8,10-trien-14-one, is a non-selective opioid receptor antagonist (Lenz et al., 1986). In the clinical setting, parenteral naloxone is used to reverse life-threatening opioid agonist-induced respiratory depression (Diego et al., 2011). However, as naloxone crosses the blood-brain-barrier, it also reverses centrally mediated analgesia (Diego et al., 2011).

After oral administration, the bioavailability of naloxone is very low at 2% due to extensive first-pass metabolism which makes it possible to obtain a highly localized opioid antagonist action in the gastrointestinal tract whilst sparing the centrally mediated opioid analgesic effects of oral oxycodone (Leppert, 2010; Diego et al., 2011). The negligible oral bioavailability of naloxone is exploited in an oral prolonged-release tablet that contains oxycodone in combination with naloxone in a fixed 2:1 ratio resulting in less constipation and less laxative consumption relative treatment with oxycodone alone (Leppert, 2010).

The oxycodone plus naloxone oxycodone tablet is available in four tablet strengths; 5/2.5 mg, 10/5 mg, 20/10 mg and 40/20 mg oxycodone/naloxone respectively (Leppert, 2010).

8. Conclusion

Moderate to severe acute and chronic pain continues to be managed with opioid analgesics according to the principles succinctly summarized by Steps 2 and 3 of the WHO 3-step Analgesic Ladder. Weak opioid analgesics are added to non-opioid analgesics for the management of moderate pain with adjuvants added if pain has a neuropathic component. For moderate to severe pain, strong opioid analgesics are recommended with the addition of non-opioids and adjuvants, as required.

9. References

Argoff, C.E., Silvershein, D.I. (2009) A comparison of long- and short-acting opioids for the treatment of chronic noncancer pain: tailoring therapy to meet patient needs. *Mayo Clin Proc* 84: 602-12.

Armstrong, S.C., Wynn, G.H., Sandson, N.B. (2009) Pharmacokinetic drug interactions of synthetic opiate analgesics. *Psychosomatics* 50: 169-76.

Bader, S., Jaroslawski, K., Blum, H.E., Becker, G. (2011) Opioid-induced constipation in advanced illness: safety and efficacy of methylnaltrexone bromide. *Clin Med Insights Oncol* 5: 201-11.

Backlund, M., Lindgren, L., Kajimoto, Y., Rosenberg, P.H. (1997) Comparison of epidural morphine and oxycodone for pain after abdominal surgery. *J Clin Anesth* 9: 30-35.

Boerner, U. (1975) The metabolism of morphine and heroin and man. *Drug Metab Rev* 4: 39-73.

Bruera, E., Sloan, P., Mount, B., Scott, J., Suarez-Almazor, M. (1996) A randomized, double-blind, double-dummy, crossover trial comparing the safety and efficacy of oral sustained-release hydromorphone with immediate-release hydromorphone in patients with cancer pain. Canadian Palliative Care Clinical Trials Group. *J Clin Oncol* 14: 1713-1717.

Bruera, E., Belzile, M., Pituskin, E., Fainsinger, R., Darke, A., Harsanyi, Z., Babul, N., Ford, I. (1998) Randomized, double-blind, cross-over trial comparing safety and efficacy of oral controlled-release oxycodone with controlled-release morphine in patients with cancer pain. *J Clin Oncol* 16: 3222-3229.

Buehner, U., Broadbent, J.R., Chesterfield, B. (2011) Remifentanil patient-controlled analgesia for labour: a complete audit cycle. *Anaesth Intensive Care* 39: 666-70.

Cachia, E., Ahmedzai, S.H. (2011) Transdermal opioids for cancer pain. *Curr Opin Support Palliat Care* 5: 15-19.

Caraco, Y., Sheller, J., Wood, A.J. (1997) Pharmacogenetic determinants of codeine induction by rifampin: the impact on codeine's respiratory, psychomotor and miotic effects. *J Pharmacol Exp Ther* 281: 330-6.

Chang, G., Chen, L., Mao, J. (2007) Opioid tolerance and hyperalgesia. *Med Clin North Am* 91: 100-211.

Clemens, K.E., Mikus, G. (2010) Combined oral prolonged-release oxycodone and naloxone in opioid-induced bowel dysfunction: review of efficacy and safety data in the treatment of patients experiencing chronic pain. *Expert Opin Pharmacother* 11: 297-310.

Davis, M.P., Walsh, D. (2001) Methadone for relief of cancer pain: a review of pharmacokinetics, pharmacodynamics, drug interactions and protocols of administration. *Support Care Cancer* 9: 73-83.

Davis, M.P., Varga, J., Dickerson, D., Walsh, D., LeGrand, S.B., Lagman, R. (2003) Normal-release and controlled-release oxycodone: pharmacokinetics, pharmacodynamics and controversy. *Support Care Cancer* 11: 84-92.

Davis, M.P. (2005) Buprenorphine in cancer pain. *Support Care Cancer,* 13, 878-87.

Diego, L., Atayee, R., Helmons, P., Hsiao, G., von Gunten, C.F. (2011) Novel opioid antagonists for opioid-induced bowel dysfunction. *Expert Opin Investig Drugs* 20: 1047-56.

Dunbar, P.J., Chapman, C.R., Buckley, F.P., Gavrin, J.R. (1996) Clinical analgesic equivalence for morphine and hydromorphone with prolonged PCA. *Pain* 68: 265-270.

Egan, T.D., Lemmens, H.J., Fiset, P., Hermann, D.J., Muir, K.T., Stanski, D.R., Shafer, S.L. (1993) The pharmacokinetics of the new short-acting opioid remifentanil (G187084B) in healthy adult male volunteers. *Anesthesiology* 79: 881-92.

Ehret, G.B., Desmeules, J.A., Broers, B. (2007) Methadone-associated long QT syndrome: improving pharmacotherapy for dependence on illegal opioids and lessons learned for pharmacology. *Expert Opin Drug Saf* 6: 289-303.

Eisenberg, E., Marinangeli, F., Birkhahn, J., Paladini, A., Varrassi, G. (2005) Time to Modify the Analgesic Ladder. *Pain: Clinical Updates,* XIII.

Etropolski, M., Kelly, K., Okamoto, A., Rauschkolb, C. (2011) Comparable efficacy and superior gastrointestinal tolerability (nausea, vomiting, constipation) of tapentadol compared with oxycodone hydrochloride. *Adv Ther* 28: 401-17.

Evans, H.C., Easthope, S.E. (2003) Transdermal buprenorphine. *Drugs* 63: 1999-2001.

Fine, P.G., Portenoy, R.K. Ad hoc expert panel on evidence review and guidelines for opioid rotation (2009) Establishing "best practices" for opioid rotation: conclusions of an expert panel. *J Pain Symptom Manage* 38: 418-25.

Fishman, S.M., Wilsey, B., Mahajan, G., Molina, P. (2002) Methadone re-incarnated: novel clinical applications with related concerns. *Pain Med* 3, 339-348.

Foss, J.F., Fisher, D.M., Schmith, V.D. (2008) Pharmacokinetics of alvimopan and its metabolite in healthy volunteers and patients in postoperative ileus trials. *Clin Pharmacol Ther* 83: 770-6.

Gardner, J.S., Blough, D., Drinkard, C.R., Shatin, D., Anderson, G., Graham, D., Alderfer, R. (2000) Tramadol and seizures: a surveillance study in a managed care population. *Pharmacotherapy* 20: 1423-1431.

Gilman, A.G., Goodman, L.S., Gilman, A. (1980) *Opioid Analgesics and Antagonists,* New York, Macmillan.

Grond, S., Sablotzki, A. (2004) Clinical pharmacology of tramadol. *Clin Pharmacokinet* 43: 879-923.

Guay, D.R. (2010) Oral hydromorphone extended-release. *Consult Pharm* 25: 816-28.

Hair, P.I., Keating, G.M., Mckeage, K. (2008) Transdermal matrix fentanyl membrane patch (matrifen): in severe cancer-related chronic pain. *Drugs* 68: 2001-9.

Harris, D.S., Mendelson, J.E., Lin, E.T., Upton, R.A., Jones, R.G. (2004) Pharmacokinetics and subjective effects of sublingual buprenorphine, alone or in combination with naloxone: lack of dose proportionality. *Clin Pharmacokinet* 43: 329-340.

Hartrick, C.T. (2009) Tapentadol immediate release for the relief of moderate-to-severe acute pain. *Expert Opin Pharmacother* 10: 2687-96.

Hasselstrom, J., Sawe, J. (1993) Morphine pharmacokinetics and metabolism in humans. Enterohepatic cycling and relative contribution of metabolites to active opioid concentrations. *Clin Pharmacokinet* 24: 344-54.

Heiskanen, T., Kalso, E. (1997) Controlled-release oxycodone and morphine in cancer related pain. *Pain* 73: 37-45.

Heiskanen, T., Olkkola, K.T., Kalso, E. (1998) Effects of blocking CYP2D6 on the pharmacokinetics and pharmacodynamics of oxycodone. *Clin Pharmacol Ther* 64: 603-611.

Horn, E., Nesbit, S.A. (2004) Pharmacology and pharmacokinetics of sedatives and analgesics. *Gastrointest Endosc Clin N Am* 14: 247-268.

Iskedjian, M., Iver, S, Lawrence Librach, S., Wang, M., Farah, B., Berbari, J. (2011) Methylnaltrexone in the treatment of opioid-induced constipation in cancer patients receiving palliative care: willingness-to-pay and cost-benefit analysis. *Pain Symptom Manage* 41: 104-115.

Johnson, R.E., Fudala, P.J., Payne, R. (2005) Buprenorphine: considerations for pain management. *J Pain Symptom Manage* 29: 297-326.

Kadiev, E., Patel, V., Rad, P., Thankachan, L., Tram, A., Weinlein, M., Woodfin, K., Raffa, R.B., Nagar, S. (2008) Role of pharmacogenetics in variable response to drugs: focus on opioids. *Expert Opin Drug Metab Toxicol* 4: 77-91.

Kalso, E., Poyhia, R., Onnela, P., Linko, K., Tigerstedt, I., Tammisto, T. (1991) Intravenous morphine and oxycodone for pain after abdominal surgery. *Acta Anaesthesiol Scand* 35: 642-646.

Karuppiah, S., Farrah, R. (2011) Alvimopan (entereg) for the treatment of postoperative ileus. *Am Fam Physician* 83: 978-9.

King, S., Forbes, K., Hanks, G.W., Ferro, C.J., Chambers, E.J. (2011) A systematic review of the use of opioid medication for those with moderate to severe cancer pain and renal impairment: a European Palliative Care Research Collaborative opioid guidelines project. *Palliat Med* 25: 525-52.

Kirchheiner, J., Schmidt, H., Tzvetkov, M., Keulen, J.T., Lotsch, J., Roots, I., Brockmoller, J. (2007) Pharmacokinetics of codeine and its metabolite morphine in ultra-rapid metabolizers due to CYP2D6 duplication. *Pharmacogenomics J* 7: 257-65.

Knotkova H, Fine PG, Portenoy RK (2009) Opioid rotation: the science and the limitations of the equianalgesic dose table. *J Pain Symptom Manage* 38: 426-39.

Krantz, M.J., Lewkowiez, L., Hays, H., Woodroffe. M.A., Robertson, A.D., Mehler, P.S. (2002) Torsade de pointes associated with very-high-dose methadone. *Ann Intern Med* 137: 501-4.

Kucukemre, F., Kunt, N., Kaygusuz, K., Kiliccioglu, F., Gurelik, B., Cetin, A. (2005) Remifentanil compared with morphine for postoperative patient-controlled analgesia after major abdominal surgery: a randomized controlled trial. *Eur J Anaesthesiol* 22: 378-85.

Lalovic, B., Phillips, B., Risler, L.L., Howald, W., Shen, D.D. (2004) Quantitative contribution of CYP2D6 and CYP3A to oxycodone metabolism in human liver and intestinal microsomes. *Drug Metab Dispos* 32: 447-454.

Lalovic, B., Kharasch, E., Hoffer, C., Risler, L., Liu-Chen, L.Y., Shen, D.D. (2006) Pharmacokinetics and pharmacodynamics of oral oxycodone in healthy human subjects: role of circulating active metabolites. *Clin Pharmacol Ther* 79: 461-79.

Latta, K.S., Ginsberg, B., Barkin, R.L. (2002) Meperidine: a critical review. *Am J Ther* 9: 53-68.

Lee, Y.S., Park, Y.C., Kim, J.H., Kim, W.Y., Yoon, S.Z., Moon, M.G., Min, T.J. (2011) Intrathecal hydromorphone added to hyperbaric bupivacaine for postoperative pain relief after knee arthroscopic surgery: a prospective, randomised, controlled trial. *Eur J Anaesthesiol* May 10; Epub ahead of print.

Lennernas, B., Hedner, T., Holmberg, M., Bredenberg, S., Nystrom, C., Lennernas, H. (2005) Pharmacokinetics and tolerability of different doses of fentanyl following sublingual administration of a rapidly dissolving tablet to cancer patients: a new approach to treatment of incident pain. *Br J Clin Pharmacol* 59: 249-53.

Lenz, G.R., Evans, S.M., Walters, D.E., Hopfinger, A.J. (1986) *Opiates*. Academic Press, Orlando, USA.

Leong, W.L., Sng, B.L., Sia, A.T. (2011) A comparison between remifentanil and meperidine for labor analgesia: a systematic review. *Anesth Analg* 113: 818-25.

Leow, K.P., Smith, M.T., Williams, B., Cramond, T. (1992) Single-dose and steady-state pharmacokinetics and pharmacodynamics of oxycodone in patients with cancer. *Clin Pharmacol Ther* 52: 487-495.

Leppert, W. (2010) The role of opioid receptor antagonists in the treatment of opioid-induced constipation: a review. *Adv Ther* 27: 714-30.

Liu, .SS., Bae, J.J., Bieltz, M., Wukovits, B., Ma, Y. (2011) A prospective survey of patient-controlled epidural analgesia with bupivacaine and clonidine after total hip replacement: A pre- and postchange comparison with bupivacaine and hydromorphone in 1,000 patients. *Anesth Analg* 2011 Aug 4 [Epub ahead of print].

Macintyre, P.E., Loadsman, J.A., Scott, D.A. (2011) Opioids, ventilation and acute pain management. *Anaesth Intensive Care* 39: 545-58.

Mancini, I., Lossignol, D.A., Body, J.J. (2000) Opioid switch to oral methadone in cancer pain. *Curr Opin Oncol* 12: 308-313.

Manfredi, P.L., Fole,y K.M., Payne, R., Houde, R., Inturrisi, C.E. (2003) Parenteral methadone: an essential medication for the treatment of pain. *J Pain Symptom Manage,* 26, 687-8.

Marinella, M.A. (1997) Meperidine-induced generalized seizures with normal renal function. *South Med J* 90: 556-8.

Mather. L.E., Smith, M.T. Opioid analgesics – clinical pharmacology and adverse effects. In: *Opioids in Pain Control – Basic and Clinical Aspects,* C. Stein (Ed.), Cambridge University Press, pp 188-211, 1999.

Mayet, S., Gossop, M., Lintzeris, N., Markides, V., Strang, J. (2011) Methadone maintenance, QTc and torsade de pointes: who needs an electrocardiogram and what is the prevalence of TQc prolongation? *Drug Alcohol Rev* 30: 388-96.

Mercadante, S., Arcuri, E. (2004) Opioids and renal function. *J Pain* 5: 2-19.

Mercadante, S., Caraceni, A. (2011) Conversion ratios for opioid switching in the treatment of cancer pain: a systematic review. *Palliat Med* 25: 504-15.

Mesolella, M., Lamarca, S., Galli, V., Ricciardiello, F., Cavaliere, M., Iengo, M. (2004) Use of Remifentanil for sedo-analgesia in stapedotomy: personal experience. *Acta Otorhinolaryngol Ital* 24: 315-20.

Michna, E., Blonsky, E.R., Schulman, S., Tzanis, E., Manley, A., Zhang, H., Iver, S., Randazzo, B. (2011) Subcutaneous methylnaltrexone for treatment of opioid-induced constipation in patients with chronic, nonmalignant pain: a randomized controlled study. *J Pain* 12: 554-62.

Milne, R.W., Nation, R.L., Somogyi, A.A. (1996) The disposition of morphine and its 3- and 6-glucuronide metabolites in humans and animals, and the importance of the metabolites to the pharmacological effects of morphine. *Drug Metab Rev* 28: 345-472.

Modesto-Lowe, V., Brooks, D., Petry, N. (2010) Methadone deaths: risk factors in pain and addicted populations. *J Gen Intern Med* 25: 305-9.

Moore, A., Collins, S., Carroll, D., McQuay, H. (1997) Paracetamol with and without codeine in acute pain: a quantitative systematic review. *Pain* 70: 193-201.

Moore, R.A., Derry, S., McQuay, J.H., Wiffen, P.J. (2011) Single dose oral analgesics for acute postoperative pain in adults. *Cochrane Database Syst Rev* Sep7;9:CD008659.

Murray, A., Hagen, N.A. (2005) Hydromorphone. *J Pain Symptom Manage* 29 (Suppl): S57-S66.

Narabayashi, M., Saijo, Y., Takenoshita, S., Chida, M., Shimoyama, N., Miura, T., Tani, K., Nishimura, K., Onozawa, Y., Hosokawa, T., Kamoto, T., Tsushima, T. (2008) Opioid rotation from oral morphine to oral oxycodone in cancer patients with intolerable adverse effects: an open-label trial. *Jpn J Clin Oncol* 38: 296-304.

Ng, T.K., Cheng, B.C., Chan, W.S., Lam, K.K., Chan, M.T. (2011) A double-blind randomised comparison of intravenous patient-controlled remifentanil with intramuscular pethidine for labour analgesia. *Anaesthesia* 66: 796-801.

Nielsen, C.K., Ross, F.B., Lotfipour, S., Saini, K.S., Edwards, S.R., Smith, M.T. (2007) Oxycodone and morphine have distinctly different pharmacological profiles: radioligand binding and behavioural studies in two rat models of neuropathic pain. *Pain* 132: 289-300.

Nielsen, C.K., Ross, F.B., Smith, M.T. (2000) Incomplete, asymmetric, and route-dependent cross-tolerance between oxycodone and morphine in the Dark Agouti rat. *J Pharmacol Exp Ther* 295: 91-9.

Nissen, L.M., Tett, S.E., Cramond, T., Williams, B., Smith, M.T. (2001) Opioid analgesic prescribing and use – an audit of analgesic prescribing by general practitioners and The Multidisciplinary Pain Centre at Royal Brisbane Hospital. *Br J Clin Pharmacol* 52: 693-8.

Pasero, C. (2005) Fentanyl for acute pain management. *J Perianesth Nurs* 20: 279-84.

Peng, P.W., Sandler, A.N. (1999) A review of the use of fentanyl analgesia in the management of acute pain in adults. *Anesthesiology* 90: 576-99.

Picard, N., Cresteil, T., Djebli, N., Marquet, P. (2005) In vitro metabolism study of buprenorphine: evidence for new metabolic pathways. *Drug Metab Dispos* 33: 689-95.

Pick, C.G., Peter, Y., Schreiber, S., Weizman, R. (1997) Pharmacological characterization of buprenorphine, a mixed agonist-antagonist with kappa 3 analgesia. *Brain Res* 744: 41-46.

Plummer, J.L., Gourlay, G.K., Cmielewski, P.L., Odontiadis, J., Harvey, I. (1995) Behavioural effects of norpethidine, a metabolite of pethidine, in rats. *Toxicology* 95: 37-44.

Poulsen, L., Brosen, K., Arendt-Nielsen, L., Gram, L.F., Elbaek, K., Sindrup, S.H. (1996) Codeine and morphine in extensive and poor metabolizers of sparteine: pharmacokinetics, analgesic effect and side effects. *Eur J Clin Pharmacol* 51: 289-95.

Poyhia, R., Seppala, T., Olkkola, K.T., Kalso, E. (1992) The pharmacokinetics and metabolism of oxycodone after intramuscular and oral administration to healthy subjects. *Br J Clin Pharmacol* 33: 617-621.

Quigley, C. (2002) Hydromorphone for acute and chronic pain. *Cochrane Database Syst Rev* CD003447.

Reimann, W., Hennies, H.H. (1994) Inhibition of spinal noradrenaline uptake in rats by the centrally acting analgesic tramadol. *Biochem Pharmacol* 47: 2289-93.

Reutens, D.C., Stewart-Wynne, E.G. (1989) Norpethidine induced myoclonus in a patient with renal failure. *J Neurol Neurosurg Psychiatry* 52: 1450-1.

Riley, J., Ross, J.R., Gretton, S..K, A'hern, R., Du Bois, R., Welsh, K., Thick, M.(2007) Proposed 5-step World Health Organization analgesic and side effect ladder. *European Journal of Pain Supplements* 1: 23-30.

Robinson, S.E. (2002) Buprenorphine: an analgesic with an expanding role in the treatment of opioid addiction. *CNS Drug Rev* 8: 377-90.

Rotshteyn, Y., Boyd, T.A., Yuan, C.S. (2011) Methylnaltrexone bromide: research update of pharmacokinetics following parenteral administration. *Expert Opin Drug Metab Toxicol* 7: 227-35.

Schiller, L.R. (1995) Review article: anti-diarrhoeal pharmacology and therapeutics. *Aliment Phrmacol Ther* 9: 87-106.

Simopoulos, T.T., Smith, H.S., Peeters-Asdourian, C., Stevens, D.S. (2002) Use of meperidine in patient-controlled analgesia and the development of a normeperidine toxic reaction. *Arch Surg* 137:84-8.

Slatkin, N.E. (2009) Opioid switching and rotation in primary care: implementation and clinical utility. *Curr Med Res Opin* 25: 2133-50.

Smith, M.T., Wright, A.W., Williams, B.E., Stuart, G., Cramond, T. (1999) Cerebrospinal fluid and plasma concentrations of morphine, morphine-3-glucuronide, and morphine-6-glucuronide in patients before and after initiation of intracerebroventricular morphine for cancer pain management. *Anesth Analg* 88: 109-16.

Smith, M.T. (2000) Neuroexcitatory effects of morphine and hydromorphone: evidence implicating the 3-glucuronide metabolites. *Clin Exp Pharmacol Physiol* 27: 524-8.

Smith, M.T. (2008) Differences between and combinations of opioids re-visited. Curr Opin *Anaesthesiol* 21: 596-601.

Somogyi, A.A., Barratt, D.T., Coller, J.K. (2007) Pharmacogenetics of opioids. *Clin Pharmacol Ther* 81: 429-44.

South, S.M., Smith, M.T (2001) Analgesic tolerance to opioids. *Pain – Clinical Updates* 9: 1-4.

Stanley, T.H. (2005) Fentanyl. *J Pain Symptom Manage* 29: S67-71.

Stroumpos, C., Manolaraki, M., Paspatis, G.A. (2010) Remifentanil, a different opioid: potential clinical applications and safety aspects. *Expert Opin Drug Saf* 9: 355-64.

Subrahmanyam, V., Renwick, A.B., Walters, D.G., Price, R.J., Tonelli, A.P., Lake, B.G. (2001) Identification of cytochrome P-450 isoforms responsible for cis-tramadol metabolism in human liver microsomes. *Drug Metab Dispos* 29: 1146-1155.

Swegle, J.M., Logemann, C. (2006) Management of common opioid-induced adverse effects. *Am Fam Physician* 74: 1347-54.

Terlinden, R., Kogel. B,Y., Englberger, W., Tzschentke, T.M. (2010) In vitro and in vivo characterization of tapentadol metabolites. *Methods Find Exp Clin Pharmacol* 32: 31-8.

Trescot, A.M., Datta, S., Lee, M., Hansen, H. (2008) Opioid pharmacology. *Pain Physician* 11: S133-53.

Tzschentke, T.M., De Vry, J., Terlinden, R., Hennies, H.H., Lange, C., Strassburger, W., Haurand, M., Kolb, J., Schneider, J., Buschmann, H., Finkam, M., Jahnel, U., Friedrichs, E. (2006) Tapentadol HCl. *Drugs Future* 31: 1053–61.

Tzschentke, T.M., Christoph, T., Kogel, B., Schiene, K., Hennies, H.H., Englberger, W., Haurand, M., Jahnel, U., Cremers, T.I., Friderichs, E., De Vry, J. (2007) (-)-(1R,2R)-3-(3-dimethylamino-1-ethyl2-methyl-propyl)-phenol hydrochloride (tapentadol HCl): a novel mu-opioid receptor agonist/norepinephrine reuptake inhibitor with broad-spectrum analgesic properties. *J Pharmacol Exp Ther* 323: 265-76.

Vadivelu, N., Timchenko, A., Huang, Y., Sinatra, R. (2011) Tapentadol extended-release for treatment of chronic pain: a review. *J Pain Res* 4: 211-8.

Vissers, K.C., Besse, K., Hans, G., Devulder, J., Morlion, B. (2010) Opioid rotation in the management of chronic pain: where is the evidence? *Pain Pract* 10: 85-93.

Volpe, D.A., McMahon Tobin, G.A., Mellon, R.D., Katki, A.G., Parker, R.J., Colatsky, T., Kropp, T.J., Verbois, S.L. (2011) Uniform assessment and raking of opioid mu receptor binding constants for selected opioid drugs. *Regul Toxicol Pharmacol* 59: 385-90.

Wade, W.E., Spruill, W.J. (2009) Tapentadol hydrochloride: a centrally acting oral analgesic. *Clin Ther* 31: 2804-18.

Walsh, S.L., Preston, K.L., Stitzer, M.L., Cone, E.J., Bigelow, G.E. (1994) Clinical pharmacology of buprenorphine: ceiling effects at high doses. *Clin Pharmacol Ther* 55: 569-80.

Walsh, D. (2005) Advances in opioid therapy and formulations. *Support Care Cancer* 13: 138-144.

Wee, B. (2008) Chronic cough. *Curr Opin Support Palliat Care* 2: 105-109.

World Health Organisation (1986) *Cancer Pain Relief.* Geneva: WHO.

Wright, A.W., Mather, L.E., Smith, M.T. (2001) Hydromorphone-3-glucuronide: a more potent neuro-excitant than its structural analogue, morphine-3-glucuronide. *Life Sci* 69: 409-420.

Zhou, S.F. (2009) Polymorphism of human cytochrome P450 2D6 and its clinical significance: part I. *Clin Pharmacokinet* 48: 689-723.

Zollner, C., Stein, C. (2007) Opioids. *Handb Exp Pharmacol* 177: 31-63.

Zwisler, S.T., Enggaard, T.P., Mikkelsen, S., Brosen, K., Sindrup, S.H. (2010) Impact of the CYP2D6 genotype on post-operative intravenous oxycodone analgesia. Acta Anaesthesiol Scand 54: 232-40.

15

The Role of Opioid Analgesics in the Treatment of Pain in Cancer Patients

Wojciech Leppert
Chair and Department of Palliative Medicine,
Poznan University of Medical Sciences, Poznan,
Poland

1. Introduction

Cancer pain treatment is based on the analgesic ladder, established in 1986 by the World Health Organization (WHO; see Fig. 1) (WHO, 1996). Cancer pain management guidelines in Europe are based on EAPC (European Association for Palliative Care) recommendations. Oral morphine is recommended by the Expert Working Group of the EAPC at the third step of the WHO analgesic ladder, which comprises additional opioids (i.e. oxycodone, fentanyl, buprenorphine, methadone, and hydromorphone) for the treatment of moderate-to-severe pain intensity (Hanks et al., 2001). The use of an analgesic ladder should be individualized with an appropriate application of supportive drugs (laxatives and antiemetics) for the prevention and treatment of opioid adverse effects (Leppert, 2009a) and nonpharmacological measures, such as radiotherapy and invasive procedures (nerve blockades and neurolytic blocks) (Eidelman et al., 2007).

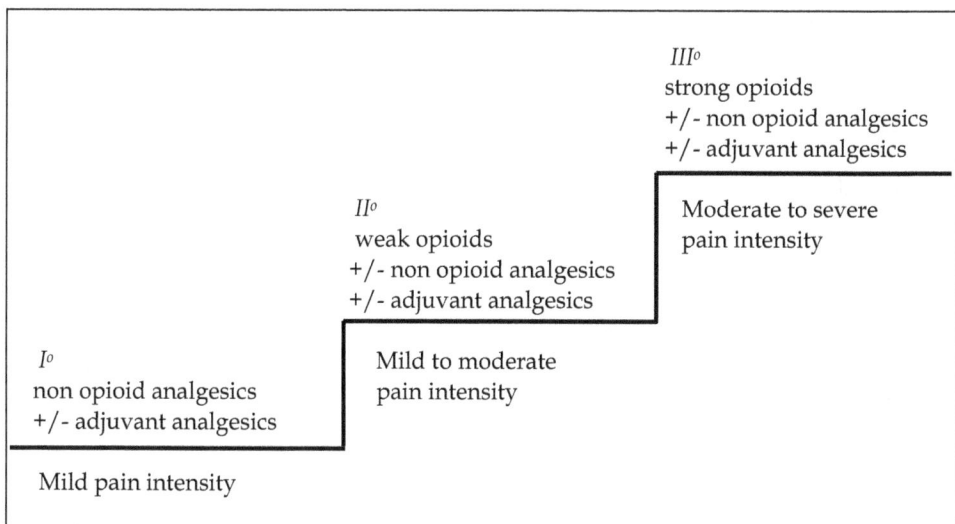

Fig. 1. World Health Organization three-step analgesic ladder

Each step of the WHO analgesic ladder: nonopioids (analgesics for mild pain, step 1 analgesics), weak opioids (analgesics for mild to moderate pain, step 2 opioid analgesics), and strong opioids (opioids for moderate-to-severe pain intensity, step 3 opioid analgesics) may be accompanied with adjuvant analgesics (coanalgesics), which can enhance opioid analgesia. In patients with bone pain, opioids may be combined with non-steroidal anti-inflammatory drugs (NSAIDs), glucocorticoids, and bisphosphonates along with local or systemic radiotherapy (Lussier et al., 2004). In patients with very severe neuropathic pain, a combination of opioids and NMDA (N-methyl D-aspartate)-receptor antagonists (e.g. ketamine) are recommended (Leppert, 2010a). Patients with neuropathic pain along with opioids may also receive anticonvulsants, and antidepressants (Bennett, 2011). Other drug groups used in patients with neuropathic pain component comprise local anesthetics and antiarrhytmics (Freynhagen & Bennett, 2009). Opioid analgesics should be supplemented with spasmolytics in patients with visceral colicky pain, especially in the course of bowel obstruction (Ripamonti et al., 2008).

2. Opioids for mild to moderate pain (weak opioids, step 2 opioid analgesics)

2.1 Tramadol

Tramadol displays opioid properties and acts on neurotransmission of noradrenalin and serotonin. Both enantiomers act synergistically and improve analgesia without increasing adverse effects. Tramadol is metabolized in the liver and excreted by the kidneys. The main metabolite is O-desmethyltramadol (M1), which displays analgesic activity with a higher affinity to μ-opioid receptors than the parent compound; (+)-M1 has 300 to 400 times greater affinity to μ-opioid receptors than tramadol and (-)-M1 mainly inhibits noradrenalin reuptake. Apart from O,N-didesmethyltramadol (M5, which has weak analgesic activity) and M1, other metabolites are inactive (Leppert and Mikolajczak, 2011). The elimination half-life of tramadol is 5 to 6 hours and that if M1 is 8 hours. During oral administration, 90% of tramadol is excreted by the kidneys and 10% in feces. Patients with renal impairment show a decreased excretion of tramadol and M1. In patients with advanced cirrhosis, there is a decrease in tramadol metabolism with decrease of hepatic clearance and increase in blood serum levels. In these patients, elimination half-life is increased 2.5-fold. The starting dose of immediate-release (IR) tramadol is 25 to 50 mg every 4 to 6 hour and that of controlled-release (CR) tablets or capsules is 50 to 100 mg twice daily; the daily dose should not exceed 400 mg (Dickman, 2007).

Patients devoid of CYP2D6 activity (poor metabolizers) need a tramadol dose higher by 30% than those with normal CYP2D6 activity (extensive metabolizers) (Stamer et al., 2003). Tramadol analgesia depends on CYP2D6 genotype, with less analgesia in poor metabolizers being associated with lack of (+)-M1 formation (Stamer et al., 2007). Genotyping is helpful in patients with duplication of CYP2D6 gene (ultrarapid metabolizers [UM]) who are at greater risk to develop tramadol adverse effects. Tramadol metabolism through CYP2D6 may cause interactions with drugs inhibiting this enzyme (eg, cimetidine and ranitidine).

Serotonin syndrome has been reported in patients taking selective serotonin reuptake inhibitors (SSRIs) in conjunction with tramadol or opioids (Gnanadesigan et al., 2005). SSRIs (eg, fluoxetine, paroxetine, and, to less extent, sertraline) used in conjunction with tramadol may cause serotonin syndrome because SSRIs inhibit tramadol metabolism and increase serotonin level; generally, they should not be coadministered with tramadol. Serotonin syndrome may appear with monoamine oxidase (MAO) inhibitors, olanzapine, risperidone, venlafaxine and mirtazapine (Davies and Glare, 2009).

The inhibition of tramadol metabolism to (+)M1 may attenuate tramadol analgesia. For example, coadministration of ondansetron (selective 5-HT_3 [hydroxytryptamine] receptor antagonist) blocks spinal 5-HT_3 receptors and competitively inhibits CYP2D6 although recent studies did not confirm such interaction (Rauers et al., 2010). Tramadol analgesia also may be impaired by coadministration of carbamazepine, which accelerates tramadol and M1 metabolism. Concomitant administration of tricyclic antidepressants increases the risk of seizures. Tramadol should be avoided in patients with history of epilepsy. In rats and mice, concomitant administration of tramadol and β-blocker and the 5-$HT_{1A/1B}$ antagonist pindolol enhances analgesia (Leppert, 2009b).

Respiratory depression is rare in the chronic use of tramadol. When it does occur, respiratory depression is connected with the opioid mode of tramadol action, so naloxone should be administered. For example, respiratory depression was reported in a cancer patient with renal impairment (creatinine clearance 30 mL/min) and with UM genotype after renal carcinoma resection. As respiratory symptoms appeared more than 10 hours after the first tramadol dose, the accumulation of M1 was the cause. The patient recovered after intravenous (IV) naloxone bolus administration (0.4 mg). This case highlights that tramadol should not be prescribed in patients with UM genotype and renal impairment (Stamer et al., 2008).

2.2 Codeine

Codeine is a methylated morphine derivative that is found naturally, along with morphine, in the poppy seed. Codeine displays analgesic and antitussive activity. Codeine is available as IR and CR formulations but also in the form of paracetamol combined preparations. IR codeine is administered every 4-6 h in chronic pain with a starting single dose of about 30 mg. The daily doses of dihydrocodeine and codeine usually do not exceed 240 mg and 300 mg, respectively; when these analgesics are ineffective, opioids for moderate-to-severe pain (strong opioids) are introduced.

Codeine is metabolized in the liver and its bioavailability is 30% to 40% after oral administration. After oral administration of codeine, maximal plasma concentration is attained within 1 to 2 hours with plasma half-life of 2.5 to 3.5 hours and analgesia maintained for 4 to 6 hours (IR formulations). Codeine is partially metabolized to morphine and its metabolites and to codeine metabolites norcodeine (NORC) and codeine-6-glucuronide (C-6-G) (Lötsch et al., 2006). The analgesic effect of codeine is about equal to 1/10th of morphine analgesia. Polymorphism of CYP2D6 is responsible for the formation of morphine, and its metabolites may affect codeine analgesia. Other codeine metabolites, C-6-G predominantly, also display analgesic activity and contribute to codeine analgesia (Vree et al., 2000). In healthy volunteers, codeine is metabolized to C-6-G (81.0% ± 9.3%), NORC (2.16% ± 1.44%), morphine (0.50% ± 0.39%), morphine-3-glucuronide (M-3-G; 2.10% ± 1.24%), morphine-6-glucuronide (M-6-G; 0.80% ± 0.63%), and normorphine (NORM; 2.44% ± 2.42%). The half-life of codeine is 1.47 hours ± 0.32 hours, and that of C-6-G is 2.75 hours ± 0.79 hours. The plasma AUC of C-6-G is about tenfold higher than that of codeine. Protein binding of codeine and C-6-G in vivo is 56.1% ± 2.5% and 34.0% ± 3.6%, respectively (Vree & Verwey-van Wissen, 1992).

Lötsch et al. explored the contributions from codeine and its metabolites to central nervous analgesic effects independent from O-demethylation of codeine to morphine. A pharmacokinetic/pharmacodynamic fit of the miotic effects by use of morphine as the only active compound was most significantly ($P < 0.0001$) improved when C-6-G as a second active moiety was added. CYP2D6-dependent formation of morphine does not explain exclusively the central nervous effects of codeine, and C-6-G is the most likely additional active moiety with possible contribution of NORC and the parent compound (Lötsch et al., 2006).

Gasche et al. depicted a patient who received oral codeine in a daily dose of 75 mg (25 mg three times a day) and who, after 4 days of treatment, experienced respiratory depression. The patient recovered after IV administration of naloxone (0.4 mg). The cause of the symptoms was CYP2D6 UM phenotype. The patient was concomitantly treated with clarithromycin and voriconazole, both known inhibitors of CYP3A4. This together with CYP2D6 gene duplication led to increased morphine formation. Blood concentrations of M-3-G and M-6-G were substantially elevated, also due to renal failure (Gasche et al., 2004). Recent reports (Kircheiner et al., 2007; Voronov et al., 2007) indicate that there is a significant risk of respiratory depression in infants whose mothers with CYP2D6 UM and UGT2B7•2/•2 genotypes taking codeine during breastfeeding (Madadi et al., 2009b). Guidelines for maternal codeine use during breastfeeding were issued in Canada (Madadi et al., 2009a) but it seems safer not to use codeine and substitute it with other analgesics in this patient group. Apart from morphine glucuronides, codeine and its metabolites (C-6-G and NORC) also contribute to codeine analgesic effects (Lötsch et al., 2006).

2.3 Dihydrocodeine

Dihydrocodeine (DHC) is a semi synthetic analogue of codeine. Apart from analgesic and antitussive activity, DHC also is used in the treatment of opioid addiction. After subcutaneous (sc) administration of DHC, 30 mg, analgesia is similar to that induced by 10 mg of morphine. After parenteral administration, DHC is twice as potent as codeine. Bioavailability of DHC after oral administration is 20%, which indicates that its analgesia after oral administration is slightly stronger than that of codeine (bioavailability after oral administration equals 30%–40%). After oral administration of DHC, the maximal serum concentration appears after 1.7 hours, plasma half-life varies 3.5 to 5.5 hours, and analgesia lasts 4-6 hours. DHC pharmacokinetics was assessed in 12 extensive metabolizers of CYP2D6 (Ammon et al., 1999). They received a single oral DHC dose of 60 mg, then after 60 hours, they were treated for 3 days with 60 mg dosed twice daily; for the next 3 days with 90 mg twice daily; and for 3 subsequent days 120 mg twice daily. In the 60 to 120 mg DHC dose range, pharmacokinetics of DHC and dihydromorphine (DHM) displayed linear characteristics: area under the curve (AUC), c_{max} (maximum serum concentration), and c_{ssmin} (minimum serum concentration at steady state) for both compounds increased depending on the drug dose (Rowell et al., 1983). Even though DHM displays higher affinity (about 100-fold) to the μ-opioid receptors and exhibits higher analgesic activity in comparison to the parent compound, the role of DHM and its glucuronides in DHC analgesia has not been unequivocally established. The starting dose of IR DHC is usually 30 mg every 4 to 6 hours, and that of CR tablets is 60 mg twice daily (Leppert, 2010b).

Renal clearance and the clearance to DHC metabolites, glucuronidation, and O-demethylation to dihydrocodeine-6-glucuronide (DHC-6-G) and DHM, respectively, are not dose dependent, which indicates that metabolism and excretion of DHC and its metabolites are also not dose dependent. Moreover, the ratio of DHC to DHM for AUC does not change depending on the dose, which suggests a lack of saturation effect of the O-demethylation process of DHC to DHM depending on CYP2D6 in patients normally metabolizing the substrates of this enzyme. Pharmacokinetic parameters were similar after single and multiple doses of 60 mg of DHC (Ammon et al., 1999). Single-dose and multiple-dose pharmacokinetics of IR and CR DHC formulations provide support for a twice-daily dosage schedule of CR DHC. DHC is metabolized in the liver to main metabolites: DHM, DHC-6-G, and nordihydrocodeine (NORDHC). NORDHC is further glucuronidated to NORDHC-6-glucuronide and O-demethylated to nordihydromorphine (NDHM). DHM undergoes glucuronidation to dihydromorphine-3-glucuronide (DHM-3-G) and dihydromorphine-6-glucuronide (DHM-6-G) and N-demethylation to NDHM. It may be concluded that DHC undergoes the first pass effect after oral administration, which is connected with the formation of significantly higher amount of metabolites after oral than after parenteral administration (Rowell et al., 1983). Studies performed to date (Schmidt et al., 2003; Webb et al., 2001) indicate that DHC analgesia is independent of CYP2D6 activity (Leppert and Majkowicz, 2010).

3. Opioids for moderate to severe pain (strong opioids, step 3 opioid analgesics)

3.1 Morphine

Morphine is the standard drug for the treatment of moderate to severe cancer pain and is a comparator for other strong opioids (Caraceni et al., 2011). This is predominantly due to large clinical experience and different routes of morphine administration (eg, oral, SC, IV, intrathecal, topical). Morphine is a hydrophilic opioid and a pure opioid agonist that acts predominantly through the activation of μ-opioid receptors (Flemming, 2010). Plasma half-life of IR formulations equals 2 to 3 hours and the bioavailability after oral morphine administration equals about 30% to 40%. Morphine undergoes glucuronidation; thus, there is little risk of pharmacokinetic interactions with other drugs.

The active metabolite responsible for analgesia is morphine-6-glucuronide (M-6-G). The accumulation of morphine and M-6-G may cause nausea and vomiting, sedation, and finally, respiratory depression. Morphine-3-glucuronide (M-3-G) is devoid of analgesic properties but may be responsible for neurotoxic effects and opioid hyperalgesia (paradoxical pain) (Gretton & Riley, 2008). The main drawback of morphine is the fact that M-3-G and M-6-G may accumulate especially in patients with renal impairment and renal failure, leading to possible intense adverse effects associated with accumulation of metabolites. In severe pain syndromes a change from oral to parenteral or intrathecal route of morphine administration may be beneficial. In case of renal problems, a switch from morphine to other opioids, such as fentanyl, methadone, or buprenorphine, is recommended. Similar to other opioids, morphine often causes constipation; therefore, the use of laxative prophylaxis is recommended. Common morphine adverse effects and possible management possibilities are showed in Table 1.

Numerous oral CR formulations of morphine, designed for 12-hour and 24-hour administration, were developed (Ridgway et al., 2010). Local administration of morphine prevents systemic adverse effects. The starting daily dose of oral morphine is usually 20 to 30 mg (for opioid-naïve patients) or 40 to 60 mg (for patients unsuccessfully treated with weak opioids) (Ripamonti et al., 2009). The dose of parenteral (SC or IV) morphine is one third of the morphine oral dose (Donnelly et al., 2002).

Adverse effect	Symptomatology	Treatment	Comments
Gastric stasis	Epigastric fullness, nausea	Metoclopramide 10 mg t.i.d.	If the symptom persists a switch to alternative opioid may be useful
Nausea/vomiting induced by vestibular stimulation	Symptoms appear on movement	Promethazine or cyclizine 25 mg t.i.d.	If intractable consider levomepromazine
Constipation	Flatulence, abdominal pain painful bowel movements,	Stool softener (macrogol or lactulose) plus stimulant (senna or bisacodyl). If no effect rectal measures or methylnaltrexone	If no effect consider switch to transdermal fentanyl or transdermal buprenorphine
Sedation	Drowsiness	Reduce dose of morphine, consider methylphedindate 5-10 mg o.d.-b.d.	May be caused by co-administered medications e.g. neuroleptics, benzodiazepines, antidepressants and co morbidities (hepatic/renal failure). Consider opioid switch
Neurotoxicity/ cognitive failure	Hyperalgesia, allodynia, myoclonic jerks/agitation, hallucinations	Reduce dose of morphine, haloperidol – 1 – 2 mg b.d. or risperidone 1 – 2 mg o.d.-b.d.	If no improvement consider opioid switch

Table 1. Common adverse effects of morphine and management possibilities

3.2 Oxycodone

Oral oxycodone is along with oral morphine recommended as a first choice opioid analgesic for the treatment of moderate to severe cancer-related pain (King et al., 2011). It is a semi synthetic thebaine derivative, a strong opioid that displays a significant affinity to κ-opioid receptors along with agonistic effect mediated by μ-opioid receptors. Limited cross-tolerance is observed between oxycodone and morphine in rats and in clinical studies (Maddocks et al, 1996). In comparison to morphine, oxycodone possesses lower affinity to μ-opioid receptors and similar lipid solubility. Oxycodone permeates the blood–brain barrier very quickly, which may explain its stronger analgesic effect in comparison to other opioids. Oxycodone does not display immunosuppressive effects in experimental studies. It has high oral bioavailability (60%–87%); the plasma half-life is 2 to 3 hours after IV administration, 3 hours after treatment with IR oral solution, and 8 hours after CR tablets. The bioavailability of rectal administration is similar to oral route (61%), but it displays greater variability.

Oxycodone is metabolized in the liver primarily to noroxycodone through CYP3A4 and, to a much less extent, to oxymorphone via CYP2D6. Noroxycodone is metabolized to noroxymorphone through CYP2D6, and oxymorphone is metabolized to noroxymorphone by CYP3A4. However, analgesia observed after oxycodone administration relies primarily on the parent compound. Noroxycodone has 17% of the potency of oxycodone. Oxymorphone, in spite of high affinity for μ-opioid receptors, is produced in very small amounts. Noroxymorphone is produced in a significant amount and displays significant affinity for opioid receptors. However, the blood–brain barrier is extremely impermeable to noroxymorphone; thus, its role in analgesia is negligible. Low blood–brain barrier permeability is also characteristic of noroxycodone and oxymorphone (Leppert, 2010c).

In patients with liver cirrhosis and hepatic diseases, the oxycodone dose should be reduced by half. Oxycodone is excreted through the kidneys. In patients with renal insufficiency, the oxycodone dose also should be reduced. In patients with renal failure, the oxycodone half-life is prolonged and ranges from 1.8 to 26 hours. The elimination of noroxycodone and oxymorphone also is impaired in patients with renal failure. CYP2D6 polymorphism probably does not influence oxycodone analgesia and adverse effects. Sertraline minimally inhibits CYP2D6 and intensifies adverse effects of oxycodone (eg, hallucinations, tremors), whereas fluoxetine and quinidine (significant CYP2D6 inhibitors) do not intensify oxycodone adverse effects. Oxycodone reduces oral bioavailability of cyclosporine by half. In healthy patients, rifampin, a CYP3A4 inducer, greatly decreased oral and IV oxycodone AUC by 86% and 53%, respectively ($P < 0.001$), and modestly reduced analgesia and increased plasma metabolite-to–parent compound ratios for noroxycodone and noroxymorphone ($P < 0.001$) (Nieminen et al., 2009). A pharmacodynamic interaction of oxycodone with other drugs acting on the central nervous system, such as benzodiazepines, neuroleptics, and antidepressants, may intensify oxycodone adverse effects, especially sedation, and respiratory depression may be intensified in the case of patients who are more sensitive to opioids.

3.3 Hydromorphone

Oral hydromorphone is an alternative to oral morphine and oral oxycodone as a first choice opioid analgesic for the treatment of moderate to severe cancer pain (Pigni et al, 2011). Hydromorphone has about 5 to 10 times more potent analgesic effect than morphine and similar pharmacodynamic properties. Hydromorphone analgesia is mainly due to μ-opioid–receptor agonist effects; it also features some affinity for δ- but not for κ-opioid receptors (Murray & Hagen, 1995). After hydromorphone administration, analgesia lasts for about 4 to 6 hours and the plasma half-life is about 2.5 hours; sustained-release oral preparations provide analgesia for 12-24 hours (Gardner-Nix & Mercadante, 2010).

The drug is metabolized mainly to hydromorphone-3-glucuronide that is devoid of analgesic activity and may accumulate in patients with renal failure; it may induce neurotoxic adverse effects to larger extent than the respective morphine metabolite (morphine-3-glucuronide) (Wright et al., 2001). Hydromorphone in small amount is also metabolized to 6-hydroxy-hydromorphone, but its role is unknown. Due to glucuronidation, the risk of hydromorphone pharmacokinetic interactions with other drugs seems to be low (Sarhill et al., 2001). Adverse effects are similar to those of morphine; however, hydromorphone less frequently induces nausea and vomiting, constipation, itching, and probably more slowly develops tolerance to analgesia (Wirz et al., 2008). In comparative studies conducted in cancer patients with pain hydromorphone displays similar analgesic efficacy to morphine (Miller et al., 1999) and oxycodone (Hagen and Babul, 1997).

Hydromorphone is especially useful for patients requiring high opioid doses via parenteral route due to strong analgesic effects and increased solubility that enables the possibility administering small volumes of the drug in SC injections.

3.4 Fentanyl
Fentanyl is a lipophilic opioid, μ-opioid–receptor agonist, with analgesic effect about 100 times more potent than that of morphine. In chronic pain treatment, transdermal fentanyl (TF) patches are applied, usually on the upper trunk. There are five types of patches that release 12, 25, 50, 75, and 100 μg/h equal to approximately 0.3, 0.6, 1.2, 1.8, and 2.4 mg fentanyl dose per day, respectively. Patches are changed every 72 hours. Patients need access to short-acting opioid preparations (i.e. oral or parenteral morphine, buccal fentanyl tablets, oral transmucosal fentanyl citrate [OTFC] or fentanyl spray) during TF therapy to effectively manage breakthrough pain episodes. Fentanyl is metabolized mainly to inactive norfentanyl; thus, it may be used in patients with renal impairment. Because the fentanyl metabolic pathway is through CYP3A4, the drugs inhibiting or inducing this enzyme should be avoided. Caution is recommended when using drugs metabolized via CYP3A4. In comparison to morphine, the advantages of TF include milder constipation, nausea, and drowsiness (Ahmedzai & Brooks, 1997).

When starting TF in opioid-naive or strong opioid–naïve patients, one patch at a dose of 12 and 25 μg/h is recommended, respectively. TF also may be used in opioid switch, especially in patients treated with morphine who suffer from intractable constipation. In an open-label study of 16 patients with cancer pain unable to take oral opioids, TF was effective and well tolerated (Leppert et al., 2000). A good analgesic effect was achieved in 11 patients, with a partial effect in an additional 2 patients. TF was effective and well-tolerated in patients formerly treated with weak opioids that did not provide satisfactory analgesia (Vielvoye-Kerkmeer et al., 2000). The indications for TF include patients' preferences, intense constipation during morphine treatment, morphine intolerance, nausea, and vomiting. TF should not be used in patients with unstable pain syndromes, especially with neuropathic pain component due to the long plasma half-life (20 h) of the drug, which hinders quick and effective dose titration. Fentanyl may be successfully used by other routes (e.g. SC, IV, intranasal inhaled, buccal) in the treatment of breakthrough pain (Slatkin et al., 2008).

3.5 Buprenorphine
Buprenorphine is a partial μ-opioid–receptor agonist and κ-receptor antagonist. A ceiling analgesic effect may be obtained at high doses (ie, 15 mg); however, such high doses are not used in clinical practice. The analgesic potency of buprenorphine is about 100 times greater than oral morphine (Likar et al., 2008). Buprenorphine may be administered sublingually due to low oral bioavailability at doses 0.2 to 0.8 mg, usually 3 times daily. It also may be administered by parenteral route (SC or IV).

Buprenorphine is metabolized to the active metabolite norbuprenorphine via CYP3A4. The parent compound and norbuprenorphine undergo glucuronidation; thus, the risk of pharmacokinetic interactions with other drugs is low. Compared with morphine, buprenorphine less frequently induces constipation, nausea, and vomiting, which is probably associated with higher lipophilicity. Buprenorphine is mainly excreted with feces (2/3) and 1/3 of the drug is excreted with urine therefore, it may be used in patients with renal failure. Respiratory depression is rare; however, when the symptom appears, naloxone injection should be administered at a dose of 2 mg, followed by continuous infusion (4 mg/h). Buprenorphine displays antihyperalgesic activity and may be successfully used in the treatment of neuropathic pain (Mercadante et al., 2007).

Buprenorphine is administered in transdermal patches (TB) releasing 35, 52.5, and 70 µg/h, which corresponds to 0.8, 1.2, and 1.6 mg/d, respectively. The patches are changed every 84 to 96 hours. In some countries, patches releasing 5 and 10 µg/h, changed weekly, are available. The starting dose for strong opioid–naïve patients is usually one patch of 35 µg/h. However, opioid-naive patients and those with renal or hepatic impairment may start with a dose of 17.5 µg/h. The treatment is usually well-tolerated. At doses up to 140 µg/h, TB does not display ceiling analgesia (Kress, 2009). Breakthrough pain may be treated with sublingual buprenorphine tablets or with IR morphine administered by oral or parenteral route (Mercadante et al., 2006).

3.6 Methadone

Methadone is a synthetic opioid and a racemate of dextrorotatory (S-methadone) and levorotatory (D-methadone) isomers. Methadone activates µ, κ, and Δ receptors (D-methadone); it displays moderate antagonistic effect to NMDA receptors (both enantiomers) and strongly inhibits the reuptake of serotonin and noradrenalin in the central nervous system (S-methadone). In high doses, methadone blocks potassium channels required for rapid cardiac muscle repolarization, which may explain the risk of developing ventricular arrhythmia.

Methadone is administered mostly to patients with cancer pain who undergo opioid switch; usually methadone is given every 8 hours. In comparison to morphine, 10 times less demand for laxatives and 2 times less nausea and vomiting were observed. Methadone may be administered as the first strong opioid to patients who have been treated with opioids for moderate pain or to opioid-naïve patients (the starting dose is usually 3–5 mg every 8 h) (Ripamonti et al., 1998) although EAPC recommends methadone as the second or the third-line opioid. Methadone can be administered to patients with renal impairment. It has weak immunosuppressive effect and does not suppress the functioning of natural killer cells. Methadone is tenfold less expensive than the CR morphine and 25-fold cheaper than TF.

Methadone is a highly lipophilic and basic drug with a high distribution volume (4.1 ± 0.65 L/kg) and a high affinity to tissues, where it cumulates after multiple administrations (in brain, lung, liver, gut, kidney, and muscles). The high affinity to tissues together with a gradual, retarded release to plasma is the cause of a prolonged half-life. The bioavailability of the drug after oral administration oscillates between 70% and 90%. The half-life is about 24 hours, but it occurs in the range of 8 to 120 hours. Analgesia lasts for 6 to 12 hours. A stable level is reached within 2 to 4 days. Methadone is metabolized mostly via liver enzymes, but also in the intestine wall via N-demethylation to inactive metabolites. The main enzyme responsible for methadone N-demethylation is CYP3A4 with a lesser CYP1A2 and CYP2D6 involvement and a significant CYP2B6 role. The drug is excreted mainly via the alimentary tract, but also through kidneys (depending on the urine pH). In chronic renal disease, methadone does not accumulate; in severe renal failure, a dose reduction may be considered. Methadone is not eliminated in the process of hemodialysis. Methadone is more difficult to use than other opioids due to complicated pharmacokinetics, numerous drug interactions, and possible QT prolongation; therefore, it should be used by physicians experienced in chronic pain management (Leppert, 2009c).

3.7 Tapentadol

Tapentadol chloride ([-]-[1*R*,2*R*]-3-[3-Dimethylamino-1-ethyl-2-methyl-propyl]-phenol hydrochloride) is an opioid with two analgesic mechanisms: agonist of μ-opioid receptors with 50 times less affinity than morphine, and inhibition of norepinephrine reuptake (Tzschentke et al., 2007). Bioavailability after oral administration is over 30%, the drug is metabolized to inactive metabolites through glucuronidation and excreted via kidneys (Kneip et al., 2008). In experimental studies tapentadol is effective in the treatment of neuropathic pain and in inflammatory pain. In clinical studies conducted in patients with low back pain, those with postoperative pain, and those with osteoarthritis, IR tapentadol at doses 50, 75, and 100 mg had more favorable adverse-effects profiles with less intense gastrointestinal adverse effects (ie, nausea, vomiting, constipation) in comparison to IR oxycodone at doses 10 and 15 mg. Clinical studies on tapentadol use in patients with cancer pain are ongoing.

4. Conclusions

Opioids are usually effective when administered alone or with adjuvant analgesics. The traditional WHO step-by-step approach should be used individually, based on the clinical assessment of pain type and intensity. Patients with severe pain intensity should use strong opioids (opioids for moderate-to-severe pain) without climbing up the analgesic ladder. Opioids may be combined with nonopioid analgesics and adjuvant analgesics appropriate for a given pain type. Understanding important attributes of commonly used opioids can help assist selection.

In case of lack of efficacy of orally or transdermally administered opioids, it may be beneficial to change the route of administration to parenteral or intrathecal (Enting et al., 2002). Another possibility is opioid switch that may improve analgesia and reduce adverse effects (Mercadante & Bruera, 2006). A good example may be patients suffering from severe constipation who may benefit when switching from morphine to TF (Ahmedzai & Brooks, 1997) and from codeine or DHC to tramadol (Leppert & Majkowicz, 2010). A newer approach is the concomitant use of two opioids, although little evidence supports such procedure (Fallon & Laird, 2011). Future studies may address genetic disposition responsible for individual patients' response to opioid analgesics (Lötsch et al., 2009).

5. References

Ahmedzai S, Brooks D. Transdermal Fentanyl versus Sustained-Release Oral Morphine in Cancer Pain: Preference, Efficacy and Quality of Life. J Pain Symptom Manage1997; 13: 254 – 261.

Ammon S, Hofmann U, Griese EU, Gugeler N, Mikus G. Pharmacokinetics of dihydrocodeine and its active metabolite after single and multiple oral dosing. Br J Clin Pharmacol 1999; 48: 317-322.

Benett MI. Effectiveness of antiepileptic or antidepressant drugs when added to opioids for cancer pain: a systematic review. Palliat Med 2011; 25: 553-559.

Caraceni A, Pigni A, Brunelli C. Is oral morphine still the first choice opioid for moderate to severe cancer pain? A systematic review within the European Palliative Care Research Collaborative guidelines project. Palliat Med 2011; 25: 402-409.

Davies MP, Glare P. Tramadol. In: Opioids in cancer pain. Second Edition; Davies MP, Glare P, Quigley C, Hardy JR. Eds. Oxford, Oxford University Press 2009, pp. 99-118.

Dickman A. Tramadol: a review of this atypical opioid. Eur J Palliat Care 2007; 14: 181-185.

Donnelly S, Davis MP, Walsh D, Naughton M. Morphine in cancer pain management: a practical guide. Support Care Cancer 2002; 10: 13 - 25.

Eidelman A, White T, Swarm RA: Interventional therapies for cancer pain management: important adjuvants to systemic analgesics. J Natl Compr Canc Netw 2007; 5: 753-760

Enting RH, Oldenmenger WH, van der Rijt CCD, Wilms EB, Elfrink EJ, Elswijk I, Sillevis Smitt PAE. A Prospective Study Evaluating the Response of Patients with Unrelieved Cancer Pain to Parenteral Opioids. Cancer 2002; 94: 3049 - 3056.

Fallon MT, Laird BJA. A systematic review of combination step III opioid therapy in cancer pain: An EPCRC opioid guideline project. Palliat Med 2011; 25: 597-603.

Flemming K. The Use of Morphine to Treat Cancer-Related Pain: A Synthesis of Quantitative and Qualitative Research. J Pain Symptom Manage 2010; 39: 139 - 154.

Freynhagen RJ, Benett MI. Diagnosis and management of neuropathic pain. BMJ 2009; 339: 391-395.

Gardner-Nix J, Mercadante S. The Role of OROS® Hydromorphone in the Management of Cancer Pain. Pain Pract 2010; 10: 72-77.

Gasche Y, Daali Y, Fathi M. et al. Codeine Intoxication Associated with Ultrarapid CYP2D6 Metabolism. N Engl J Med 2004; 351: 2827-2831.

Gnanadesigan N, Espinoza RT, Smith R, Israel M, Reuben DB. Interaction of serotonergic antidepressants and opioid analgesics: is serotonin syndrome going undetected? J Am Med Dir Assoc 2005; 6: 265-269

Gretton S, Riley J. Morphine metabolites: a review of their clinical effects. Eur J Palliat Care 2008; 15: 110 - 114.

Hagen NA, Babul N. Comparative clinical efficacy and safety of a novel controlled-release oxycodone formulation and controlled-release hydromorphone in the treatment of cancer pain. Cancer 1997; 79: 1428-1437.

Hanks GW, de Conno F, Cherny N, Hanna M, Kalso E, McQuay HJ, Mercadante S, et al. Expert Working Group of the Research Network of the European Association for Palliative Care: Morphine and alternative opioids in cancer pain: the EAPC recommendations. Br J Cancer 2001; 84: 587-593.

King SJ, Reid C, Forbes K, Hanks G. A systematic review of oxycodone in the management of cancer pain. Palliat Med 2011; 25: 454-470.

Kirchheiner J, Schmidt H, Tzetkov M, Keulen J-T, Lötsch J, Roots I, Brockmöller J. Pharmacokinetics of codeine and its metabolite morphine in ultra-rapid metabolizers due to CYP2D6 duplication. Pharmacogenomics J 2007; 7: 257-265.

Kneip C, Terlinden R, Beier H, Chen G. Investigations Into the Drug-Drug Interaction potential of tapentadol in Human Liver Microsomes and fresh Human Hepatocytes. Drug Metabol Lett 2008; 2: 67-75.

Kress HG. Clinical update on the pharmacology, efficacy and safety of transdermal buprenorphine. Eur J Pain 2009; 13: 219 - 230.

Leppert W, Luczak J, Gorzelinska L, Kozikowska J. Research from the Palliative Care Department in Poznan on treatment of neoplasm pain with Durogesic (transdermal fentanyl) (Polish). Przegl Lek 2000; 57: 59 - 64.

Leppert W, Majkowicz M. The impact of tramadol and dihydrocodeine treatment on quality of life of patients with cancer pain. Int J Clin Pract 2010; 64: 1681 – 1687.

Leppert W, Mikolajczak P. Analgesic Effects and Assays of Controlled-Release Tramadol and O-desmethyltramadol in Cancer Patients with Pain. Curr Pharmaceut Biotechnol 2011; 12: 306 – 312.

Leppert W. Dihydrocodeine as an analgesic for the treatment of moderate to severe chronic pain. Curr Drug Metab 2010; 11: 494-506.

Leppert W. Progress in pharmacological pain treatment with opioid analgesics (Polish). Wspolcz Onkol 2009; 13: 66-73.

Leppert W. Role of oxycodone and oxycodone/naloxone in cancer pain management. Pharmacol Rep 2010; 62: 578 – 591.

Leppert W. The role of ketamine in the management of neuropathic cancer pain – a Polish experience. Proceedings of the 3rd International Congress on Neuropathic pain, NeuPSIG, Athens (Greece), May 27 – 30, 2010, Ed. Christopher D. Wells. Medimond International Proceedings 2010, pp. 199 – 203.

Leppert W. The role of methadone in cancer pain treatment – a review. Int J Clin Pract 2009; 63: 1095 – 1109.

Leppert W. Tramadol as an analgesic for mild to moderate cancer pain. Pharmacol Rep 2009; 61: 978-992.

Likar R, Krainer B, Sittl R. Challenging the equipotency calculation for transdermal buprenorphine: four case studies. Int J Clin Pract 2008; 62: 152 – 156.

Lötsch J, Geisslinger G, Tegeder I. Genetic modulation of the pharmacological treatment of pain. Pharmacol Ther 2009; 124: 168-184.

Lötsch J, Skarke C, Schmidt H, Rohrbacher M, Hofmann U, Schwab M, Geisslinger G. Evidence for morphine-independent central nervous opioid effects after administration of codeine: Contribution of other codeine metabolites. Clin Pharmacol Ther 2006; 79: 35-48.

Lussier D, Huskey AG, Portenoy RK. Adjuvant Analgesics in Cancer Pain Management. Oncologist 2004; 9: 571-591.

Madadi P, Moretti M, Djokanovic N, Bozzo P, Nulman I, Ito S, Koren G. Guidelines for maternal codeine use during breastfeeding. Can Fam Phys 2009; 55: 1077-1078.

Madadi P, Ross CJD, Hayden MR, Carleton BC, Gaedigk A, Leeder JS, Koren G. Pharmacogenetics of Neonatal Opioid Toxicity Following Maternal Use of Codeine During Breastfeeding: A Case-Control Study. Clin Pharmacol Ther 2009; 85: 31-35.

Maddocks I, Somogyi A, Abbott F, Hayball P, Parker D. Attenuation of morphine-induced delirium in palliative care by substitution with infusion of oxycodone. J Pain Symptom Manage1996; 12: 182–189.

Mercadante S, Bruera E. Opioid switching: a systematic and critical review. Cancer Treat Rev 2006; 32: 304 – 315.

Mercadante S, Ferrera P, Villari P. Is there a ceiling effect of transdermal buprenorphine? Preliminary data in cancer patients. Support Care Cancer 2007; 15: 441 – 444.

Mercadante S, Villari P. Ferrera P. et al. Safety and effectiveness of intravenous morphine for episodic breakthrough pain in patients receiving transdermal buprenorphine. J Pain Symptom Manage 2006; 32: 175 – 179.

Miller MG, McCarthy N, O'Boyle CA et al. Continuous subcutaneous infusion of morphine vs. hydromorphone: a controlled trial. J Pain Symptom Manage 1999; 18: 9 – 16.

Murray A, Hagen NA. Hydromorphone. J Pain Symptom Manage 1995; 29 (Suppl): S57 – S66.

Nieminen TH, Hagelberg NM, Saari TI, Pertovaara A, Neuvonen M, Laine K, Neuvonen PJ, Olkkola KT. Rifampin Greatly Reduces the Plasma Concentrations of Intravenous and Oral Oxycodone. Anesthesiology 2009; 110: 1371-1378.

Pigni A, Brunelli C, Caraceni A. The role of hydromorphone in cancer pain treatment: a systematic review. Palliat Med 2011; 25: 471-477.

Rauers NI, Stuber F, Lee E.-H. et al. Antagonistic Effects of Ondansetron and Tramadol? A Randomized Placebo and Active Drug Controlled Study. J Pain 2010; 11: 1274-1281.

Ridgway D, Sopata M, Burneckis A, Jespersen L, Andersen C. Clinical Efficacy and Safety of Once-Daily Dosing of a Novel, Prolonged-Release Oral Morphine Tablet Compared With Twice-Daily Dosing of a Standard Controlled-Release Morphine Tablet in Patients With Cancer Pain: A Randomized, Double-Blind, Exploratory Crossover Study. J Pain Symptom Manage 2010; 39: 712 – 720.

Ripamonti C, Groff L, Brunelli C, Polastri D, Stavrakis A, De Conno F. Switching From Morphine to Oral Methadone in treating Cancer Pain: What Is the Equianalgesic Dose Ratio? J Clin Oncol 1998; 16: 3216 – 3221.

Ripamonti CI, Campa T, Fagnoni E, Brunelli C, Luzzani M, Maltoni M, De Conno F. on behalf of MERITO Study Group. Normal-release Oral Morphine Starting Dose in Cancer Patients With Pain. Clin J Pain 2009; 25: 386-390.

Ripamonti CI, Easson AM, Gerdes H. Management of malignant bowel obstruction. Eur J Cancer 2008; 44: 1105 – 1115.

Rowell FJ, Seymour RA, Rawlins MD. Pharmacokinetics of Intravenous and Oral Dihydrocodeine and its Acid Metabolites. Eur J Clin Pharmacol 1983; 25: 419-424.

Sarhill N, Walsh D, Nelson KA. Hydromorphone: pharmacology and clinical applications in cancer patients. Support Care Cancer 2001; 9: 84 – 96.

Schmidt H, Vormfelde SV, Walchner-Bonjean M. et al. The role of active metabolites in dihydrocodeine effects. Int J Clin Pharmacol Ther 2003; 41: 95-106.

Slatkin NE, Xie F, Messina J, Segal TJ. Fentanyl Buccal Tablet for Relief of Breakthrough Pain in Opioid-Tolerant Patients With Cancer-Related Chronic Pain. J Support Oncol 2008; 5: 327 – 334.

Stamer U, Musshoff F, Kobilay M, Madea B, Hoeft A, Stuber F. Concentrations of Tramadol and O-desmethyltramadol Enantiomers in Different CY2D6 Genotypes. Clin Pharmacol Ther 2007; 82: 41-47.

Stamer U, Stuber F, Muders T, Musshoff F. Respiratory Depression with Tramadol in a Patient with Renal Impairment and CYP2D6 Gene Duplication. Anesth Analg 2008; 107: 926–929.

Stamer UM, Lehnen K, Höthker F, Bayerer B, Wolf S, Hoeft A, Stuber F. Impact of CYP2D6 genotype on postoperative tramadol analgesia. Pain 2003; 105: 231-238.

Tzschentke TM, Christoph T, Kögel B. et al. (-)-(1R,2R)-3-(3-Dimethylamino-1-ethyl-2-methyl-propyl)-phenol Hydrochloride (Tapentadol HCl): a Novel µ-Opioid Receptor Agonist/Norepinephrine Reuptake Inhibitor with Broad-Spectrum Analgesic Properties. J Pharmacol Exp Ther 2007; 323: 265 – 276.

Vielvoye-Kerkmeer APE, Mattern C, Uitendaal MP. Transdermal Fentanyl in Opioid-Naive Cancer Pain Patients: An Open Trial Using Transdermal Fentanyl for the Treatment of Chronic Cancer Pain in Opioid-Naive Patients and a Group Using Codeine. J Pain Symptom Manage 2000; 19: 185 - 192.

Voronov P, Przybylo HJ, Jagannathan N. Apnea in a child after oral codeine: a genetic variant – an ultra-rapid metabolizer. Pediatric Anesthesia 2007; 17: 684-687.

Vree TB, van Dongen RTM, Koopman-Kimenai PM. Codeine analgesia is due to codeine-6-glucuronide, not morphine. Int J Clin Pract 2000; 54: 395-398.

Vree TB, Verwey-van Wissen CP. Pharmacokinetics and metabolism of codeine in humans. Biopharm Drug Disp 1992; 13: 445-460.

Webb JA, Rostami-Hodjegan A, Abdul-Manap R, Hofmann U, Mikus G, Kamali F. Contribution of dihydrocodeine and dihydromorphine to analgesia following dihydrocodeine administration in man: a PK-PD modelling analysis. Br J Clin Pharmacol 2001; 52: 35-43.

Wirz S, Wartenberg HC, Nadstawek J. Less nausea, emesis, and constipation comparing hydromorphone and morphine? A prospective open-labeled investigation on cancer pain. Support Care Cancer 2008; 16: 999 – 1009.

World Health Organization: Cancer Pain Relief and Palliative Care. Geneva: World Health Organization, 1996.

Wright AW, Mather LE, Smith MT. Hydromorphone-3-glucuronide: a more potent neuro-excitant than its structural analogue, morphine-3-glucuronide. Life Sci 2001; 69: 409-420

16

Pain Management and Costs of a Combination of Oxycodone + Naloxone in Low Back Pain Patients

R. Rychlik, K. Viehmann, D. Daniel, P. Kiencke and J. Kresimon
Institute of Empirical Health Economics, Burscheid,
Germany

1. Introduction

In industrial nations, low back pain (lbp) is one of the leading causes of physical limitation. It is also a main source of incapacitation, suffering and expense. According to the national institute of neurological disorders and stroke in the US, LBP accounts for more sick leave and disability than any other medical condition. In Germany, life time prevalence of LBP reaches up to 84 %, with the highest rate for people aged between 35 and 55. According to the German Health Report of the year 2002, the costs of rehabilitation and early retirement amounted to more than 15 billion € , and direct and indirect cost of illness up to 26 billion EURO. Thus the effective management of low back pain is a major health and economic concern.

In a minority of patients presenting for evaluation in a primary care setting, lbp can be reliably attributed to a specific underlying pathology, such as malignancy, vertebral compression fracture or inflammatory/infectious processes. The majority, 80-90%, of patients present primary or non-specific lbp. There is little documented knowledge of possible causes of non-specific lbp. Risk factors are probably related to genetic predisposition, lifestyle (e.g., overweight, lack of physical activity), physical strain and psychological distress.

Opioid analgesics are well established in the treatment of severe pain conditions and have internationally gained a strong position as a potent daily pain treatment option. Many physicians are still apprehensive about the administration of opioids within a continuous therapy, due to potential drug abuse and possible adverse effects, such as impaired gastrointestinal functioning.

To achieve a satisfactory balance between analgesia and side effects, the assessment and treatment of opioid side effects are fundamental aspects of the therapy. This may increase the likelihood of a favourable treatment outcome, potentially allow higher and more efficacious opioid doses, and improve quality of life by reducing other discomforting symptoms. Economic consequences of insufficiently treated chronic lbp and treatment of potential adverse drug effects also play a significant role from the society's point of view. Additional expenses may include costs that emerge from additional obligatory treatments, hospitalization and work incapacity.

2. Primary objective

The primary objective of this health services research study was to assess the health-related quality of life and the total costs (direct and indirect) of patients in Germany suffering from chronic back pain. Therapy with oxycodone + naloxone[1] was compared to therapy with other strong opioids (WHO-step III opioids).

Main aims are:

- Health related quality of life over a period of one year – patients on therapy with oxycodone + naloxone compared to therapy with other WHO-step III opioids.
- Costs for the pain therapy and therapy of AE/ADR in in- and out-patients.
- Patients' inability to work, days off work compared between both cohorts.
- The incidence of early retirement due to chronic back pain and the average age of these patients.

3. Secondary objective

The secondary objective of the study was to evaluate the data for effectiveness under daily routine conditions of the therapy with oxycodone + naloxone or other WHO-step III opioids (strong opioids).

Main issues were:

- The long-term effectiveness of treatment of chronic back pain under daily routine conditions with oxycodone + naloxone or other strong opioids (WHO-step III opioids).
- Frequency of the administration of rescue-medication (drugs additionally taken once only, as an emergency treatment of pain) under therapy with oxycodone + naloxone compared to other strong opioids (WHO-step III opioids).

4. Methods

In order to portray the actual costs ("true costs") incurred for patients suffering from chronic back pain, data had to be documented under daily routine conditions ("real-world-design"). Therefore, a cohort study design was chosen. Two cohorts were observed: Patients in the first cohort were treated with oxycodone + naloxone (cohort 1). Patients in the second cohort were treated with another WHO-step III opioid (cohort 2). In accordance with the statistical analysis plan, each participating physician was asked to document five patients per cohort. Because of the non-interventional study design, individual site-specific imbalances due to the cohort recruitment will be discussed from a statistical point of view.

4.1 Patient population

Opioid-naive and opioid-pretreated female and male adults (> 18 years) who suffered from chronic back pain below the costal arch and above the gluteal groove, who require a round-a-clock-treatment with WHO-step III opioids, were considered. Patients with cancer pain, herniated vertebral disks, or pain caused by an accident, were excluded. Patients who recently started therapy with oxycodone + naloxone or another WHO-step III opioid were also considered, as well as patients, who were switched from a WHO-step

---

[1] Targin®

II to a WHO-step III opioid or from one WHO-step III opiod to another WHO. The change of therapy was not allowed to be correlated to the study. Consequently, patients treated with oxycodone + naloxone or other WHO-step III opioids were eligible for the study.

For all patients, the summary of product characteristics (SPC) was considered with regard to patient's safety and need to perform daily activities.

Patients not treated according to the SPC were excluded from the study.

4.2 Inclusion and exclusion criteria

- Therapy with oxycodone + naloxone or another WHO-step III opioid was documented for all patients over an observation period of approximately twelve months, including prescription and administration of the medication (regular daily administration, period of administration).
- Patients were informed about the study and agreed to participate by signing and dating the informed consent form.
- Patients were able to comprehend the language as well as the contents of the study materials (patient information, informed consent form and patient questionnaires).
- Patients suffered from chronic back pain below the costal arch and above the gluteal groove.
- Patients with tumor pain, herniated vertebral disks, or pain caused by an accident, were excluded.
- Patients were more than 18 years old.
- oxycodone + naloxone or another WHO-step III opioids were not contraindicated.
- Female patients were neither pregnant nor breastfeeding.

Patients were excluded from the study if any of the following applied:

- A contraindication to the planned treatment regime occurred.
- The patient withdrew his/her consent to participate in the study.
- Newly diagnosed pregnancy.
- Administration of oxycodone + naloxone or another WHO-step III opioid was not in accordance with the specifications of the SPC.

4.3 Duration and conduct of the study
4.3.1 Study sites and number of patients

200 general practitioners and orthopedics, some of them specializing in pain therapy, should be achieved to participate at in this nation-wide, multi-center, non-interventional study. As stated in the observational plan, the enrolment of 2,000 patients (10 patients per physician, 5 patients per cohort) with chronic back pain was required to document patients at baseline (V1), after one week (V2), four weeks (V3), six months (V4) and after 12 months.

4.3.2 Time schedule

Screening and recruitment of the participating physicians were conducted by the Institute of Empirical Health Economics (IfEG) prior to the start of the study. IfEG CRAs started to visit the physicians´ medical centers in September 2008. Patients were enrolled by the physicians and observed for one year. Documentation started according to the project schedule after the patients had signed the informed consent form (ICF). An interim analysis was scheduled approximately six months after the beginning of the observation period. The study-report was due three months after last patient last visit (LPLV).

4.3.3 Patient information and informed consent form (ICF)
Prior to their participation, patients had to sign the ICF. The patient information describes the objectives, contents and risks of the study. Furthermore, the patients were informed that withdrawal from the observational study was possible at any point in time without further consequences. The patient obtained a copy of the patient information and the ICF. The physician is obligated to keep the signed ICF records at least for 15 years.

4.3.4 Documentation of treatment
Socio-demographic data, the clinical variables regarding progress of the disease, as well as the treatment costs incurred for the attending physician were documented on standardized case report forms (CRF). All consultations during the observation period due to chronic back pain were documented. The consultations took place as they would within the scope of the treatment of chronic back pain and no study-specific visits were indicated. Physicians sent the completed CRF by postal service to IfEG.

4.3.5 Documentation by patients
During the observation period, patients actively participated in the documentation by completing standardized health-related quality of life questionnaires (SF-36 v2 Health Survey) at four points in time. Visits took place every quarter and the quality of life questionnaires were completed during the visits.
Intensity of pain and stool consistency was recorded daily for the first four weeks, followed by recording every two weeks on patient diaries.
The patients also completed standardized questionnaires regarding constipation and the pain intensity of the last seven days during each consultation.

4.4 Variables
The variables considered for this report are described in the following sections.

4.4.1 Socio-demographic and administrative variables
The following data were collected regarding at the first visit (V1):
* gender
* date of birth (month/year)
* height
* weight
* ethnic group
* patient's ability to comprehend the patient information and informed consent
* family status
* educational school level and training level
* status of occupation
* status of ability to work (and correlation with chronic back pain)
* exemption from additional payments
* type of health insurance
* physicians' specialization and additional pain therapy qualifications

4.4.2 Clinical variables
The following clinical data were collected at V1:
- diagnosis of chronic back pain (back pain causing disease)
- concomitant diseases
- medical pre-treatment outside of pain therapy
- assessment of previous pain therapy prior to enrolment (by physician and patient)
- other disorders apart from pain indication experienced within the last week before the beginning of observational study (separately for opioid-naive patients and opioid-pretreated patients)
- previous and current drug therapy for chronic back pain treatment
- change/adjustment/withdrawal of therapy with oxycodone + naloxone or another opioid of WHO-step III
- dosage and application times of the therapy with oxycodone + naloxone or another opioid of WHO-step III
- concomitant medication
- rescue-medication
- assessment of pain, intensity of pain and general mobility of the patient (patient diary)
- average period of analgesia experienced by the patient

4.4.3 Variables of costs
The following variables of costs were included in the cost calculation. For all costs, a causal correlation to the underlying chronic back pain had to exist. Costs for the treatment of adverse events or adverse drug reactions were also included.
- ambulatory treatment costs (consultations including house calls, emergency treatments and medical specialist consultation) contributable to chronic back pain
- type (trade name and active ingredient) and amount (number of packages and package size) of prescribed and recommended drugs
- non-medicinal therapies
- inability to work within the last twelve months before the start and during the observation period
- early retirement
- reduction in earning capacity
- hospitalizations
- other medicinal interventions
- remedies and medical devices
- consultations at other physicians
- emergency treatments
- additional acquisitions or measures taken (e.g. conversion of an apartment)

4.5 Quality of life questionnaires
4.5.1 Quality of life questionnaires (SF-36 v2 Health Survey)
The SF-36 is a multi-purpose, short-form health survey with 36 questions. It provides an 8-scale profile of functional health and well-being scores, as well as a psychometrically-based physical and mental health summary and a preference-based health utility index. It is a

generic measure, as opposed to surveys that target a specific age, disease, or treatment group [16].

The taxonomy has three levels: (1) items; (2) eight scales with 2-10 items each; and (3) two summaries. All but one of the 36 items (self-reported health transition) are used to score the eight SF-36 scales. Each item is used in scoring only one scale.

The SF-36 has the following composition:

- Physical Functioning
- Role-Physical
- Physical Pain
- General Health
- Vitality
- Social Functioning
- Role-Emotional
- Mental Health

The calculations (pole reversal and recalibration of items, missing values, and transformation of scales) of the SF-36-subscales and the physical and mental summation scales are performed with the SSPS-program by Mogens Trab Damsgaard. The SSPS-program is described in the SF-36 manual. The totals from the 8 subscales are subsequently transformed to a percentage scale (co-domain 0-100). Norm-based scoring (NBS) algorithms are introduced for all eight scales and employ a linear T-score transformation with mean = 50 and standard deviation = 10. The weightings of subscales within summation scales are performed with the weight factor used in the American standard sample.

The SF-36 was completed for V1, V3 (after 4 weeks), V4 (after 6 months) and V5 (after 12 months).

4.5.2 Brief Pain Inventory Short Form (BPI-SF)

The Brief Pain Inventory is a standardized method applied for self assessment of pain and its outcomes in an abbreviated form. This inventory encompasses numeric rating scales for pain intensity and reduction in pain contributable to the treatment, as well as a graphic picture. Emphasise is placed on sensory pain components and the documentation of pain-related impairments.

The sum scale for pain intensity contains four questions: to most severe, minimum, and average pain severity experienced during the last 24 hours and at that moment (range 0-10 points per questions, total range 0-40 points). An increase in point score implies an increase in pain.

The sum scale for pain-related impairment consists of seven questions to self assessment of impairment in the daily routine (activity, mood, movement, occupation, relationships, sleep and vitality) within the last 24 hours (range 0-10 points per question, total range 0-70 points).

Cumulative values for pain intensity and pain-related impairment were calculated. An increase in cumulative values implies an increase in pain.

The third factor evaluated pain relief due to the analgesic therapy expressed as a percentage from the baseline value.

The BPI-SF was completed for V1 (beginning), V3 (after 4 weeks), V4 (after 6 months) and V5 (after 12 months).

4.6 Statistical analysis
4.6.1 Data entry
A data entry template for the complete documentation was designed by IfEG by using the program Oracle 11.1.06G. Data entry was conducted successively after CRFs were received.

4.6.2 Handling of dropouts
Patients were defined as dropouts if they were enrolled although the population criteria were not fulfilled, andif they did not receive any study-related medication. Dropouts were completely excluded from the effectiveness analysis.

Withdrawal patients were defined as patients who also include those patients who discontinued the therapy with oxycodone + naloxone or another WHO-step III opioid before the end of the observation period, withdrew their consent, or who became pregnant during the observation period. These patients are included in the effectiveness and efficacy analysis and are not considered to be dropouts, unless the therapy with oxycodone + naloxone or another WHO-step III opioid was administered for less than three months

4.6.3 Study population
The following populations were defined before data analysis:
- Safety-Population (SP): all patients who were included in the observational study and attended at least one follow-up visit
- Intent-to-Treat-Population (ITT-P): all patients for whom at least one examination regarding effectiveness (pain and bowel function) was conducted
- Per-Protocol-Population (PPP): all patients for whom all quarter and all BPI-SF assessment were completely documented

For the Per-Protocol-Population, only the CRFs completed for the whole observation period were considered, whereas for the Intent-To-Treat-Population, all available data were considered. Data in this paper refer to safety-population and intent-to-treat population only.

4.6.4 Statistical analysis
The data analyses are conducted with the software PASW 18.0 for Windows, as well as MS-Excel 2007 and MS-Access 2007. The evaluation is descriptive, based on the character of the documentation. An inferential statistic is performed for the comparison of the cohorts.

5. Analysis and results

5.1 Description of the study population
A total of 1.013 patients from 134 physicians were entered into the database (figure 1). 43 patients had to be excluded from the analysis: Of these, 24 patients did not receive any study-related medication and for 19 patients the physicians did not complete documentation to the end of the study. Therefore, 970 patients were included in the safety population (SP) comprising 583 patients from the cohort "oxycodone + naloxone" (cohort 1) and 371 from the cohort "other WHO-step III opioids" (cohort 2). No cohort classification was possible for 16 patients, because these patients did not take any strong opioid (oxycodone + naloxone or

other WHO-step III opioids). 560 cohort 1 and 364 cohort 2 patients were feasible for the Intent-To-Treat-Population. For the Per-Protocol-Population, 569 patients were included: 345 of cohort 1 and 224 of cohort 2.

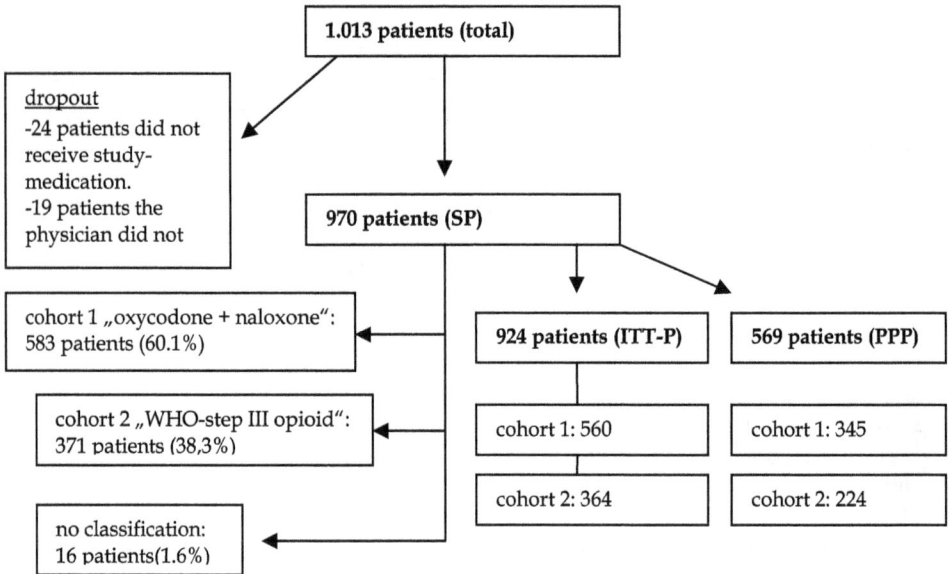

Fig. 1. Organigram of the study population

The majority of the patients were female (~60%) which refers to the epidemiological distribution in Germany within an aging population: the average age was around 64 years and by this most patients had been retired or were of least unable to work. Only 20% of the patients were employed (Table 1).

	cohort 1		cohort 2		
	N	rate	N	rate	p-value
female	350	62,5%	221	60,7%	P= 0,585
male	210	37,5%	143	39,3%	
age	560	63,4	364	64,9	p = 0,084
employed	121	21,6%	62	17,0%	p = 0,088
number of days off work 12 months before inclusion	81	75,0	40	95,4	p = 0,496

Table 1. Gender and age of the population

Almost all patients were classified as caucasians, more than half of the patients were married and app. 50% had an educational level above secondary general school. Less than 7% were ensured privately.

At visit 1 924 days off work in the last year were documented for both cohorts (560 in cohort 1). 17% of the included patients reported a reduction in earning capacity. 14,6% in cohort 1 and 16,8% in cohort 2 had been retired early due to chronic back pain.

Nearly 45% (!) of all patients reported a poor effectiveness of the applied pain therapies.

During the course of the study both physicians and patients assessed a higher effectiveness increase in cohort 1 compared to cohort 2. This refers also to tolerability.

5.2 Quality of life
5.2.1 SF-36

Figure 2 shows the results of the SF-36 evaluation for physical health.

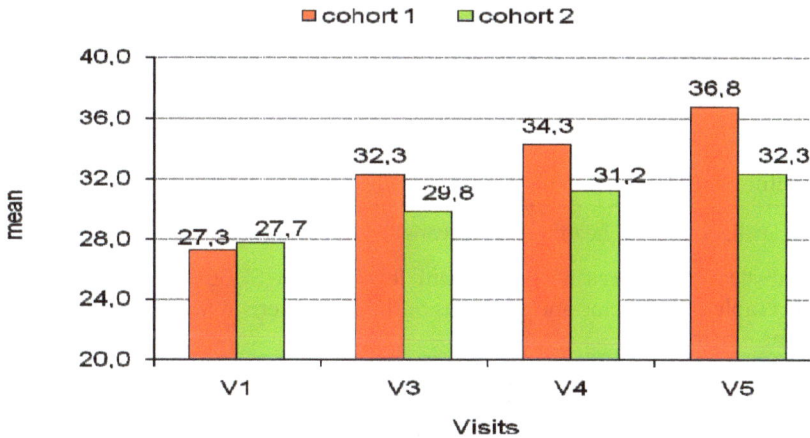

	cohort 1			cohort 2			
	number	mean	SD	number	mean	SD	p-value
Standardized physical health	356	9,65	10,29	244	4,55	8,90	p < 0,001

Fig. 2. Standardized physical health SF-36 (means)

The difference between the physical health of cohort 1 compared to cohort 2 were significant for the periods V5>V3, V3>V1, V4 >V1 and V4>V1 but not for V4>V3 and V5>V4. The results for both cohorts indicate a continuous improvement, which was more pronounced in cohort 1. This result is also mirrored by the data on standardized mental health (Figure 3).

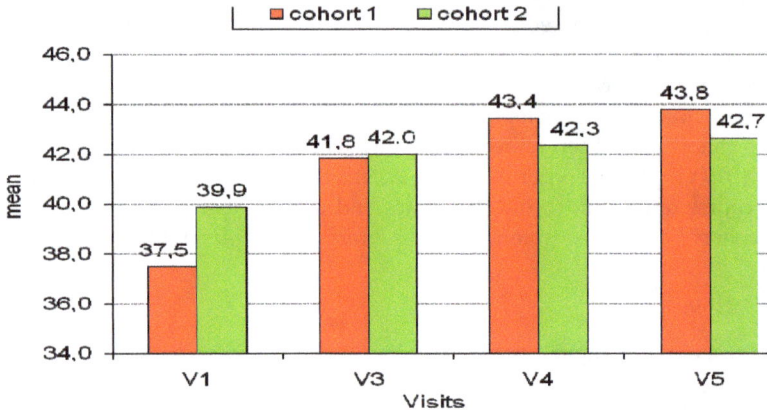

Fig. 3. Standardized mental health SF-36 (means)

	cohort 1			cohort 2			
	number	mean	SD	number	mean	SD	p-value
Standardized mental health	356	6,34	12,82	244	2,58	12,33	p < 0,001

In total statistical power reached significant level for all SF-36 positions except "Role-emotional" (Table 2). All items and positions of the SF-36 were in favour of the combination of oxycodone + naloxone.

SF-36 Positions	cohort 1			cohort 2			p-value
	number	mean	SD	number	mean	SD	
1 Physical function	392	23,09	29,79	272	8,52	26,36	< 0,001
2 Role-physical	370	31,28	44,62	261	16,44	41,15	< 0,001
3 Bodily Pain	379	25,66	25,97	263	11,97	19,10	< 0,001
4 General health	375	13,32	22,64	257	6,16	17,76	< 0,001
5 Vitality	376	16,21	22,64	261	5,77	18,69	< 0,001
6 Social functioning	377	19,46	28,50	263	6,65	25,91	< 0,001
7 Role-emotional	363	22,87	56,34	252	14,02	54,19	0,057
8 Mental health	376	15,13	22,88	261	6,27	19,75	< 0,001

Table 2. Summary of SF-36 positions

5.2.2 Brief Pain Inventory Short Form (BPI-SF)

The Brief Pain Inventory Short Form (BPI-SF) contains numeric rating scales for pain intensity and pain impairment as well as for pain relief. Fig. 4 shows the differences between the total scores of pain intensity. Significant differences were found between cohort 1 and cohort 2 at V5, V4 and V3 compared to V1. Significant differences were also determined for the time periods V3 to V5 and V3 to V4.

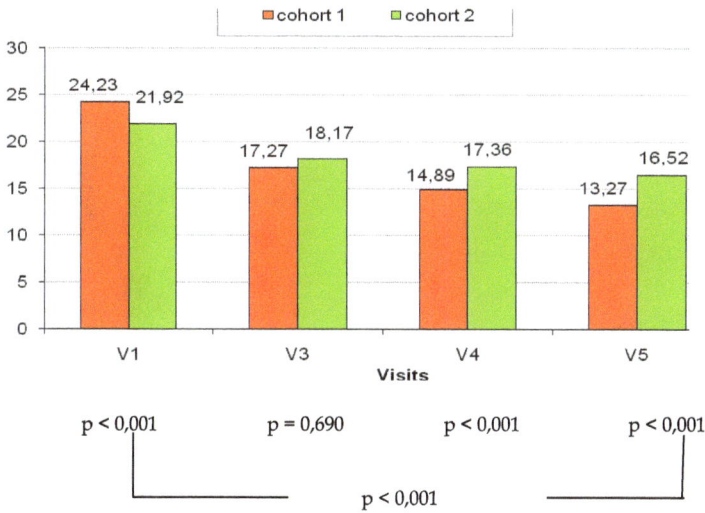

Fig. 4. Sum scale of pain intensity (means)
Brief Pain Inventory (BPI-Shortform)

Worst pain in the last 24 hours decreased in cohort 1 more over all periods than in cohort 2 although worst pain was significantly higher in cohort 1 at baseline (V1).
After 12 months (V5) both cohorts revealed highly significant differences (Fig. 5).

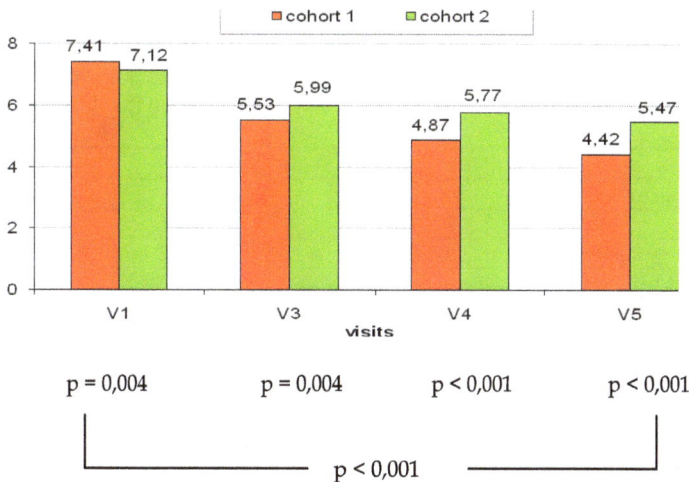

Fig. 5. Worst pain in the last 24 hours (means)
Brief Pain Inventory (BPI-Shortform)

Pain relief treatments or medications administered were also recorded. The patients had to mark the percentage that represents how much pain relief they have experienced (0%=no relief, 100%=complete relief). The pain relief of cohort 1 patients compared to cohort 2 was significant at V1 (p < 0.001) and at V5 (p = 0.001). At visit 1 the pain relief on average amounted to 39.2 % in cohort 1 and to 46.02 % in cohort 2. At the end of the study (V5) the averaged pain relief was 64.2 % in cohort 1 and 58.9 % in cohort 2 (Fig. 6).

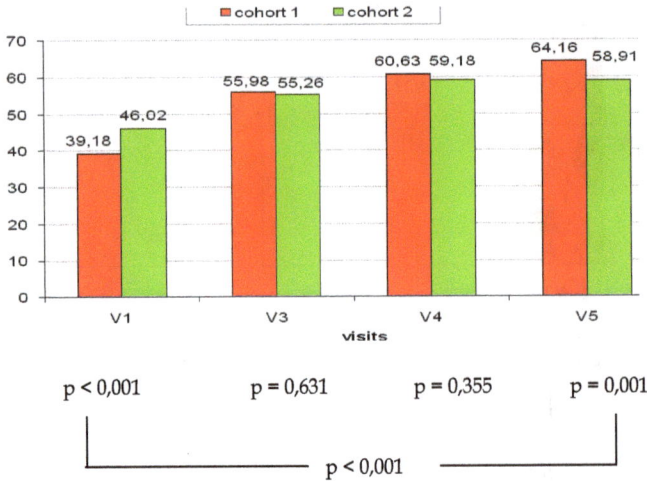

Fig. 6. Pain relief (means)
Brief Pain Inventory (BPI-Shortform)

6. Costs

Annual average direct costs of 2,403.45 € accumulated per patient in cohort 1 and 2,772.98 € per patient in cohort 2. The difference in annual average costs was not significant (p = 0.195). The approximately 13 % lower amount incurred in cohort 1 can be attributed to drug expenses, emergency treatment and hospitalisation/rehabilitation. The differences between both cohorts were significant for co-medication (p < 0.001) and rescue-medication (p = 0.021) (Tab. 3).

cost category	total	cohort 1	cohort 2
out-patient treatment	477,03 €	481,79 €	469,71 €
drug expenses	1.653,73 €	1.532,69 €	1.839,93 €
oxycodone + naloxone	812,17 €	1.270,16 €	107,57 €
opioid WHO-III	611,68 €	65,04 €	1.452,67 €
comedication	211,51 €	181,83 €	257,16 €
rescue medication	18,37 €	15,67 €	22,54 €
remedies	34,20 €	31,07 €	39,03 €
non-medical therapy	54,95 €	53,11 €	57,79 €
emergency treatments	64,76 €	52,57 €	83,52 €
hospitalization/rehabilitation	264,35 €	252,22 €	283,01 €
direct costs	2.549,02 €	2.403,45 €	2.772,98 €

Table 3. Direct costs categories

Fig. 7 shows the indirect costs for the cohorts. Higher averaged indirect costs per patient were calculated for cohort 2. The higher indirect costs resulted from higher costs due to reduction in earning capacity. Approximately 26 % less costs were documented for cohort 1 patients than for cohort 2 patients in this part of indirect costs.

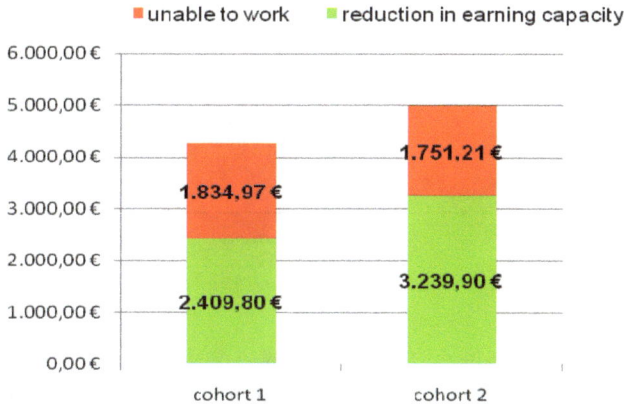

Fig. 7. Indirect cost categories for the cohorts

The incremental cost-effectiveness ratio (ICER) represents the ratio between the differences in treatment costs (ΔC) and treatment effects (ΔE) for cohort OXN and cohort "other strong opioids". It presents the cost of an additional effect unit. The ICER was tested against the main parameters (Tab. 4).

parameter	cohort 1		cohort 2		ICER	$\Delta C/\Delta E$
	ΔE	CER	ΔE	CER		
direct costs (C)	2,403 €		2,773 €		---	-370 €
SF-36 (physical health)	9.65	249 €	4.55	610 €	-72 €	-370 €/5.10
SF-36 (mental health)	6.34	379 €	2.58	1,074 €	-98 €	-370 €/3.76
BPI-SF (pain relief)	24.14	100 €	12.44	223 €	-32 €	-370 €/11.7
CER: Cost-Effectiveness Ratio; ICER: Incremental Cost-Effectiveness Ratio						

Table 4. Cost-effectiveness ratio

The following formula was used for the calculation of the incremental cost-effectiveness ratio:

$$ICER = \frac{\text{(costs of cohort OXN)-(costs of cohort "other strong opioids")}}{\text{(effect of cohort OXN)-(effect of cohort "other strong opioids")}} = \frac{\text{cost difference}}{\text{effect difference}}$$

$$ICER = \frac{\overline{C}_{\text{cohort OXN}} - \overline{C}_{\text{cohort "other strong opioids"}}}{\overline{E}_{\text{cohort OXN}} - \overline{E}_{\text{cohort "other strong opioids"}}} = \frac{\Delta \overline{C}}{\Delta \overline{E}}$$

Negative values were calculated for the ICER of the main parameters, which implies more effectiveness at a lower price for the alternative therapy with Oxycodone + Naloxone (Fig. 8).

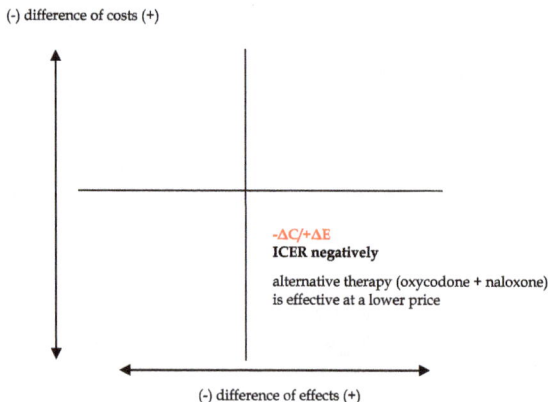

Fig. 8. Cost-effectiveness area

7. Conclusion

As a final conclusion it can be stated that patients of cohort 1 (oxycodone + naloxone) experienced a better quality of life and less back pain after twelve months compared to patients of cohort 2 (other WHO-step III opioids). According to the cost effectiveness-analysis therapy with oxycodone + naloxone is more effective and generates lower costs than cohort 2. These results and findings should be confirmed by a randomized, blinded controlled trial.

8. References

[1] http://www.ninds.nih.gov/disorders/backpain/detail-backpain.htm, stand 16.06.2008
[2] Arzneimittelkommission der deutschen Ärzteschaft: Therapieempfehlungen der Arzneimittelkommission der deutschen Ärzteschaft: Kreuzschmerzen. Arzneiverordnung in der Praxis; 3. Auflage 2007.
[3] Diemer W, Burchert H: Chronische Schmerzen – Kopf- und Rückenschmerzen, Tumorschmerzen. Gesundheitsberichterstattung. Heft 7 (2002)
[4] Roth SH, Fleischmann RM, Burch FX et al.: Around-the-clock, Controlled-Release Oxycodone Therapy for Osteoarthritis-Related Pain. Arch Intern Med. 160, 853-860 (2000)
[5] Furlan AD, Sandoval JA, Mailis-Gagnon A et al.: Opioids for Chronic Noncancer Pain: A Metaanalysis of Effectiveness and Side Effects. CMAJ. 174 (11), 1589-1594 (2006)
[6] Panchal SJ, Müller-Schwefe P, Wurzelmann JI: Opioid-Induced Bowel Dysfunction: Prevalence, Pathophysiology and Burden. Int J Clin Pract. 61 (7), 1181-1187 (2007)
[7] Rote Liste Win®, Ausgabe 2007/I, Version 3.3
[8] http://www.gelbe-liste.de (12/2007)
[9] http.//kbv.de/ebm2009/ebmgesamt.htm
[10] http://www.e-bis.de/ebm/; http://e-bis.de/goae/defaultFrame.htm
[11] http://drg.uni-muenster.de/de/webground/m.webground.php?menu=6
[12] Average of 2, 100 hospitals based on data oft he TK, stand 21.19.2009; http://www.tk-online.de
[13] Schulenburg JM et al. Deutsche Empfehlung zur gesundheitsökonomischen Evaluation – dritte und aktualisierte Fassung. Gesundh ökon Qual manag. 12, 285-290 (2007)
[14] RVaktuell. 11, 470 (2006)

Permissions

The contributors of this book come from diverse backgrounds, making this book a truly international effort. This book will bring forth new frontiers with its revolutionizing research information and detailed analysis of the nascent developments around the world.

We would like to thank Gabor B. Racz, MD, FIPP, ABIPP, for lending his expertise to make the book truly unique. He has played a crucial role in the development of this book. Without his invaluable contribution this book wouldn't have been possible. He has made vital efforts to compile up to date information on the varied aspects of this subject to make this book a valuable addition to the collection of many professionals and students.

This book was conceptualized with the vision of imparting up-to-date information and advanced data in this field. To ensure the same, a matchless editorial board was set up. Every individual on the board went through rigorous rounds of assessment to prove their worth. After which they invested a large part of their time researching and compiling the most relevant data for our readers. Conferences and sessions were held from time to time between the editorial board and the contributing authors to present the data in the most comprehensible form. The editorial team has worked tirelessly to provide valuable and valid information to help people across the globe.

Every chapter published in this book has been scrutinized by our experts. Their significance has been extensively debated. The topics covered herein carry significant findings which will fuel the growth of the discipline. They may even be implemented as practical applications or may be referred to as a beginning point for another development. Chapters in this book were first published by InTech; hereby published with permission under the Creative Commons Attribution License or equivalent.

The editorial board has been involved in producing this book since its inception. They have spent rigorous hours researching and exploring the diverse topics which have resulted in the successful publishing of this book. They have passed on their knowledge of decades through this book. To expedite this challenging task, the publisher supported the team at every step. A small team of assistant editors was also appointed to further simplify the editing procedure and attain best results for the readers.

Our editorial team has been hand-picked from every corner of the world. Their multi-ethnicity adds dynamic inputs to the discussions which result in innovative outcomes. These outcomes are then further discussed with the researchers and contributors who give their valuable feedback and opinion regarding the same. The feedback is then collaborated with the researches and they are edited in a comprehensive manner to aid the understanding of the subject.

Apart from the editorial board, the designing team has also invested a significant amount of their time in understanding the subject and creating the most relevant covers. They scrutinized every image to scout for the most suitable representation of the subject and create an appropriate cover for the book.

The publishing team has been involved in this book since its early stages. They were actively engaged in every process, be it collecting the data, connecting with the contributors or procuring relevant information. The team has been an ardent support to the editorial, designing and production team. Their endless efforts to recruit the best for this project, has resulted in the accomplishment of this book. They are a veteran in the field of academics and their pool of knowledge is as vast as their experience in printing. Their expertise and guidance has proved useful at every step. Their uncompromising quality standards have made this book an exceptional effort. Their encouragement from time to time has been an inspiration for everyone.

The publisher and the editorial board hope that this book will prove to be a valuable piece of knowledge for researchers, students, practitioners and scholars across the globe.

List of Contributors

Jen-Kun Cheng
Mackay Memorial Hospital/Mackay Medical College, Taiwan

Kambiz Hassanzadeh and Esmael Izadpanah
Kurdistan University of Medical Sciences, Sanandaj, Iran

Pradeep K. Dhal, Diego A. Gianolio and Robert J. Miller
Drug and Biomaterial R&D, Genzyme Corporation – A Sanofi Company, Waltham, MA, USA

Austin B. Yongye and Karina Martínez-Mayorga
Torrey Pines Institute for Molecular Studies, Port Saint Lucie, FL, USA

Igor Ukrainets
National University of Pharmacy, Ukraine

Matthew S. Alkaitis
Neuroscience Center at Dartmouth, Dartmouth Medical School, USA Nuffield Department of Clinical Laboratory Sciences, John Radcliffe Hospital, UK

Christian Ndong and Russell P. Landry III
Neuroscience Center at Dartmouth, Dartmouth Medical School, USA Department of Anesthesiology, Dartmouth-Hitchcock Medical Center, USA

Joyce A. DeLeo and E. Alfonso Romero-Sandoval
Neuroscience Center at Dartmouth, Dartmouth Medical School, USA. Department of Anesthesiology, Dartmouth-Hitchcock Medical Center, USA. Department of Pharmacology and Toxicology, Dartmouth-Hitchcock Medical Center, USA

Kevin L. Wininger
Orthopedic & Spine Center, Columbus, Ohio, USA Otterbein University, Westerville, Ohio, USA

Joseph Baker
Cappagh National Orthopedic Hospital, Ireland

G. Ulufer Sivrikaya
Sisli Etfal Training and Research Hospital, Department of 2nd Anesthesiology and Reanimation, Istanbul, Turkey

Stephen D. Lucas, Linda Le-Wendling and F. Kayser Enneking
Department of Anesthesiology, University of Florida College of Medicine, Gainesville, Florida, USA

Antigona Hasani, Hysni Jashari, Valbon Gashi and Albion Dervishi
University Clinical Center of Kosova, Department of Anesthesiology and Department of Pediatric Surgery, Prishtina, Republic of Kosova

Semra Calimli, Ahmet Topal, Atilla Erol, Aybars Tavlan and Seref Otelcioglu
Selcuk University, Meram Medical Faculty, Turkey

Mario Dauri, Ludovica Celidonio, Sarit Nahmias, Eleonora Fabbi, Filadelfo Coniglione and Maria Beatrice Silvi
Department of Anesthesia and Intensive Care Unit, Tor Vergata University, Rome, Italy

Wei H. Goh
Centre for Integrated Preclinical Drug Development, the University of Queensland, St. Lucia Campus, Brisbane, Queensland

Maree T. Smith
Centre for Integrated Preclinical Drug Development, the University of Queensland, St. Lucia Campus, Brisbane, Queensland School of Pharmacy, the University of Queensland, Australia

Wojciech Leppert
Chair and Department of Palliative Medicine, Poznan University of Medical Sciences, Poznan, Poland

R. Rychlik, K. Viehmann, D. Daniel, P. Kiencke and J. Kresimon
Institute of Empirical Health Economics, Burscheid, Germany

www.ingramcontent.com/pod-product-compliance
Lightning Source LLC
Chambersburg PA
CBHW070725190326
41458CB00004B/1040

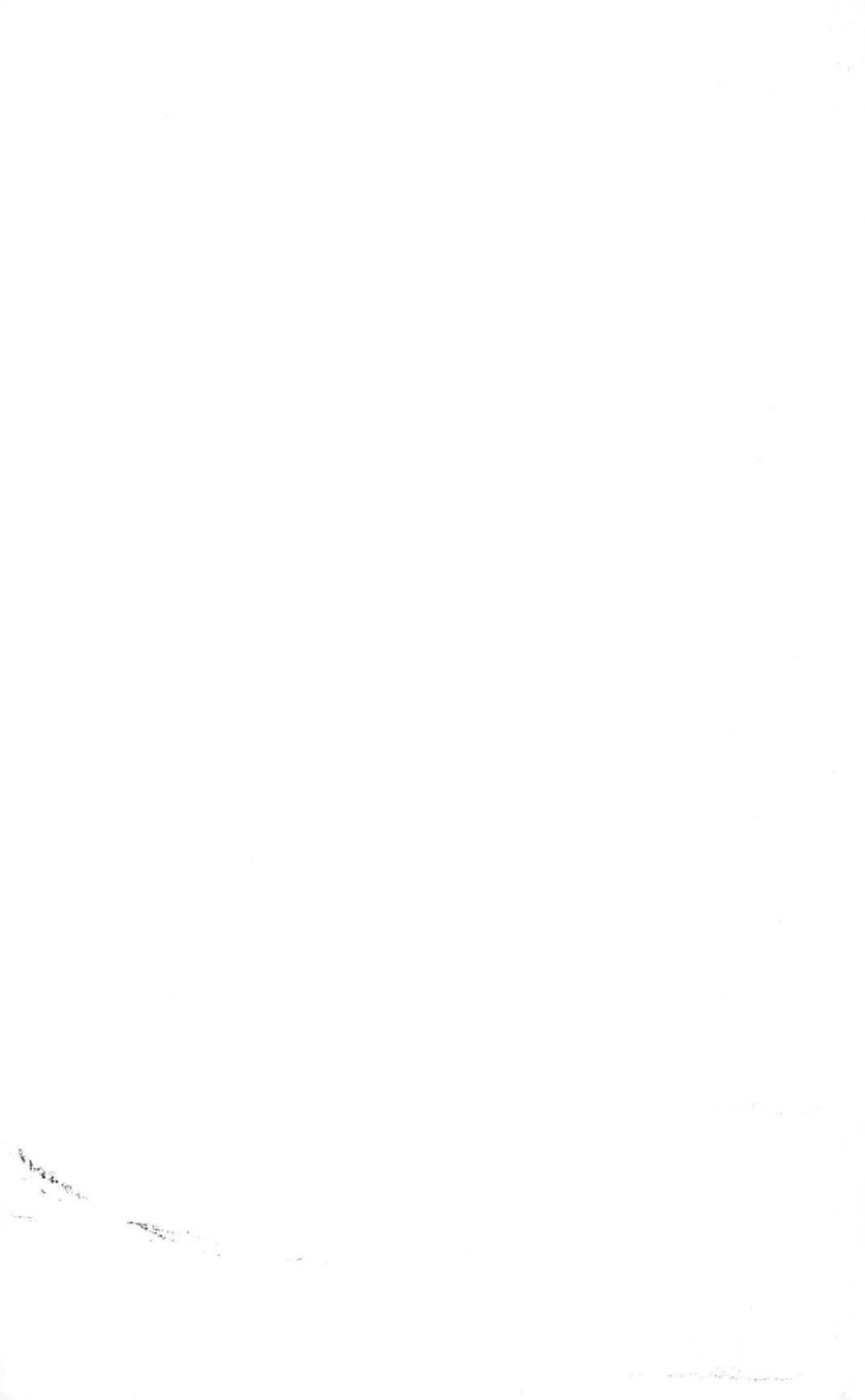